Practical Food Microbiology

EDITED BY

Diane Roberts

BSc, PhD, CBiol, FIBiol, FIFST
Former Deputy Director, Food Safety Microbiology Laboratory
Public Health Laboratory Service
Central Public Health Laboratory
61 Colindale Avenue
London
NW9 5HT
UK

D1556089

Melody Greenwood

BSc, MPhil, CBiol, FIBiol, FIFST, MRCSHC
Director of Wessex Environmental Microbiology Services
Public Health Laboratory Service
Level B, South Laboratory Block
Southampton General Hospital
Southampton
SO16 6YD
UK

THIRD EDITION

Blackwell
Publishing

© 2003 by Blackwell Publishing Ltd

Blackwell Publishing Inc., 350 Main Street, Malden, Massachusetts 02148-5018, USA

Blackwell Publishing Ltd, Osney Mead, Oxford OX2 0EL, UK

Blackwell Publishing Asia Pty Ltd, 550 Swanston Street, Carlton, Victoria 3053, Australia

Blackwell Verlag GmbH, Kurfürstendamm 57, 10707 Berlin, Germany

First published by the Public Health Laboratory Service (as in-house manual) 1986
Second edition 1995
Third edition 2003 Blackwell Publishing Ltd

Library of Congress Cataloging-in-Publication Data

Practical food microbiology/
edited by Diane Roberts, Melody Greenwood.—3rd ed.
        p.   ;   cm.
  Includes bibliographical references and index.
  ISBN 1-40510-075-3 (alk. paper)
  1. Food—Microbiology.
  [DNLM: 1. Food Microbiology. QW 85 P895 2002]
  I. Roberts, Diane, Ph.D.   II. Greenwood, Melody.
  QR115 .P73 2002
  664′.001′579—dc21
                                      2002011930
ISBN 1-40510-075-3

A catalogue record for this title is available from the British Library

Set in 9/13 pt Stone Serif by SNP Best-set Typesetter Ltd., Hong Kong
Printed and bound in Bodmin, Cornwall by MPG Books

Commissioning Editor: Maria Kahn
Editorial Assistant: Elizabeth Callaghan
Production Editor: Fiona Pattison
Production Controller: Kate Wilson

For further information on Blackwell Publishing, visit our website:
www.blackwellpublishing.com

Contents

Acknowledgements

The editors gratefully acknowledge assistance in the revision of this manual received from colleagues both within the PHLS and elsewhere.

The section on legislation, previously prepared by Professor Richard Gilbert, has been revised and expanded by Dr Christine Little of the PHLS Environmental Surveillance Unit at the Communicable Diseases Surveillance Centre, Colindale. Chris has also given invaluable help in updating references to food law, microbiological standards and guidelines throughout the entire manual. The appendix on examination of food from suspected food poisoning incidents has been revised and expanded by Professor Eric Bolton, currently Director of the PHLS Food Safety Microbiology Laboratory, Colindale. Information relating to canned foods and the examination of both the contents and the can structure has been reviewed and updated by David Shorten of Crown Cork and Seal, Wantage, Oxfordshire.

Section 9, dealing with the testing of shellfish, is new to this edition of the manual. It has been prepared by Melody Greenwood with the support of Dr David Lees, Rachel Rangdale and Dr Ron Lee from the Centre for the Environment, Fisheries and Aquaculture Science (CEFAS), Weymouth.

Revision of the remainder of the manual has been shared between the two editors and they are grateful for the help and support of colleagues in their respective laboratories, in particular Dr Caroline Willis at Wessex Environmental Microbiology Services, PHLS Southampton, for her help with producing colour plates, and Medical Illustration Department, Southampton University Hospitals NHS Trust.

The editors also wish to recognize the contributions of groups and individuals who were instrumental in producing earlier editions of the manual: The members of the PHLS Food Methods Working Group*, chaired by Dr William Hooper, who produced the 1986 laboratory benchbook version and the various contributors† who provided material for the 1995 edition published by the PHLS.

The guidance and support from the PHLS Communications Unit is also acknowledged, especially that of Kalpna Kotecha.

*PHLS Food Methods Working Group 1986: Dr WL Hooper, Mr GK Bailey, Dr RAE Barrell, Mr C Barwis, Dr C Dulake, Mr SJ Line, Dr JA Pinegar, Dr D Roberts, Miss JM Watkinson.

†Contributors to the 1995 edition: Dr H Appleton, Dr P Burden, Dr DP Casemore, Mr G Chance, Dr JV Dadswell, Dr TJ Donovan, Mr J Gibson, Dr RJ Gilbert, Ms MH Greenwood, Dr WL Hooper, Dr SL Mawer, Dr D Roberts, Dr GM Tebbutt, Mrs JM Thirlwell.

Introduction

Eating habits in the western world today bear little resemblance to those of our grandparents and those who lived in the earlier part of the twentieth century. The science and technology of food production, processing and distribution has developed dramatically. With the aid of more rapid transport, by land, sea and air, an almost limitless range of food, in greater quantities than ever, from all over the world, is available from retail outlets for home preparation or 'eating out' at restaurants, fast food establishments and other food service premises. Less and less food is prepared now from fresh, locally produced basic ingredients as described in the older cookery books. Even when a basic recipe is used many of the ingredients will have been produced and processed in locations far from the place of final preparation, service and consumption.

This advancement in food availability and range, while it has satisfied the appetite of the consumer and introduced new tastes and eating experiences, has also been a cause of some concerns. These relate to whether the food is a benefit to the customer or whether it may be injurious to health. Consumers are concerned about both the nutritional composition of foods and the use of new ingredients and additives, new processes, and methods of packaging and storage that may result in a proliferation of microorganisms. The latter part of the twentieth century has seen an increase in the number of reports of food-borne illness, in the UK and other countries, that have been regarded by many as totally unacceptable. Vast quantities of food are consumed every day and the risk of illness or other adverse effects from contamination or inappropriate processing may be relatively small; even so, governments, such as that in the UK, have been forced to take action to improve food safety. In 2000 an independent food safety watchdog, the Food Standards Agency, was set up in the UK to protect the public's health and consumer interests in relation to food. The Agency has a number of targets which include: reduction of food-borne illness by 20% by improving food safety throughout the food chain; helping people to eat more healthily; making labelling more honest and informative; promoting best practice within the food industry; improving the enforcement of food law and earning people's trust by what they do and how they do it. Readers are directed to the Agency's website (see Appendix D) for further details on how they are proceeding. Subsequently a European Food Standards Agency has also been established.

For more than half a century the Public Health Laboratory Service (PHLS) has provided both microbiological advice and scientific expertise in the examination of food and water and the environment of their production. This service has been provided primarily for those who enforce the food law, the local and port health authorities and their environmental health departments and officers.

The scope of the laboratory work falls into a number of categories. An important element for the safeguarding of public health is the investigation of food that is a cause of complaint from a consumer, or in consequence of human illness attributed to the consumption of suspect food. Another public health function is the routine monitoring of food offered for sale as an independent check on the safety of food marketed within the territories of port health and local authorities. Routine monitoring or surveillance has in recent years received increasing attention because of the heightened awareness of the potential problems associated with food by the general public and official government bodies. Such routine testing increasingly incorporates planned surveillance of specific products deemed to present a potential risk or about which there is little documented information available. This surveillance can be initiated at a number of levels from the European Union (EU) through government departments or agencies, through local environmental health liaison groups to the PHLS as a whole or to a group of laboratories. The information gained from such planned surveillance is invaluable in the formulation of guidance to food producers and food law enforcers. The experience of the PHLS network of laboratories in providing a food, water and environmental service in England and Wales is not only wide ranging over almost every conceivable type of food, but also provides a foundation for the development and use of methodology appropriate to the needs of those charged with the promotion of health and protection from health risks associated with food.

The purpose of this manual is to assist those who are called upon to examine food or who seek to assess the findings of a microbiological examination of food. The majority of the methods described are used extensively in the PHLS, are published as PHLS standard operating procedures (SOPs) and form the basis of the methodology documented for accreditation of laboratories by the United Kingdom Accreditation Service (UKAS). Most methods are based on the corresponding standard methods produced by ISO/CEN/BSI. Laboratories are therefore examining food in a standard manner that is of value when the results are assessed in the context of risk to the consumer. This standard approach is also of importance in relation to the European single market. Official Control laboratories (those that examine food for the purposes of enforcing the food law) must be accredited, use standard methods and must also challenge their procedures by participation in a proficiency testing or external quality assessment scheme.

It is emphasized that the paramount objective in undertaking a food examination is to ensure that what the consumer eats is safe, or as safe as can be expected in the condition in which it is presented. The methods in this manual are appropriate for foods at point of consumption and it may be perceived that there is a bias towards the detection of pathogenic organisms or potential pathogens with lesser attention being given to the natural flora of the food material. Problems do arise from such microbial spoilage, but it rarely causes human illness. Visual inspection and observation of smell and taste will, in many instances, cause rejection of a food without recourse to microbiological examination.

The microbiological examination of food undertaken by food processors or manufacturers is usually performed for a reason entirely different to that of a laboratory that has a regulatory function. Food suppliers need to know that their products meet a specification that will ensure that the food will still be acceptable at the end of the expected shelf-life. The criteria used to assess food at production premises are more rigorous than those used to assess a ready-to-eat food at the point of sale. Apart from food that has received a sterilizing process in a sealed container, all other food undergoes microbial change over time. Such change is due to the normal ecology of living organisms that multiply, produce potentially toxic by-products and die at a rate that will depend on the environment. Temperature, water activity (a_w), pH, availability of oxygen and of nutrients, and effects of different food ingredients or additives all determine the changes that occur in a food at any point in time. In the past, the approaches adopted by the quality controller in a food factory and the public health microbiologist investigating food in a possible food-borne incident were thought to have little bearing on each other. However, these spheres of activity have moved much closer together. Quality control is increasingly being required to demonstrate freedom from harmful organisms while the public health or clinical laboratory needs to be able to assess the whole range of microbial activity in a food in order to determine whether a pathogen can compete with and outgrow the natural flora.

Prepared cooked, chilled or frozen food is produced in such large quantities and is so widely distributed that the economic loss to the food industry in the event of a major food poisoning outbreak would be enormous. There would also be additional costs to the nation in lost working days and, in serious cases, medical care. Some legislation, such as the community controls imposed at EU level which have to be implemented into the domestic food law of member states, and also domestic legislation such as the UK Food Safety Act 1990, are designed to take into account international attitudes to food control. Early vertical EC Directives that are product-specific have included microbiological criteria that relate to the point of production. More recently there has been a move towards risk assessment and application of hazard analysis critical control point (HACCP) procedures, whereby the process is controlled by monitoring of specific critical processing points. Thus microbiological monitoring of the product is only required for verification purposes. Microbiological criteria suitable for products in international trade fall somewhere between those applicable at point of production and those applicable at the end of shelf-life. In order to give guidance on the interpretation of the results of examination of foods at point of sale, the PHLS has produced guidelines for ready-to-eat foods using the data accumulated from many years of routine monitoring and surveillance studies of such foods (see Section 2).

The aim of this manual is to act as a reference for the selection of suitable test methods for a number of types of food. The methods chosen can be performed in most food laboratories with readily available materials and equipment.

For further information the reader is referred to the bibliography in Appendix D, and for guidelines to the appendix to Section 2.

The structure of this manual

This manual is structured to take the reader through the various steps in the microbiological examination of food. It begins by outlining why there is a need for such examination and the legislation, both from the EU and within the UK, which relates to the various food products (Sections 1 and 2). Section 3 discusses individual foods and the problems with which they are associated, then lists the tests relevant to their examination and the microbiological criteria available for particular food products.

Sections 4 to 6 give details on methods of sampling of foods and laboratory tests for enumeration, enrichment and isolation of food-borne microorganisms with particular mention of quality control and calculation of results. The microbiological methods relating to dairy products, eggs and shellfish are dealt with separately in Sections 7, 8 and 9 respectively. Legislation for dairy products lays down detailed methods for examination that are generally specific for that group of foods, thus a single section has been devoted to those methods. Similarly, the methods given in Section 8 for the examination of eggs, in-shell and bulk, are product-specific and differ in some respects from the general methods described in earlier sections. Section 9 is devoted to the examination of molluscan shellfish and includes details of sample preparation in addition to specific methods of examination. The more common biochemical tests necessary in the steps towards confirming the identity of organisms isolated from food are described in Section 10.

Supplementary information such as safety notes, procedural hints and worked examples, is included at various points in the methods in Sections 4–10. This information is highlighted in the text with boxes.

There are four appendices, A to D. Appendix A is a quick reference guide to the microbiological tests. The table provides a summary of the information provided in Sections 3, 7, 8 and 9, concerning the laboratory tests for specific foods. It serves as a rapid guide to the appropriate food heading and the type of test that should be considered. Once the food heading and range of tests have been identified then reference can be made to the more detailed information available elsewhere in this manual. In Section 3, which deals with schedules for the examination of foods, the tests have been divided into three groups: statutory, recommended and supplementary. These groups are identified in the quick reference guide by symbols for ease of recognition.

Appendix B discusses the steps to be taken in the examination of food from suspected food poisoning incidents with a brief summary of features of the most common agents. Appendix C lists UK reference facilities and PHLS EQA schemes, while Appendix D lists a number of useful texts on food microbiology and food safety and the website addresses of a number of organizations and agencies that can provide helpful information.

1 Indications for sampling and interpretation of results

1.1 Risk assessment and hazard analysis

Almost all international food trade legislation is focused on assessing and managing risks from food. It is now a legal obligation in the European Union (EU) for food processors to identify any steps in their activities that are critical in ensuring food safety and to ensure that adequate safety procedures are implemented, maintained and reviewed [1]. The risk assessment of the food production process should identify and characterize the hazards in the process, assess the exposure and characterize the risks [2]. Hazard analysis critical control point (HACCP) principles should then be used to identify the critical control points to control the risks in order to form the basis of product safety management systems (Section 2). Sampling for microbiological testing is an important part of the risk assessment as it can be used to monitor the efficacy of the control systems but end product testing cannot be relied upon as a means of assuring food safety.

1.2 Indications for sampling

Foods are sampled principally for the following reasons:
- Checks on hygienic production and handling techniques.
- Quality control and shelf-life performance.
- Suspicion of being the cause of food poisoning or as a result of consumer complaint.
- Verification of the quality of imported food.

Most quality control testing will be done by, or at the request of, the manufacturer whose interest is to demonstrate to the wholesaler, retailer or customer a quality product and, if possible, the product's superiority over competitors' products. With increasing need to label foods with a 'use-by' date, the setting of criteria to be satisfied throughout the declared shelf-life has become commonplace. Sampling for quality control purposes can be predetermined and structured in such a way that minor variations within batches of single products can be detected quickly so that modification can be made before any noticeable change occurs that might alter consumer preference. In large manufacturing premises this might entail sampling at the beginning and end of a production run and at other times such as at the time of despatch from the factory and at the end of shelf-life under simulated retail conditions. Other food producers may adopt intermittent spot checks, while small producers are more likely to rely on process control without microbiological tests.

Independent checks on the hygienic production of a product and examination for evidence of poor storage and handling technique as part of the overall assessment of food placed on retail sale are desirable for further quality assurance and to help assure consumer safety. For these purposes, sampling needs to be targeted quite specifically if any useful data are to be collected. Organized surveys over limited time periods involving one specific product or type of product from certain types of shop or catering establishment and the use of a standard technique for examination will produce data that can be compared with those obtained in a similar manner elsewhere and on other occasions. Uniformity of approach is essential or wrong conclusions can be drawn. For example, results expressed as 'present' or 'absent' are of no value unless the quantity of food examined is stated. Numerical counts of colony forming units may vary quite considerably unless the dilution method, culture media and temperature of incubation employed on each occasion are the same. Checks on product hygiene and consumer acceptability can only properly be assessed with full possession of the product history. Food taken from shop display after in-house slicing and weighing may not be the same as that sampled whole and, within limits, the wider the range of organisms sought and quantified the better a food examiner can form an opinion about the food. Criteria used to assess a product at the end of shelf-life are often assumed to be applicable to the food 'as eaten', but storage conditions between purchase and consumption may also affect test results.

Sampling in cases of suspected food poisoning will be directed specifically at the food consumed by the complainant. Every effort should be made to sample the remains of the suspect food even if this means its retrieval from the refuse bin. Other food from the same meal, even if it is not the suspect ingredient, will be of next greatest value followed by other batches of food obtainable from the same catering establishment or supplier. If the causal food poisoning organism is known, examination can be limited to a search for that organism, thereby conserving laboratory resources. Further guidance is given in Appendix B.

Examination of food imported into the EU is performed to ensure that the food is of equivalent quality to food produced within the Union. When possible this is judged against criteria contained in EU legislation. In some instances, when a problem is identified in certain areas of the world, a commission decision will direct the examination of specific food items from those areas and the parameters to be tested.

In designing a sampling plan it is most important that all who are concerned with the collection and submission of the samples, the laboratory staff and those who will be involved in interpretation of results, are consulted at an early stage. The objectives need to be clearly defined and understood to avoid wasted time and effort. There are limitations with all microbiological tests and these have to be taken into consideration before any action can be taken following a report from the laboratory. Many investigations involving pathogenic organisms will be concerned primarily with presence or absence of the organism in a defined amount of sample. This represents a 'two-class' plan, where in a given number of samples, n, a certain number will show the unacceptable presence of the test organism.

With some examinations for pathogenic organisms, and particularly in quality assessment studies where results are expressed in terms of colony counts, it is more usual to allow some latitude in results that marginally exceed the desired maximum count denoting satisfactory or acceptable limits and/or quality. In these instances it is appropriate to designate a permitted range that depends on the type of food and the situation. A full explanation of the principles and specific applications of sampling for microbiological analysis may be found in the publication of the International Commission on Microbiological Specifications for Foods (ICMSF) [3]. The sampling plan and tests may be selected as appropriate to the particular case or according to the circumstances related to the nature and treatment of the food that influence the potential hazards with which it is associated.

Where a rigid 'two-class' plan is not essential, use can be made of a 'three-class' plan that accepts a proportion of sample units whose test results fall between unequivocal acceptability and rejection. In devising a plan for a particular food it is necessary to set values for n, m, M and c where:

- n is the number of sample units comprising the sample;
- m is the threshold value for the number of bacteria; the result is considered satisfactory if the number of bacteria in all sample units does not exceed this value;
- M is the maximum value for the number of bacteria; the result is considered unsatisfactory if the number of bacteria in one or more sample units is equal to or greater than this value;
- c is the number of sample units where the bacterial count may be between m and M.
- The sample is considered acceptable if the bacterial counts of the other sample units are equal to or less than the value of m. For practical purposes, n is frequently given a value of five, and c a value of one or two.

Although there are some European Community (EC) directives that specify both standard and guideline criteria for certain foods, European legislation is now mainly focused on good manufacturing practice and the need for businesses to adopt HACCP principles to help ensure safe food production. Emphasis should be placed on the education of those who handle food as good hygiene is a prerequisite for safe food. The quality of basic food materials and scrupulous attention to hygiene and working practices are far more important than bacteriological checks on the processed food. Structured sampling for data collection in support of HACCP systems is, however, a valuable tool when used in an informed manner.

1.3 Choice of method

Ideally, if microbiological criteria are included in food legislation or in a specification then the methods to be used for testing should be identified. The choice of method should be given careful consideration. Many of the organisms present in a food will be in a stressed condition as a result of the physical and chemical processes used in the production of that food. Freezing, drying, salting, pickling, sublethal heat treatment and extended chilling will all affect the recovery of target organisms. If the stressed organisms are then subjected to a harsh isolation protocol their recovery will be impaired and a falsely low result obtained. Some isolation methods take this into account and incorporate a resuscitation stage into the procedure. This is particularly important when attempting to recover pathogens such as *Salmonella*.

Preparation of the sample for examination should take into account the characteristics of the food product. If it is highly salted the concentration of the salt in the sample homogenate should be reduced to 2% or less to remove any inhibitory properties of the salt. Similarly if the product is highly acid or alkaline the pH of the homogenate may require adjustment to near neutrality to optimize recovery. Rehydration of dried products should be gradual to prevention the introduction of osmotic shock. These and other procedures can help maximize recovery of the target organisms from all foods examined.

Traditionally microorganisms in foods are enumerated by pour plate procedures, and these methods frequently form the basis of international standards. However these may not be ideal for recovery of stressed cells. If foods have been frozen or subjected to extensive chilling the temperature of the molten agar (*c.* 45°C) may result in further stress to the contaminating organisms. Many of the target organisms in foods either prefer or require aerobic conditions for growth. The restriction of oxygen in the depths of the agar in a plate may impede or prevent their growth. In the UK surface colony count methods are generally preferred for enumeration as they do not have these drawbacks and in addition have the convenience of being able to use pre-poured plates. However, surface methods of enumeration restrict the size of the inoculum and this may affect the limit of detection.

For certain organisms such as *Salmonella* that cause gastroenteritis their very presence in a food is significant. In addition, the levels present may be very low. In these cases it is necessary to use presence/absence procedures rather than relying on enumeration techniques for detection. Presence/absence procedures allow the examination of larger portions of sample, typically 25 g, by use of liquid enrichment procedures in nutrient and selective media formulated to optimize the recovery of the target organism in the presence of other naturally occurring food microflora.

It should be clear from the above that the method used for each target organism sought in a food should be tailored to maximize the likelihood of recovery of that organism. In this way the microbiologist can have confidence that if the target organism is not detected it is likely to be a true result.

1.4   Interpretation of results

The interpretation of results in food microbiology is perhaps the most difficult and complex aspect of the examination process. Not only is it often impossible to make a definitive judgement owing to absence of supporting information but the precision and reproducibility of many microbiological tests may vary. Microorganisms in non-sterile food are in a dynamic environment in which multiplication and death of different species at differing rates means that the result of a test can only be valid for a single point in time. Colony counts alone can be misleading if bacterial growth has ceased whereas toxins already produced will persist. Staphylococcal enterotoxin survives the drying process in the manufacture of powdered milk and has caused confusion when reliance has been placed on culture results alone. It is sometimes not appreciated that homogeneity is rare in food and so the results obtained for one portion can be very different from those for another even if the samples have been taken in close proximity within the same batch. A variation in the viable counts of organisms will be apparent even in fluid foods such as soups and gravies if not homogenized in the laboratory before the test sample is taken. However, aerobic colony counts alone can be extremely valuable in the food manufacturing industry as the technique is straightforward and acceptance or rejection decisions can be made on variance from the norm for any one product when sampled regularly at the same point under the same conditions.

In regulatory control or hazard monitoring, colony counts obtained through random sampling can only form a small part of the overall assessment of the product. The number of pathogenic or potentially pathogenic organisms in a sample has a far greater significance but results depend on the food and the time at which it was sampled. Food that is sterilized in a can will remain sterile until the can is opened. Environmental contaminants may then be introduced and their numbers will vary according to the storage conditions, temperature and degree of handling both before the point of sale and after. Interpretation therefore requires cognizance both of the observed results and of the history of the food up to its receipt at the laboratory. Laboratory results alone make interpretation difficult unless the presence of an obligate pathogen such as *Salmonella* spp. has been demonstrated.

It is likely that the results of tests involving a search for indicator organisms such as members of the Enterobacteriaceae will only allow an informed judgement to be made, for example, about the adequacy of heat treatment or the level of post-processing contamination that has taken place. The presence of faecal organisms such as *Escherichia coli* means that either they have always been in the product or they have been acquired at a later stage during processing, handling or storage. Their presence indicates the need for further investigation. Their absence gives some degree of assurance but cannot guarantee the absence of pathogens of faecal origin such as *Salmonella*. Even absence of target pathogens in tests specific for them only provides a degree of probability of absence in the whole batch of food (see ICMSF [3]). It is therefore essential that a food producer does not rely on end product testing alone but uses it in conjunction with good manufacturing practice and sound HACCP procedures.

Often the simplest approach is to proceed initially with definitive tests for specific pathogens. It is known that *Salmonella* infection is the commonest hazard in food of animal origin. It will certainly not be possible to subject a whole batch of the food to examination for this organism. A degree of assurance is only obtained when tests on uniform quantities of representative samples of the food by standard methods prove negative.

1.5 The laboratory report

The value of a laboratory report can, at best, only match the quality of the sample and the accompanying information. Comparisons can only be made between reports from different laboratories or on different occasions if the reporting methods are standardized. A standardized report form assists in this respect. The report should include a description of the food itself and observations on the physical condition of the sample. The results of general and indicator tests and those concerning specific organisms should relate to a specified mass or volume of the food. For the majority of quantitative tests it is convenient to relate the presence or absence of the organism sought to 1 g or 1 mL of test sample even if the actual quantity examined is different. Knowledge of the precise quantity of test sample is essential for calculating colony counts.

When interpretation of a laboratory report is required for referee purposes, such as in a court of law, it is vital that the documentation provides an uninterrupted record of the progress of the sample through the laboratory. The qualifications, status and role of recognized food examiners in the UK have now been established [4]. In order to ensure the continuity of evidence, the following documents and information should be available:

- The date, time and place of sampling recorded by the sampling officer.
- Verification of the custody of the sample during transit to the laboratory and the conditions of storage during transport.
- Signatures that acknowledge transfer of the sample to a member of the laboratory staff.
- Records of conditions of storage in the laboratory.
- Records of the members of staff performing all the stages of testing and the conditions prevailing during the tests.
- Records of all results obtained and how they were derived.
- The certificate of examination issued by the food examiner based on this accurate laboratory documentation.

1.6 Criteria

Before a sampling programme is embarked upon the criteria to be adopted in the interpretation of the results need to be agreed between the parties concerned. This avoids a great deal of useless investigation and wasted financial outlay. For these reasons it is not possible to give criteria that are applicable in all situations. Each investigation needs its own assessment by qualified and experienced personnel. The interpretation of statutory tests with 'pass' or 'fail' end point criteria has to be undertaken with care since microorganisms are living entities that cannot be assessed in finite terms in the way that chemical analysis allows.

In 1992 the Public Health Laboratory Service (PHLS) published guidelines for microbiological acceptability of some ready-to-eat foods [5]. This was in response to requests from Environmental Health Officers, consumer organizations and government agencies for help in the furtherance of improving knowledge about the safety of food. Apart from setting proscriptive limits for certain pathogens, the guidelines recommend ranges of bacterial colony counts for a number of different types of food which allow the division of results into four different levels of quality. These range from 'satisfactory' quality to 'unacceptable, potentially hazardous' quality. The guidelines have no formal status and refer only to 'ready-to-eat' food sampled at point of sale, but they do reflect the opinions of experienced workers with access to a wealth of published and unpublished data collected over half a century by the PHLS. These guidelines have been updated and expanded twice since 1992 on the basis of comments received from microbiologists and Environmental Health Officers and accumulation of further data derived from routine samples and targeted, structured surveys. Modification and extension of their scope is made periodically in response to any suggestions or criticism. The PHLS guidelines current at the time of publication of this manual are summarized in Section 2.

The Institute of Food Science and Technology has also published microbiological criteria [6] that are applicable to a wide range of foods. These criteria adopt a two-tier approach, the levels expected as a result of good manufacturing practice and the maximum levels that are acceptable at any point in the shelf-life of a food.

In food microbiology there is no rule of thumb that provides an interpretation in all circumstances. Each food must be considered individually taking into account all the relevant factors including the ingredients, process, type of packaging, conditions of storage and the likely remaining shelf-life.

1.7 References

1 European Commission. Council Directive 93/43/EEC on the hygiene of foodstuffs. *Off J Eur Communities* 1993; **L175**: 1–11.
2 Mitchell RT. *Practical Microbiological Risk Analysis*. Oxford: Chandos Publishing Ltd, 2000.

3   International Commission on Microbiological Specifications for Foods. *Microorganisms in Foods. 2. Sampling for Microbiological Analysis: Principles and Specific Applications.* 2nd edn. Oxford: Blackwell Scientific, 1986.

4   Great Britain. *Statutory Instrument 1990 No. 2463. The Food Safety (Sampling and Qualifications) Regulations 1990.* London: HMSO, 1990.

5   Gilbert RJ. Provisional microbiological guidelines for some ready-to-eat foods sampled at point of sale: notes for PHLS Food Examiners. *PHLS Microbiol Dig* 1992; **9**: 98–9.

6   Bell C, Greenwood M, Hooker J, Kyriakides A, Mills R. *Development and Use of Microbiological Criteria for Foods.* London: Institute of Food Science and Technology, 1999.

2 Legislation, codes of practice and microbiological criteria

2.1 UK legislation: the Food Safety Act 1990

The Food Safety Act, the main provisions of which came into effect on 1 January 1991, provides the basic framework for all food legislation throughout the UK. Its primary aim is to strengthen and update the previous food legislation to achieve the highest possible standards of food safety and consumer protection throughout the food chain. The main feature of the Act is the number of enabling powers that it contains. This allows ministers to make further regulations to implement food safety measures and to produce codes of practice to bring about more consistent standards of enforcement. Food is broadly defined under the Act to include virtually anything that is eaten, drunk or sold as a food product; the definition also includes water, which was not covered under previous food legislation.

There were a number of reasons why a new Food Safety Act was required [1]:

- Existing legislation, which had been consolidated in the Food Act 1984, but not fully revised since 1938, had not kept pace with the rapid advances in food technology, and changes in eating habits and shopping patterns.
- There were gaps in the existing legislation.
- The major changes of approach to food law brought about by the European Community (EC) harmonization programme required a change in the UK food law to make the implementation of EC legislation easier.
- The considerable concern in the late 1980s within the government and the general public about the increasing incidence of food-borne infection, particularly associated with *Campylobacter* spp., *Salmonella* spp. (especially *S.* Enteritidis phage type 4) and *Listeria monocytogenes*.

Some features of the Act in relation to food microbiology are as follows.

Section 8 Selling food not complying with food safety requirements

Paragraph (2)

This key provision of the Act makes it an offence to sell food that does not comply with food safety requirements. Food fails to comply if:

- it has been rendered injurious to health;
- it is unfit for human consumption; or
- it is so contaminated, whether by extraneous matter or otherwise, that it would not be reasonable to expect it to be used for human consumption in that state. This would, for example, include food being affected by mould that does not necessarily make it injurious or unfit.

The element of 'contamination' was not included in previous legislation, under which possession of contaminated food was not an offence unless it was sold to the purchaser's prejudice; that is, the food was not of the nature, substance and quality demanded. Contamination therefore will permit prosecutions to be brought solely on the results of the microbiological examination or chemical analysis of food.

Paragraph (3)

Under previous legislation it was difficult to deal with a batch of food that was believed to be unfit. Under the present Act if any part of a batch of food fails to comply with food safety requirements, then the whole batch will be presumed not to comply until the contrary is proved. This power mirrors the policy of reputable manufacturers to withdraw an entire consignment if some products are found to be contaminated.

Section 9(2 & 4) Detention of suspect food

The powers to inspect and seize food are largely the same as under previous legislation except that authorized officers may detain food for 21 days to allow microbiological examination or chemical analysis to be performed to establish whether it complies with food safety requirements. These powers also apply to food that is thought 'likely to cause food poisoning or any disease communicable to humans'.

Section 13 Emergency control orders

This section provides ministers with the power to issue emergency control orders to prohibit the sale of food where there is an imminent risk of injury to health. This power will be used where voluntary procedures, following the issue of food hazard warnings, are unlikely to be effective, for example the sale of a widely distributed contaminated canned food.

Section 16(1b) Provision for microbiological standards

Provision may be made by regulations for securing that food is fit for human consumption and meets such microbiological standards (whether going to the fitness of food or otherwise) as may be specified by or under the regulations. This allows for the introduction of mandatory microbiological standards for specified foods.

Section 17(1) Enforcement of Community provisions

This section provides ministers the power, by regulations, to make such provision with respect to food, food sources or contact materials as appears to them to be called for by any EC obligation. This will permit the enforcement of any Community provisions for microbiological standards for foods.

Section 28(2) Food examiners

The Act recognizes the role of the food examiner to perform the new statutory function of microbiological examination of food. In this task the role of the food examiner will correspond to that of the public analyst who has a long-standing remit to carry out statutory analysis (chemical) of food samples. Food examiners therefore are the individuals to whom an enforcement officer is required to submit any sample taken for enforcement purposes (i.e. where it may be introduced as evidence in any court proceedings under the Act) if the officer considers the sample should undergo microbiological examination. The purpose of this legislation is to ensure that the microbiological examination of food is carried out to a high standard and (by specifying their necessary qualifications) to ensure that the competence of food examiners when asked to give an expert view during legal proceedings against a food producer/retailer is not open to question.

Qualifications for food examiners are prescribed in the Food Safety (Sampling and Qualifications) Regulations 1990, which came into force on 1 January 1991. There is no single qualification to denote the requisite academic attainment and practical experience of a food examiner, and the regulations allow a wide range of academic or professional qualification in conjunction with 3 years relevant experience. An important element of the Regulations is the provision of certificates by examiners relating to the microbiological results of examination of samples submitted to them. Food examiners are expected to provide written opinion and observation, if deemed appropriate, on the safety and quality of food samples submitted to their laboratories for examination under the Regulations. The certificates are legal documents and can be used as evidence in legal proceedings.

Section 40 Codes of practice

Ministers may issue codes of practice to guide food authorities on the execution and enforcement of the Act and subsequent legislation made under it. The objective of issuing codes of practice is to ensure more even and consistent standards of enforcement across the UK. These documents are not legally binding but food authorities will be required to have regard to the guidance contained in them. However, ministers will be able to issue directions requiring food authorities to take specific action in order to conform with a code of practice and these directions will be enforceable through the courts.

Twenty codes of practice have been issued to date, some of which have been or are being updated and amended [2]. Code of Practice No. 7 (Sampling for Analysis or Examination) is of particular importance to food examiners as it gives guidance to enforcement officers for taking samples, and should help to ensure that adequate and appropriate samples are submitted for examination. Code of Practice No. 7 has recently been revised to take account of experience gained in practice.

2.2 European Community legislation

Food hygiene and food safety legislation can no longer be viewed in an exclusively national context, it is an EC-wide issue. The EC has been involved in food legislation since 1964. The pace of its development and implementation accelerated in the period to the end of 1992 prior to the completion of the single European market. However, EC food law in the run-up to the establishment of the single market in 1992 was still essentially concentrated on questions of trade and free movement of goods. Following the bovine spongiform encephalopathy (BSE) crisis the European Parliament reformed the Commission's structures for preparing food legislation and published a Green Paper on Food Law (COM(97)176) in May 1997. Its main thrust is ensuring the protection of consumers and public health and the free circulation of goods within the Single Market. The Green Paper identified six principles of EC food policy; proposed the general application of hazard analysis critical control point (HACCP) principles to all products; put forward the proposal that primary agricultural products should be included within the Product Liability Directive (85/374/EEC); and ensured that all EC laws are compatible with the new international obligations of the European Union under the World Trade Organization (WTO) Sanitary and Phytosanitary and Technical Barriers to Trade Agreements. By the end of 1997, food law issues had become such a priority that heads of government and states at their twice-yearly European Summits agreed to a Declaration on Food Safety at Luxembourg on 12–13 December 1997 [3]. In 1999, Directive 99/34/EC amended the Product Liability Directive (85/374/EEC) in that primary agricultural products are no longer exempt so as to restore consumer confidence in the safety of such products.

On 12 January 2000 the European Commission adopted a White Paper on Food Safety [4]. The Commission stated in this document that the most appropriate response to guarantee the highest EC food safety standards is the establishment of an independent European Food Authority. The White Paper also includes a comprehensive range of over 80 areas where European food law needs to be amended and improved. The new legal frame-work will cover animal feed, animal health and welfare, hygiene, contaminants and residues, novel food, additives, flavourings, packaging and irradiation. In November 2000 the European Commission put forward a proposal for a Regulation laying down the general principles of food law and establishing the European Food Authority. The European Parliament (EP) approved the creation of an independent European Food Safety Authority (EFSA) in a final agreement on 11 December 2001 so that the EFSA can start operating in the first half of 2002. 'Safety' has been added to the title of the new body through an amendment adopted by the EP. On 21 January 2001, the EFSA became a reality when the Council of Ministers adopted the key legislation that provides the legal basis for establishing the EFSA and general principles and requirements for EU food law (Regulation 2002/178/EC) [5]. The General Food Law Regulation 2002/178/EC embodies the responsibilities and obligations to be placed upon all operators in the food chain from farmers to retailers.

The EFSA will have a broad mandate, including a wide range of scientific and technical support tasks on all matters having a direct or indirect impact on food safety. The EFSA's mission therefore includes the provision of scientific opinions on all issues in relation to animal health and welfare, plant health and genetically modified organisms, without prejudice to the competence conferred to the Agency for the Evaluation for Medicinal Products (EMEA). The EFSA will also have a major task in informing the public about its activities.

Types of EC legislation

The three types of legislation within the EC are [6]:
- **Regulation**. A legal act which has general applications and is binding in its entirety and directly applicable to the citizens, courts and governments of all Member States. Regulations do not therefore have to be transferred into domestic laws and are chiefly designed to ensure uniformity of law across the Community.
- **Directive**. A binding law directed to one or more Member States. The law states objectives that the Member State(s) are required to confirm within a specified time. A directive has to be implemented by Member States by amendment of their domestic laws to comply with the stated objectives; in the UK this is being done in the form of new statutory instruments under the Food Safety Act. This process is known as 'approximation of laws' or 'harmonization' since it involves the alignment of domestic policy throughout the Community.

- **Decision**. An act which is directed at specific individuals, companies or Member States which is binding in its entirety. Decisions addressed to Member States are directly applicable in the same way as directives.

The 1985 European Commission White Paper 'Completing the Internal Market' catalogued the measures necessary to allow for the free movement of goods (including foods, services, capital and labour) which would lead to the removal of all physical, technical and fiscal barriers between Member States. Since 1 January 1993, food has moved freely within the EC with the minimum of inspection at land or sea frontiers. Harmonized rules have been adopted, applicable to all food produced in the EC, underpinned by the principle of mutual recognition of national standards and regulations for matters that do not require EC legislation [7]. Specific directives are in place for minced meat and meat preparations, live bivalve molluscs, fishery products, milk and milk products, and egg products and for the hygiene of foodstuffs. Foods entering the EC from countries outside (third countries) will be subject to EC hygiene standards. Products of animal origin will undergo a rigorous inspection on entering the EC.

2.3   Hazard analysis

There is growing acceptance throughout the EU and in many other countries of the value of HACCP principles in ensuring the microbiological safety of foods. The HACCP approach [8] is a systematic way of analysing the potential hazards of a food operation, identifying the points in the operation where the hazards may occur, and where controls over those that are important to consumer safety can be achieved. Most of the product-specific EC directives as well as the Directive on the Hygiene of Foodstuffs (93/43/EEC), place obligations on industry and food business operators to adopt HACCP principles as the basis for their product safety management systems. The advantages of the HACCP approach over a food safety control system based purely on microbiological standards is now widely recognized. Thus, the Commission proposes to consolidate and simplify existing EC food hygiene legislation [4,9]. These are expected to be implemented by 2004. The proposed consolidation adopts a unified approach to hygiene and extends the general hygiene rules and HACCP principles to cover hygiene throughout the food chain, including primary production, i.e. the 'farm-to-fork' approach to managing food safety. Responsibility of food safety will be unambiguously placed onto food producers. A fully documented HACCP plan will be required of all food producers, including caterers, regardless of size. This will include a specific monitoring programme, thereby reinforcing the own-check principle of food producers. An absolute requirement for full traceability of all foods and ingredients used in food production is also introduced, such that all food producers must keep adequate records to allow full traceability throughout the products' allotted shelf-life.

2.4 Laboratory accreditation

The mutual recognition of microbiological results obtained by different control bodies is an essential precondition to unrestricted trade in food between the Member States. Since 1 November 1998, under the terms of the Official Control of Foodstuffs Directive (89/397/EEC) and the Additional Measures Food Control Directive (93/99/EC), only Official Food Control Laboratories are allowed to examine Official Control Samples. These laboratories are accredited by their national accreditation organization according to the Euronorm (EN 45001) series of standards. The directives also require that such laboratories participate in a proficiency testing scheme. In the UK this means accreditation by the United Kingdom Accreditation Service (UKAS), and participation in a food microbiology quality assessment (proficiency testing) scheme, such as that introduced by the Public Health Laboratory Service (PHLS) in September 1991 [10]. Since this legislation was adopted the standard to which laboratories must be accredited has been changed to ISO/IEC 17025 [11].

2.5 Microbiological criteria

Several international organizations are concerned with the establishment and application of microbiological criteria for foods; these include the EU, the World Health Organization (WHO), the International Commission on Microbiological Specifications for Foods (ICMSF) and the Codex Alimentarius Commission. The purpose of establishing these criteria is to protect the health of the consumer by providing safe, sound and wholesome products, and to meet the requirements of fair practices in trade. The mere existence of criteria cannot protect consumer health *per se*; of equal, or greater, importance is the use of good manufacturing practice to ensure that undesirable organisms are eliminated as far as is practicable. Microbiological criteria can be divided under the headings:

- **Microbiological standards**. Mandatory criteria that are included in legislation or regulations; failure to comply with these can result in prosecution.
- **Microbiological specifications**. Generally contractual agreements between a manufacturer and a purchaser to check that foods are of the required quality.
- **Microbiological guidelines**. Non-mandatory criteria usually intended to guide the manufacturer and help to ensure good hygienic practice.

Ideally, any microbiological criterion for a food should include the following information:

- a statement of the microorganisms and/or toxins of concern;
- laboratory methods for their detection and quantification;
- the sampling plan;
- the microbiological limits; and
- the number of samples required to conform to these limits.

Some EC directives, e.g. those for milk and milk-based products and for fishery products, contain a mixture of mandatory (microbiological standards) and non-mandatory criteria (guidelines).

In theory, EC-based microbiological standards would provide common criteria against which the safety of food could be measured consistently. However, some Member States, including the UK, have adopted a cautious approach to defining and agreeing specific standards for particular types of foods. Currently few directives have specified microbiological standards but other directives have provisions for standards to be agreed at a later date, or where standards have been set there is scope for them to be revised. Future EU legislation may specify both microbiological criteria and the laboratory methods to be employed for checking compliance with the criteria.

The following directives include microbiological standards:
- Egg Products Directive 89/437/EEC, as amended by Directive 89/662/EEC and Directive 91/684/EEC (see Sections 3 and 8).
- Live Bivalve Molluscs Directive 91/492/EEC, as amended by Directive 97/61/EC (see Sections 3 and 9).
- Fishery Products Directive 91/493/EEC, as amended by Directive 95/71/EC and Commission Decision 93/51/EEC on the microbiological criteria applicable to the production of cooked crustaceans and molluscan shellfish (see Sections 3 and 9).
- Milk and Milk-based Products Directive 92/46/EEC (see Sections 3 and 7).
- Minced Meat and Meat Preparations Directive 94/65/EC (see Section 3).

2.6 Microbiological guidelines for some ready-to-eat foods sampled at point of sale

In the past, Environmental Health Officers frequently sought advice from their local public health laboratory on the significance of the microbiological results of food samples they had submitted for examination. In the absence of microbiological standards (UK or EC) or published guidelines for many types of foods such interpretation has had to be based on personal experience of results from a large number of such foods examined over many years. While there is no reason to doubt the soundness of such advice in the past, the need to complete formal certificates within the new legal framework suggested that structured guidance would assist those designated as food examiners within the PHLS to fulfil their obligations.

In 2000 the PHLS published the second revised guidelines on the interpretation of the results from the microbiological examination of various ready-to-eat foods sampled at point of sale (Tables 2.1 & 2.2) [12]. The guidelines were expanded to take account of experience gained of their value in practice and additional information that has become available. They are not statutory microbiological standards; they only reflect the opinion of the PHLS Advisory Committee on Food and Dairy Products and are subject to periodic revision as

Table 2.1 PHLS Guidelines for the microbiological quality of various ready-to-eat foods. Reproduced with permission of the PHLS Communicable Disease Surveillance Centre © PHLS [12].

Food category (see Table 2.2)	Criterion	Microbiological quality (cfu/g unless stated)			
		Satisfactory	Acceptable	Unsatisfactory	Unacceptable/ potentially hazardous
	Aerobic colony count* 30°C/4 h				
1		$<10^3$	10^3–$<10^4$	$\geq10^4$	N/A†**
2		$<10^4$	10^4–$<10^5$	$\geq10^5$	N/A**
3		$<10^5$	10^5–$<10^6$	$\geq10^6$	N/A**
4		$<10^6$	10^6–$<10^7$	$\geq10^7$	N/A**
5		N/A	N/A	N/A	N/A**
	Indicator organisms††				
1–5	Enterobacteriaceae‡	<100	100–$<10^4$	$\geq10^4$	N/A**
1–5	Escherichia coli (total)	<20	20–<100	≥100	N/A**
1–5	Listeria spp. (total)	<20	20–<100	≥100	N/A**
	Pathogens				
1–5	Salmonella spp.	ND			D
1–5	Campylobacter spp.	ND			D
1–5	E.coli O157 & other VTEC	ND			D
1–5	Vibrio cholerae	ND			D
1–5	Vibrio parahaemolyticus§	<20	20–<100	100–$<10^3$	$\geq10^3$
1–5	Listeria monocytogenes	<20¶	20–<100	N/A	≥100
1–5	Staphylococcus aureus	<20	20–<100	100–$<10^4$	$\geq10^4$
1–5	Clostridium perfringens	<20	20–<100	100–$<10^4$	$\geq10^4$
1–5	Bacillus cereus and other pathogenic Bacillus spp.‖	$<10^3$	10^3–$<10^4$	10^4–$<10^5$	$\geq10^5$

cfu, colony forming units; VTEC, verocytotoxin producing E.coli. D, detected in 25 g; ND, not detected in 25 g.

*Guidelines for aerobic colony counts may not apply to certain fermented foods, e.g. salami, soft cheese and unpasteurized yoghurt. These foods fall into Category 5. Acceptability is based on appearance, smell, texture and the levels or absence of indicator organisms or pathogens.

†N/A denotes not applicable.

‡Not applicable to fresh fruit, vegetables and salad vegetables.

§Relevant to seafoods only.

‖If the Bacillus counts exceed 10^4 cfu/g, the organism should be identified.

¶Not detected in 25 g for certain long shelf-life products under refrigeration.

**Prosecution based solely on high colony counts and/or indicator organisms in the absence of other criteria of unacceptability is unlikely to be successful.

††On occasions some strains may be pathogenic.

Table 2.2 Colony count categories for different types of ready-to-eat foods. Reproduced with permission of the PHLS Communicable Disease Surveillance Centre © PHLS [12].

Food group	Product	Category
Meat	Beefburgers	1
	Brawn	4
	Faggots	2
	Ham: raw (Parma/country style)	5
	Kebabs	2
	Meat meals (shepherds/cottage pie, casseroles)	2
	Meat pies (steak and kidney, pasty)	1
	Meat, sliced (cooked ham, tongue)	4
	Meat, sliced (beef, haslet, pork, poultry, etc.)	3
	Pork pies	1
	Poultry (unsliced)	2
	Salami and fermented meat products	5
	Sausages (British)	2
	Sausages (smoked)	5
	Sausage roll	1
	Scotch egg	1
	Tripe and other offal	4
Seafood	Crustaceans (crab, lobster, prawns)	3
	Herring/roll mop and other raw pickled fish	1
	Other fish (cooked)	3
	Seafood meals	3
	Molluscs and other shellfish (cooked)	4
	Smoked fish	4
	Taramasalata	4
Dessert	Cakes, pastries, slices and desserts — with dairy cream	3
	Cakes, pastries, slices and desserts — without dairy cream	2
	Cheesecake	5
	Mousse/dessert	1
	Tarts, flans and pies	2
	Trifle	3
Savoury	Bean curd	5
	Bhaji (onion, spinach, vegetable)	1
	Cheese-based bakery products	2
	Fermented foods	5
	Flan/quiche	2
	Hummus, tzatziki and other dips	4
	Mayonnaise/dressings	2
	Paté (meat, seafood or vegetable)	3
	Samosa	2
	Satay	3
	Spring rolls	3
Vegetable	Coleslaw	3
	Fruit and vegetables (dried)	3
	Fruit and vegetables (fresh)	5

Table 2.2 *continued.*

Food group	Product	Category
	Prepared mixed salads and crudités	4
	Rice	3
	Vegetables and vegetable meals (cooked)	2
Dairy	Cheese	5
	Ice-cream, milk shakes (non-dairy)	2
	Ice-lollipops, slush and sorbet	2
	Yoghurt/frozen yoghurt (natural)	5
Ready-to-eat meals	Pasta/pizza	2
	Meals (other)	2
Sandwiches and filled rolls	With salad	5
	Without salad	4
	With cheese	5

additional information becomes available. The guidelines have no formal standing or status, but:

- samples falling in the 'unsatisfactory' category indicate that further sampling may be necessary and that Environmental Health Officers may wish to undertake a detailed inspection of the premises, food production and handling processes, etc.;
- samples falling in the 'unacceptable, potentially hazardous' category might form a basis for prosecution by the Environmental Health Department.

Careful consideration should be given to the likelihood of success when embarking on a prosecution based solely on unsatisfactory levels in the absence of other unacceptable criteria. PHLS food examiners draw on their own experience and expertise in determining the advice and comments they wish to give and are required to do this when asked to give an expert opinion during legal proceedings. Provision has been made for the inclusion of microbiological standards for foods in both the Food Safety Act 1990 and in EC legislation. Although mandatory standards for more ready-to-eat foods would simplify the interpretation of results, it is preferable to concentrate resources on implementing good manufacturing practice coupled with HACCP principles and risk assessment than to increase end product testing to ensure conformity with microbiological criteria.

Other UK publications containing microbiological guidelines issued by professional and trade organizations representing the food industry are listed in the appendix below.

2.7 Appendix: UK sources of microbiological guidelines

Airline catering

Airline Caterers Technical Coordinating Committee (ACTCC). Airline catering code of good catering practice, 1990. London: ACTCC.

Biscuit, cake, chocolate and confectionery products

Biscuit, Cake, Chocolate and Confectionery Alliance (BCCCA). Hygiene code of practice in biscuit, cake, chocolate and confectionery products, 1998. London: BCCCA.

Biscuit, Cake, Chocolate and Confectionery Alliance (BCCCA). *Salmonella* and related microorganisms in cocoa, chocolate and confectionery ingredients and products: Report of the Microbiological Working Party, 1985. London: BCCCA.

Cheeses

The Creamery Proprietors' Association. Guidelines for good hygienic practice in the manufacture of soft and fresh cheeses, 1988. *Available from:* The Creamery Proprietors' Association, 19 Cornwall Terrace, London NW1 4QP.

The Specialist Cheesemakers' Association. The Specialist Cheesemakers' code of best practice, 1996. *Available from:* The Specialist Cheesemakers' Association, PO Box 448, Newcastle-under-Lyme, Staffs ST5 0BF.

Chilled and frozen foods—for catering

Department of Health. *Chilled and Frozen, Guidelines in Cook-Chill and Cook-Freeze Catering Systems.* London: HMSO, 1989.

Chilled Food Association (CFA). Guidelines for good hygienic practice in the manufacture of chilled foods, 3rd edn, 1997. London: CFA.

Cooked meats

Gaze JE, Shaw R, Archer J. *Identification and Prevention of Hazards Associated with Slow Cooling of Hams and Other Large Cooked Meats and Meat Products. Review No. 8.* Campden & Chorleywood Food Research Association (CCFRA), 1998. Chipping Campden: CCFRA.

Betts GD. *A Code of Practice for the Manufacture of Vacuum and Modified Atmosphere Packaged Chilled Foods. Guideline No. 11.* Campden & Chorleywood Food Research Association, 1996. Chipping Campden: CCFRA.

Food processing

Holah J. *Effective Microbiological Sampling of Food Processing Environments. Guideline No. 20.* Campden & Chorleywood Food Research Association, 1999. Chipping Campden: CCFRA.

Institute of Food Science and Technology (IFST). Development and use of microbiological criteria for foods, 1999. London: IFST.

Ice to cool drinks

Brewers and Licensed Retailers Association (BLRA). Ice hygiene. London: BLRA.

Ice-cream

Ice-Cream Alliance (ICA). Code of practice for the hygienic manufacture of ice-cream, revised 1995. Nottingham: ICA.

Industry guides

Industry Guide to Good Hygiene Practice. Catering Guide, revised 1997. London: Chartered Institute of Environmental Health (CIEH).

Industry Guide to Good Hygiene Practice. Retail Guide, 1997. London: CIEH.

Industry Guide to Good Hygiene Practice. Baking Guide, 1997. London: CIEH.

Industry Guide to Good Hygiene Practice. Wholesale Distributors Guide, 1998. London: CIEH.

Industry Guide to Good Hygiene Practice. Markets and Fairs Guide, 1998. London: CIEH.

Industry Guide to Good Hygiene Practice. Fresh Produce, 1999. London: CIEH.

Industry Guide to Good Hygiene Practice. Flour Milling Guide, 1999. London: CIEH.

Industry Guide to Good Hygiene Practice. Vending and Dispensing Guide Supplement (to the Catering Guide), 2000. London: CIEH.

Hospital Caterers Association. Good Practice Guide. Food service standards at ward level, 1997. Sittingbourne: Hospital Caterers Association.

Hospital Caterers Association. Hygiene Good Practice Guide. An audit tool, 1997. Sittingbourne: Hospital Caterers Association.

Chartered Institute of Environmental Health (CIEH). Hygiene on Coaches. Guidelines to ensure the safe and adequate provision of water supplies, toilet facilities and catering arrangements on board passenger coaches. *Available from:* Chadwick House Group Ltd, Chadwick Court, 15 Hatfields, London SE1 8DJ.

Milk-based powders

The Association of British Preserved Milk Manufacturers (ABPMM). Guidelines for good hygienic practice in the manufacture of milk-based products, 1987. London: ABPMM.

Sandwiches

British Sandwich Association (BSA). Code of practice on vending sandwiches, 1995. Wantage: BSA.

British Sandwich Association (BSA). Code of practice and minimum standards for sandwich bars and those making sandwiches on the premises, revised 2001. Ardington: BSA.

British Sandwich Association (BSA). Code of practice and minimum standards for sandwich manufacturers (producers), revised 2001. Ardington: BSA.

Seafish

The Sea Fish Industry Authority. Guidelines for the facilities and equipment required for handling bivalve molluscs from harvesting through to distribution to retail outlets, 1997. St Andrew's Dock, Hull: Seafish Technology.

Sous-vide processing

Betts GD. *The Microbiological Safety of Sous-vide Processing. Technical Manual No. 39.* Campden & Chorleywood Food Research Association (CCFRA), 1992. Chipping Campden: CCFRA.

Sprouted seeds, mung beans, etc.

Brown KL, Oscroft CA. *Guidelines for the Hygienic Manufacture, Distribution and Retail Sale of Sprouted Seeds with Particular Reference to Mung Beans. Technical Manual No. 25.* Campden & Chorleywood Food Research Association (CCFRA), 1989. Chipping Campden: CCFRA.

2.8 References

1 Swinson C, Rubery E, Roberts C. The Food Safety Act. *Bull R Coll Pathol* 1991; **75**: 7–10.
2 Codes of Practice published by HMSO (unless stated):
   No. 1 Responsibility for Enforcement of the Food Safety Act 1990 (ISBN 0-11-321354-9).
   No. 2 Legal Matters (ISBN 0-11-321353-0).
   No. 3 Inspection Procedures — General (ISBN 0-11-321355-7).
   No. 4 Inspection, Detention and Seizure of Suspect Food (ISBN 0-11-321350-6).
   No. 5 The Use of Improvement Notices (ISBN 0-11-321777-3).
   No. 6 Prohibition Procedures (ISBN 0-11-321349-2).
   No. 7 Sampling for Analysis or Examination (Revised October 2000), Food Standards Agency, 2000 (ISBN 0-11-321351-4).
   No. 8 Food Standards Inspection (Revised July 1996) (ISBN 0-11-321466-9).
   No. 9 Food Hygiene Inspections (Second Revision October 2000), Food Standards Agency, 2000 (ISBN 0-11-321931-8).
   No. 10 Enforcement of the Temperature Control Requirements of Food Hygiene Regulations (ISBN 0-11-321465 0).
   No. 11 Enforcement of the Food Premises (Registration) Regulations (ISBN 0-11-321478-2).
   No. 12 Quick-Frozen Foodstuffs; Division of Enforcement Responsibilities; Enforcement of Temperature Monitoring and Temperature Measurement (Revised 1994) (ISBN 0-11-321-793-5).
   No. 13 Enforcement of the Food Safety Act 1990 in Relation to Crown Premises (ISBN 0-11-321500-2).
   No. 14 Enforcement of the Food Safety (Live Bivalve Molluscs and Other Shellfish) Regulations 1992 (ISBN 0-11-321695-5).
   No. 15 Enforcement of the Food Safety (Fishery Products) Regulations 1992 and Associated Regulations (ISBN 0-11-321798-6).

No. 16 Enforcement of the Food Safety Act 1990 in Relation to the Food Hazard Warning System (Revised August 1997) (ISBN 0-11-321583-5).

No. 17 Enforcement of the Meat Products (Hygiene) Regulations 1994 ('The Regulations') (ISBN 0-11-321880-X).

No. 18 Enforcement of the Dairy Products (Hygiene) Regulations 1995 and the Dairy Products (Hygiene) (Scotland) Regulations 1995 ('The Regulations') (ISBN 0-11-321957-1).

No. 19 Qualifications and Experience of Authorized Officers and Experts (Revised October 2000), Food Standards Agency, 2000.

No. 20 Exchange of Information between Member States of the EU on Routine Food.

3   European Council. Declaration by the European Council on Food Safety, Presidency Conclusions, 12–13 December 1997. Luxembourg: European Council, 1997.

4   European Commission. *White Paper on Food Safety.* COM (1999) 719 final, 12 January 2000.
europe.eu.int/COMM/dgs/health_consumer/library/pub/pub06_en.pdf

5   Regulation 2002/178/EC of the European Parliament and of the Council of 28 January 2002 laying down the general principles and requirements of food law, establishing the European Food Safety Authority and laying down procedures in matters of food saftey. *Official Journal of the European Communities* 2002; L31/1–24.

6   Murphy C. Stages in the EC decision-making process. *PHLS Microbiol Dig* 1991; **8**: 6–8.

7   Robinson L, Murray T. The European Community and United Kingdom hygiene and safety legislation. *Bull R Coll Pathol* 1992; **77**: 20–1.

8   International Commission on Microbiological Specifications for Foods. *Microorganisms in Foods. 4. Application of the Hazard Analysis Critical Control Point (HACCP) System to Ensure Microbiological Safety and Quality.* Oxford: Blackwell Scientific, 1998.

9   European Commission. *Proposal for a regulation of the European Parliament and of the Council on the Hygiene of Foodstuffs.* COM (2000) 438 final. *Official Journal of the European Communities* 2000; C365E/43–57.

10   Van Netten P, Roberts D, Russell J, Perry SF. The PHLS Food Microbiology Quality Assessment Scheme. In: Roberts C, Kelsey MC, eds. *Microbiology, Accreditation and Quality Assessment Schemes in the UK.* Association of Medical Microbiologists 1992; **2**: 28–30.

11   ISO/IEC 17025. *General Requirements for the Competence of Testing and Calibration Laboratories.* Geneva: International Organisation for Standardization, 1999.

12   Gilbert RJ, de Louvois J, Donovan T, *et al.* Second revision of the microbiological guidelines for some ready-to-eat foods sampled at point of sale: an expert opinion from the Public Health Laboratory Service (PHLS). *Comm Dis Public Health* 2000; **3**: 163–7.

3   Schedules for examination of food

This section lists the tests that are employed in the microbiological examination of food and reproduces from published legislation and voluntary codes of practice the microbiological criteria for a number of food products.

3.1   Presentation of test schedules

A schedule of microbiological tests is given under each food heading together with background information on the potential hazards, processing, storage and transportation of the types of food to which the heading relates. The recommended methods for performing the tests are described in Sections 4–9 of this manual and are cross-referenced in the right-hand column of the schedules. The tests are listed in the schedules according to their status, i.e. statutory, recommended or supplementary (see below), and the order in which the methods appear in the subsequent sections in this manual. **The schedules are not intended to reflect the order in which the tests would be performed**.

The symbols that appear in the schedules indicate the status of the tests as follows:

Statutory test (♦)
The test is specified in UK legislation (Statutory Instruments [SI]) or in an European Community (EC) directive for which there is no comparable SI.

Recommended test (▲)
The test should be carried out routinely but there is no legal requirement to do so.

Supplementary test (■)
The test should be performed only when there is a specific reason for doing so, for example when the product has been implicated in an outbreak of illness or when storage conditions were inadequate.

3.2 Microbiological criteria

Where microbiological criteria were available for a particular product or food at the time of preparation of this manual, they are given next to the test schedule for information. The criteria were taken from legislation or from the recommendations of trade or professional organizations allied to the food industry and are subject to change. The relevant up-to-date source documents should be consulted whenever possible.

3.3 Animal feeds

Mammals and birds reared intensively require large amounts of dehydrated protein feed. This material is prepared from meat, offal, bones, blood or feathers, or combinations of these. Fish and vegetable protein may also be added. Animal proteins have a variable but often high content of salmonellae which depends on the initial contamination of the raw materials and on the hygiene of manufacture. Animals fed with contaminated feed, particularly pigs and poultry, often carry these salmonellae in their intestinal tracts, with no sign of illness. Meat from such infected animals may become contaminated during slaughter and processing, and the infection passed on to humans during subsequent poor hygiene practices during preparation or inadequate cooking and storage procedures.

Although animal feed may be heat treated during processing, there are many opportunities for recontamination. Processors (rendering plants) are required to obtain approval from the appropriate Minister (Department of Environment, Food and Rural Affairs (DEFRA)—formerly the Ministry of Agriculture Fisheries and Food (MAFF); the Scottish Office; the Welsh Office) under the Animal By-Products Order 1999 [1]. Feed has to be tested by an approved laboratory before despatch and shown to conform to the parameters listed below. A number of codes of practice have been issued for the control of *Salmonella* in animal feeding stuffs, one of the main requirements of which is the regular monitoring of the material for *Salmonella* using the same method as described for rendering plants in the Animal By-Products Order.

The bacteria in processed food may be damaged as a result of the dehydration process employed during its manufacture, and so a resuscitation step is necessary to ensure the recovery of contaminating organisms.

The sample should be tested on the day of receipt or on the 1st working day that allows the method to be completed. If the test is not begun on the day of receipt the sample must be stored in a refrigerator until required. Refrigerated samples should be left at room temperature for at least 4 h before examination. The sample should be tested in duplicate 25 g portions for *Salmonella*, five 10 g portions for Enterobacteriaceae, and for rendered material derived from high-risk material duplicate 10 g portions for *Clostridium perfringens*. Preparation of samples and methods for examination are given in detail in the Aminal By-Products Order. For *C. perfringens* the Order specifies duplicate pour plates using Shahidi Ferguson agar in a pour plate method similar to that given in Section 6.5, method 1, but also allows enumeration in duplicate exactly as described in method 1 of Section 6.5. The *Salmonella* method is a pre-enrichment and enrichment using one enrichment broth only, Rappaport Vassiliadis (RV) broth incubated at 41.5°C with plating after 24 h and 48 h onto two agar plates. Enterobacteriaceae are enumerated as described in Section 6.7 method 1 using a 1/10 dilution.

Test	Section/method
Product from rendering plants:	
◆ *Clostridium perfringens*	6.5, method 1 (with Shahidi Ferguson agar)
◆ *Salmonella* spp.	6.12 (RV only)
◆ Enterobacteriaceae	6.7, method 1
◆ The Animal By-Products Order (1999) [1]	

Microbiological criteria for animal feeds

The Animal By-Products Order (1999) [1]

In the case of rendered material derived from high-risk material—free from *Clostridium perfringens* (the sample size is equivalent to 0.2 g therefore limit is absent in 2×0.2 g).

For all samples:
Free from *Salmonella* (absent in 2×25 g samples).

Enterobacteriaceae—the sample fails if any arithmetic mean of the duplicate plates exceeds 30 (3×10^2 colony forming units (cfu)/g sample); or three or more arithmetic means are above 10 (1×10^2 cfu/g).

3.4   Baby foods

While infants are fed with milk direct from the breast there is little risk of enteric infection, but once the transition is made to a prepared food or dried milk formula the risk is greater. The immunity of infants against infective organisms is less than that of adults and undernourished or sick infants are particularly susceptible. It is important therefore that milk formulas for babies and dried, bottled or canned baby foods are of good microbiological quality.

A dried formula may be quite safe until reconstituted, whereupon contamination may be introduced and these organisms and others already present may multiply, depending on the temperature at which the product is held. Particular care is necessary in hospitals and maternity units where central milk kitchens supply prepared bottled feeds for distribution. Milk that has been sterilized in the bottle with the teat already in place (inverted) is preferred in most such situations. Similar care should be taken with the preparation and distribution of nasogastric enteral feeds for patients of all ages. Contamination of these feeds can lead to colonization and infection, particularly in immunocompromised patients. Specific advice on the preparation, administration and monitoring of feeds has been produced [2,3]. Where possible, commercially produced prepacked sterile naso-gastric feeds should be given. Sterile water should be used for the dilution of feeds, where necessary.

Dried infant milk has also been identified as a potential source of low numbers of *Enterobacter sakazaki*, an organism that can colonize neonates resulting in abdominal distension, bloody diarrhoea and, in rare cases, sepsis and meningitis [4].

Sampling plans and specifications for dry shelf-stable products, products intended for consumption after the addition of liquid, dried products requiring heating before consumption, and thermally processed products packed in hermetically sealed containers for infants have been drawn up by a committee of the Food and Agriculture Organization (FAO)/World Health Organization (WHO) [5]. Reference values for dried weaning foods and similar products to be used by debilitated consumer groups are also suggested by Mossel and colleagues [6].

The level of *Salmonella* contamination within a dried powdered formula may be so low that it may be missed by examination of only a 25 g sample. In instances where such a product has been implicated in cases of illness in infants it is recommended that multiple 25 g samples are examined from each individual container.

Thermally processed baby food may be examined as for canned food.

Test	Section/method
▲ Colony count	Section 5
▲ *Bacillus cereus*	6.2
▲ Clostridia	6.5
▲ Coliforms/*Escherichia coli*	6.6
▲ *Salmonella* spp.	6.12
▲ *Staphylococcus aureus*	6.14

Microbiological criteria for baby foods

FAO/WHO (1977) [5]

Microbiological specifications for feeds for infants and children.

Product	Organism	Standard
Dried biscuit type		
1 Plain	None	
2 Coated	Coliforms	$m=<3$, $M=20$, $n=5$, $c=2$
	Salmonella spp.	Absent in 25 g, $n=10$, $c=0$
Dried and instant products	Colony count	$m=10^3$, $M=10^4$, $n=5$, $c=2$
	Coliforms	$m=<3$, $M=20$, $n=5$, $c=1$
	Salmonella spp.	Absent in 25 g, $n=60$, $c=0$
Dried products requiring heating before consumption	Colony count	$m=<10^4$, $M=10^5$, $n=5$, $c=2$
	Coliforms	$m=10$, $M=10^2$, $n=5$, $c=2$
	Salmonella spp.	Absent in 25 g, $n=5$, $c=0$
Thermally processed products packaged in hermetically sealed containers	(a) Shall be free of microorganisms capable of growth in the product under normal non-refrigerated storage and distribution	
	(b) Shall not contain any substances originating from microorganisms in amounts which may represent a hazard to health	
	(c) If of pH greater than 4.6 shall have received a processing treatment which renders them free of viable organisms of public health significance	

n, the number of sample units; m, the threshold value for the number of bacteria (satisfactory if not exceeded); M, the maximum value for the number of bacteria (unsatisfactory if exceeded); c, the number of sample units where the bacterial count may be between m and M. (For further explanation see p. 3.)

3.5 Bakery products and confectionery

Incidents of food poisoning have occurred from bakery products, chocolate and confectionery products, but they are rare. Most of the problems with these products are associated with spoilage.

Bread

Moulds are responsible for most of the spoilage problems. The low water activity of bread effectively inhibits bacterial growth provided that the storage conditions are satisfactory. During baking the internal temperature achieved is sufficient to kill bacteria and moulds, apart from some spores. Adequate control of cooling and measures to prevent contamination after baking from slicing and wrapping machines are important. Ropiness, caused by *Bacillus* spp., may occur in a home-baked product, but is unlikely in bread produced commercially, particularly with preservatives such as acetate or propionate.

Fillings and coatings

Most of the food poisoning problems have been associated with the wide variety of fillings or coatings in or added to baked products, such as dairy or artificial creams, custard, coconut, egg products and meats and gravies. Test schedules for these products appear under separate food headings in this section.

Chocolate products

These have a low water activity and often a high fat content. Though once considered safe, chocolate products have now been implicated in a number of *Salmonella* outbreaks [7,8]. In these outbreaks the infectious dose was low and the salmonellae may have been protected from the acidity of the stomach by the high fat content of the chocolate. Soft-centred chocolates may be subject to yeast spoilage.

Following the outbreaks, in 1984 the UK Cocoa, Chocolate and Confectionery Alliance and the Cake and Biscuit Alliance set up a working party to examine the implications for the industry of chocolate contaminated with salmonellae (see Section 2.7). The working party recommended that the emphasis of control should be on preventing the conditions under which salmonellae might contaminate and grow in raw materials, process, environments and product rather than on microbiological testing. Checks to monitor batches of material were considered to be of value in providing information about commodities and in detecting gross contamination. A plan for frequency of sampling and testing for salmonellae was suggested.

Test	Section/method
▲ *Bacillus cereus* and *Bacillus* spp.	6.2
▲ Coliforms/*Escherichia coli*	6.6
▲ Enterobacteriaceae	6.7
▲ *Staphylococcus aureus*	6.14
▲ Yeasts and moulds	6.17
■ Colony count	5.3–5.6
■ *Salmonella* spp.	6.12

3.6 Brines

Bacon and ham are the most common cured meat products. The processes are similar except that sugar may be added in the curing of ham. The principal ingredients of curing solutions are sodium chloride, sodium nitrate and sodium nitrite. These, together with the pH and storage temperature, control the stability of cured meats. Salt reduces the water activity, restricting the growth of spoilage bacteria. Some types of continental sausage are cured and may also be fermented.

In the manufacture of bacon, sides of pork are injected with a freshly prepared solution of salts, often containing about 24% sodium chloride (injection brine), and then immersed in a 15% salt solution (cover brine) for 3–5 days. The cover brine is used repeatedly, with filtering and adjustment of salt concentration between curing cycles. With good management it can be used indefinitely. Dry salting or pickling of meat joints may not prevent spoilage of the deeper tissues.

The stability of curing brines is directly related to microbiological growth and activity, the activity being measured in terms of the reduction of nitrate and/or nitrite with the associated increase in pH. Routine microbiological and chemical examination of curing brines can detect loss of stability and indicate the type of treatment necessary to control the brine [9] and, subsequently, the cure of the bacon. A decrease in salt concentration and shorter immersion time in response to consumer preferences will have an effect on the stability of the product.

Injection brine should be sampled from the preparation or storage tank; cover brine from the reconstitution tank with the mixing device in operation. Direct microscopic counts provide a rapid means of control of cover brine. The presence of salt-requiring vibrios (e.g. *V. costicola*) in brines is usually indicative of 'back flow' contamination, i.e. contamination from cured meats into the curing system. These organisms are important spoilers of bacon.

Test	Section/method
Injection brine:	
▲ Colony count at 22°C	5.3–5.6
Cover brine:	
▲ Colony count at 22°C	5.3–5.6
▲ Coliforms/*Escherichia coli*	6.6
▲ *Vibrio* spp.	6.15
■ Direct microscopic count	4.6

3.7 Canned food

Canned food has been involved in enteric infection and food poisoning incidents, including cases of typhoid, botulism, salmonellosis and staphylococcal poisoning, although in relation to the large amount of canned food consumed such events are uncommon. Problems have also occurred relating to spoilage of consignments of canned food from a variety of countries.

Canned food may be of two types:
- **shelf stable**, i.e. processed to sterility or given a milder process but still expected to withstand storage at ambient temperature for at least 12 months and commonly up to 2 years or more; or
- **perishable**, i.e. given a milder or pasteurization process which permits a limited shelf-life if kept cold.

It must be understood that the heat processing of canned foods is designed to render the product shelf stable at ambient storage temperatures, a process which is referred to as 'commercial sterility'. In most instances the pack may contain residual levels of dormant spores which will not germinate and grow in the product under normal storage conditions. For low-acid foods (pH >4.5) these may be thermoduric spores of *Bacillus* spp. and *Clostridium* spp. that will not germinate below 45°C and for semi-acid and acid category foodstuffs (pH <4.5) may be mesophilic spores of *Bacillus* spp. and *Clostridium* spp. Canned cured meats may also contain mesophilic spores that are prevented from germination by the preservative salt content of the product. The microbiological examination of canned foods should be designed to isolate and identify the abnormal microflora that had led to product spoilage.

Routine quality control is the responsibility of the manufacturer and random sampling at point of sale is impractical. Imported canned products may need to be examined at point of entry to the UK if defects or spoilage develop at point of sale, or the products are implicated in human disease. Apparent swollen can spoilage may occur by chemical attack of the internal metallic surface of the container by the food; improved lacquering has reduced the likelihood of this.

Spoilage organisms may be present in a canned product as a result of inadequate heat processing or from recontamination due to leakage after processing. The results of microbial spoilage are variable. Many bacteria are fermentative and produce souring by the formation of acids. Gas may also be produced and there may be changes in the colour and texture of the product.

Heat treatment

Inadequate processing may result in spoilage by thermoduric and sometimes mesophilic spore-forming bacteria. Though rare, in the extreme it can lead to spoilage by vegetative bacteria. Thermoduric organisms generally cause fermentative spoilage and produce either acid from the available carbohydrates (certain *Bacillus* spp.) or acid and gas (certain *Clostridium* spp.). In the former, the ends of the container remain flat (so-called 'flat-sour spoilage'), and in the latter the can may swell and eventually burst.

Spoilage by mesophilic *Clostridium* spp. may be fermentative, with the production of acid and gas, or putrefactive. In the latter, the anaerobic decomposition of proteins into peptides and amino acids causes the production of foul odours due to hydrogen sulphide, ammonia, amines and other strong-smelling products. The proteolytic anaerobes grow best in weakly acidic canned food such as meat, fish and poultry. Spoilage of acidic food, with a pH of 4.5 or less, such as canned fruit or pickles, is uncommon. Yeasts or moulds may occur in incidences of serious underprocessing. Mould can raise the pH of some acidic food sufficiently to permit the growth of bacteria such as *C. botulinum*.

Some meat products, e.g. canned ham, are less palatable after severe heat processing and so are given the minimum of heat treatment. The pH and level of curing salts in the food in combination with the correct storage temperature should prevent any surviving organisms from multiplying. Vegetative cells of thermoduric bacteria are fairly heat resistant and may spoil this type of product, for example, *Enterococcus faecalis* in canned ham.

Can defects

Spoilage by vegetative bacteria or yeasts usually indicates a defect in the can structure. The negative pressure within a can after heating may allow contaminated cooling water to be drawn in if the can has defective seams. When the seams are dry the chances of contamination are slight. Often only a few cans in a batch are affected. Contamination of canned food by human pathogens, notably *Salmonella Typhi*, has occurred in this way. Adequate chlorination of the cooling water reduces the risk of contamination. The most common point of entry is the junction of the side seam and the double seams of the can lid or base. Small holes due to rust or damage can also allow bacteria to enter. For glass jar packs closed with metal lids the integrity of the sealing surface is an essential feature, especially the finish of the glass jar sealing face and the lining gasket material in the metal lid.

Test	Section/method
▲ Visual inspection/ pre-examination incubation, opening and sampling	Section 4
Stability/spoilage—routine	
▲ pH	4.5
▲ Water activity (a_w)	4.7
▲ Direct microscopic examination	4.6
▲ Colony count at 22°C, 37°C and 55°C	5.3–5.6
▲ Enrichment culture for aerobes	In a suitable liquid medium, e.g. nutrient broth
▲ Enrichment culture for anaerobes	6.5
Food poisoning or spoilage incidents	
Central core or other representative sample:	
▲ pH	4.5
▲ Direct microscopic examination	4.6
▲ Enrichment culture for aerobes	In a suitable liquid medium, e.g. nutrient broth
▲ Enrichment culture for anaerobes	6.5
Subculture of the above, when growth apparent, to appropriate agar plate media:	
▲ *Bacillus* spp.	6.2
▲ Clostridia	6.5
▲ Coliforms/*Escherichia coli*	6.6
▲ Enterobacteriaceae	6.7
▲ Lactobacilli/streptococci	6.9
▲ *Salmonella* spp.	6.12
▲ *Staphylococcus aureus*	6.14
Surface scrapings and seam swabs:	
▲ Direct plate culture	On suitable media, e.g. blood agar, nutrient agar, plate count agar
▲ Enterobacteriaceae	6.7
▲ *Escherichia coli*	6.6

Examination

Before contemplating microbiological examination of canned products it is important to obtain as much background data as possible. The International Commission on Microbiological Specifications for Foods (ICMSF) suggests that routine microbiological testing of shelf-stable canned meat products is unnecessary provided that data on processing, water supply, seam inspection and chemical composition are available and satisfactory [10].

It is important to examine cans for defects before opening them. On removal of the contents a full structural examination can be made. The extent of bacteriological tests on the contents will depend on the reason for examination. If spoilage has occurred, direct microscopy of the homogenate may give useful information about the causative organism(s) and indicate suitable parameters for examination.

3.8 Cereals and rice [11]

Food of plant origin that is used in a dried form may have undergone heat treatment to remove moisture or may have been allowed to dry naturally. The heat treatment applied is usually sufficient to eliminate vegetative cells, but sporing organisms such as *Clostridium perfringens* and *Bacillus cereus* and other *Bacillus* spp. will survive. Food in a dehydrated form may be considered safe other than risks for cross-contamination to other foods, but bacterial growth may occur once it is rehydrated.

Most samples of raw rice contain small numbers of *B. cereus*, and rice has been implicated on many occasions in outbreaks of *B. cereus* food poisoning following storage of cooked rice at ambient temperatures for long periods of time before reheating. Similarly foods containing cereal products such as flour used for thickening sauces or in meat and pastry products have been implicated in incidents of illness attributed to other species of *Bacillus*, mainly of the *B. subtilis/licheniformis* group. The *Bacillus* spores germinate and multiply during periods of storage at unsuitable temperatures. Many pathogenic organisms may be introduced to grains by exposure to human or animal contamination. Organisms present on dried food may be transferred to more sensitive food.

Pasta products are made from wheat flour, potable water and semolina or farina, and other ingredients such as egg (powdered or frozen), spinach, tomato, soya protein, vitamins and minerals may be added. A stiff dough, containing about 30% water, is extruded and dried at a temperature below that of pasteurization. Bacteria may grow rapidly during mixing and drying and pathogens may survive in the final product. Bacteria do not grow in the dry material, but there is a danger of cross contamination from the dried product to a finished moist food. Many of the organisms present in pasta will be killed during cooking. Staphylococcal enterotoxin may not be inactivated by cooking and has been implicated in food poisoning from pasta products when high levels of *S. aureus* and preformed enterotoxin were found in the pasta. Low numbers of *S. aureus* are often found in pasta products.

The most important microbial health hazard from cereal products is mycotoxins caused by the growth of moulds.

Test	Section/method
▲ Aerobic colony count	5.3–5.6
▲ Mycotoxins	Appendix C
■ *Bacillus cereus* and other *Bacillus* spp.	6.2
■ *Salmonella* spp.	6.12
■ *Staphylococcus aureus*	6.14

3.9 Coconut

Salmonellosis has been associated with the consumption of uncooked desiccated coconut. Improved preparation and drying procedures have reduced contamination of the dried product, but *Salmonella* contamination may still be found in some consignments and remains a potential hazard.

Test	Section/method
▲ *Salmonella* spp.	6.12

3.10 Dairy products

Milk is at risk of faecal contamination from the cow or other producer species and is subject to potential contamination from equipment, the environment and humans during collection and processing. Milk supports the growth of many pathogens and, before the widespread adoption of pasteurization and refrigerated storage, was a well-recognized vehicle for food poisoning. Traditionally, a dye reduction test such as the methylene blue test has been used as a simple, inexpensive indicator of product hygiene for milk, cream and ice-cream. However, quality defects with refrigerated products are commonly due to psychrotrophic bacteria that frequently show poor dye reduction activity. More useful information may be obtained by a colony count together with a coliform count and this is reflected in changes in the legislation covering milk.

The EC Milk and Milk-based Products Directive 92/46/EEC [12], that has been transposed into UK national law as the Dairy Products (Hygiene) Regulations 1995 [13], lays down health rules for the production and placing on the market of raw milk, heat treated drinking milk, milk for the manufacture of milk-based products and milk-based products intended for human consumption. The directive includes microbiological criteria for milk and also for certain types of cheese, butter and liquid, powdered and frozen milk-based products including dairy ice-cream. Microbiological limits for milk from animals other than the cow (goat, ewe, buffalo) are also specified. The legislation incorporating the directive into UK law has therefore superseded most of the previous legislation pertaining to milk and dairy products.

BS 4285 describes microbiological methods for the detection of a wide range of organisms in dairy products [14]. More recent updates of some of these methods have been issued as BS ISO or BS EN ISO documents and are cited in Section 7 of this manual. Section 7 is devoted to the examination of milk and other dairy products as they are subject to extensive testing for statutory purposes.

Cheese

Most cheese is made by the fermentation of milk. The finished product usually contains large numbers of the lactic acid producing bacteria that were used to bring about the fermentation together with moulds and bacteria used to impart traditional flavours. Fresh cheese, however, often has a low bacterial count of about 10^3 organisms/g owing to destruction of the lactic acid bacteria by heat during production of the cheese.

There are three main types of cheese:

- **Hard-pressed cheese**. Cheddar is a prime example of this type of cheese. It is made from firm, relatively dry curd that is ripened by bacteria and matured over a period of some months. Lactobacilli gradually become predominant during the ripening process. This cheese has a low water activity, low pH and a high salt content.
- **Soft cheese**. Some varieties of soft cheese are eaten fresh (e.g. Cottage, Cream) while others are ripened, usually by the action of surface moulds (e.g. Brie, Camembert). Soft cheese retains a high moisture content, has a relatively high pH and a low salt content. Some pathogens, such as *Listeria monocytogenes*, are able to multiply during the maturation period particularly in the area just below the rind or crust.
- **Blue-veined mould-ripened cheese**. The particular flavour of the final product is achieved by inoculating the cheese with moulds, such as *Penicillium* spp., that grow within the cheese (e.g. Stilton, Gorgonzola).

Pathogens present in milk used for the manufacture of cheese may survive the cheese making process and remain viable in the finished product. Most cheese is made with pasteurized milk and should not contain pathogens. Contamination of a product made with pasteurized milk may occur at various stages during manufacture.

Most ripened cheeses have a high colony count because of the presence of the lactic acid producing bacteria used to achieve fermentation of the milk. Samples taken from a soft or a mould-ripened cheese should always include the outer rind when examined for *Listeria* spp. as higher numbers of the organism are found in the rind.

The Creamery Proprietors' Association has produced a code of practice for the production of soft cheese and fresh cheese (see Section 2.7). It includes advisory microbiological guidelines, with particular reference to *Listeria* spp., on environmental routine and investigative screening.

Test	Section/method
◆ Coliforms (30°C) (guideline)	7.4, method 1
◆ *Escherichia coli* (raw milk cheese, soft cheese)	7.4, method 1
◆ *Listeria monocytogenes*	6.10
◆ *Salmonella* spp.	6.12
◆ *Staphylococcus aureus*	6.14
▲ pH	4.5
■ Colony count	Section 5, e.g. 5.3–5.6

◆ Dairy Products (Hygiene) Regulations (1995) [13]

Microbiological criteria for cheese

Dairy Products (Hygiene) Regulations (1995) [13]

The following criteria are applicable to the manufactured product on removal from the processing establishment.

Product	Organism	Standard
Cheese other than hard cheese	*Listeria monocytogenes*	Absent in 25 g, $n=5$, $c=0$ (from 5×5 g samples)
Hard cheese		Absent in 1 g, $n=5$, $c=0$
All products	*Salmonella* spp.	Absent in 25 g, $n=5$, $c=0$
Cheese made from raw or thermised milk	*Staphylococcus aureus*	$m=10^3$, $M=10^4$, $n=5$, $c=2$
Soft cheese (made from heat treated milk)		$m=10^2$, $M=10^3$, $n=5$, $c=2$
Fresh cheese		$m=10$, $M=10^2$, $n=5$, $c=2$
Cheese made from raw or thermised milk	*Escherichia coli*	$m=10^4$, $M=10^5$, $n=5$, $c=2$
Soft cheese (made from heat treated milk)		$m=10^2$, $M=10^3$, $n=5$, $c=2$
Indicator organisms—guidelines:		
Soft cheese (made from heat treated milk)	Coliforms (30°C)	$m=10^4$, $M=10^5$, $n=5$, $c=2$

n, the number of sample units; m, the threshold value for the number of bacteria (satisfactory if not exceeded); M, the maximum value for the number of bacteria (unsatisfactory if exceeded); c, the number of sample units where the bacterial count may be between m and M. (For further explanation see p. 3.)

Creamery Proprietors' Association (see Section 2.7)

Advisory microbiological guidelines for soft cheese and fresh cheese:

Pathogenic *Listeria* spp. should not be detected in 15×25 g samples per lot of end product.

Cream

Cream may be separated from raw or pasteurized milk. Cream made from pasteurized milk contains thermoduric organisms (e.g. *Bacillus* spp.) that have survived heat treatment or are post-pasteurization contaminants. In addition, raw cream may contain any of the pathogens found in raw milk. Sterilized and ultra heat treated (UHT) cream in sealed containers should not contain viable organisms. Pasteurized, sterilized and UHT cream are required to satisfy statutory tests as prescribed in the Dairy Products (Hygiene) Regulations 1995 [13]. In the past the methylene blue reduction test was used as a simple, inexpensive indicator of the hygienic quality of raw, pasteurized and clotted cream. However, anomalies did occur between the results of that test and those of colony count and coliform tests. The latter tests give more useful information and are preferred by the dairy industry. Pasteurized cream examined at the heat treatment premises is covered by the Dairy Products (Hygiene) Regulations, which imposes a coliform (30°C) test (guideline) and examination for *Salmonella* spp. and *L. monocytogenes*. There is a requirement to satisfy a phosphatase test and to give a negative peroxidase test. Sterilized and UHT cream are required to satisfy a pre-incubated plate count test as before, but the specified temperature of incubation is 30°C.

Test	Section/method
Untreated cream:	
▲ Colony count	7.2, method 1
▲ *Bacillus* spp.	6.2
▲ *Campylobacter* spp.	6.4
▲ *Listeria monocytogenes*	6.10
▲ *Salmonella* spp.	6.12
▲ *Staphylococcus aureus*	6.14
▲ Coliforms/*Escherichia coli*	7.4, method 1
■ *Brucella* spp.	6.3
■ *Yersinia* spp.	6.18
Pasteurized cream:	
◆ *Listeria monocytogenes*	6.9
◆ *Salmonella* spp.	6.12
◆ Peroxidase test	7.1, method 4
◆ Coliform test (30°C)	7.4, method 1
◆ Phosphatase test	7.4, method 7
■ Colony count	7.2, method 1
■ *Bacillus* spp.	6.2

continued

Microbiological criteria for cream

Dairy Products (Hygiene) Regulations (1995) [13]

Pasteurized cream:

Listeria monocytogenes	Absent in 1 mL
Salmonella spp.	Absent in 25 mL, $n=5$, $c=0$
Coliforms (30°C)	$m=0$, $M=5$, $c=2$
Phosphatase	Must satisfy the test
Peroxidase	Must give a negative reaction

Sterilized or UHT cream:

Colony count (30°C)*	Not more than 100 cfu/1 mL

---

*After incubation in a closed container at 30°C for 15 days.

n, the number of sample units; m, the threshold value for the number of bacteria (satisfactory if not exceeded); M, the maximum value for the number of bacteria (unsatisfactory if exceeded); c, the number of sample units where the bacterial count may be between m and M. (For further explanation see p. 3.)

Ice-cream

The Ice-cream Regulations (1959, 1963) require that ingredients used in the manufacture of ice-cream are pasteurized or sterilized and subsequently kept at a low temperature until the freezing process has begun [15,16]. The regulations make it an offence to sell or offer for sale ice-cream that has not been so treated or has been allowed to reach a temperature above −2°C without again being heat treated. Certain types of water ices and ice-lollies are exempt from the heat treatment requirements because they are sufficiently acid (pH 4.5 or less) to make such treatment unnecessary.

A modified methylene blue reduction test has been used as a crude indication of the hygienic quality of ice-cream; products that are coloured or contain additives such as fruit juices and nuts are unsuitable for the test. A combination of colony count and coliform count is commonly used in industrial quality control.

Microbiological criteria for frozen milk-based products, including ice-cream, sampled at the processing establishment, are contained in the Milk and Milk-based Products Directive 92/46/EEC [12] and the Dairy Products (Hygiene) Regulations (1995) [13]. Commercially produced ice-cream mix has an excellent safety record because heat treatment of the product has long been a statutory requirement. However, ice-cream made from basic ingredients (for example in domestic or catering premises) containing raw egg and other potentially contaminated items has been associated with incidents of food poisoning. Machines that deliver soft ice-cream require special attention with respect to regular maintenance and cleaning to prevent build up of contamination in pipes and nozzles. UHT ice-cream mix should be treated as for other UHT dairy products (milk, cream, milk-based drinks) and a colony count performed after pre-incubation of the sample at 30°C.

Test	Section/method
◆ *Listeria monocytogenes*	6.10
◆ *Salmonella* spp.	6.12
◆ *Staphylococcus aureus*	6.14
◆ Coliforms (30°C) (guideline)	7.4, method 1
◆ Colony count (30°C) (guideline)	7.4, method 8
■ *Bacillus* spp.	6.2
■ *Escherichia coli*	7.4, method 1 or 6.6
UHT mix:	
▲ Colony count (30°C)*	7.3, method 1

◆ Dairy Products (Hygiene) Regulations (1995) [13]
*After pre-incubation at 30°C for 15 days.

Microbiological criteria for ice-cream

Dairy Products (Hygiene) Regulations (1995) [13]

Criteria for frozen milk-based products:

Listeria monocytogenes	Absent in 1 g
Salmonella spp.	Absent in 25 g, $n=5$, $c=0$
Coliforms (30°C) (guideline)	$m=10$, $M=100$, $n=5$, $c=2$
Staphylococcus aureus	$m=10$, $M=100$, $n=5$, $c=2$
Colony count (30°C) (guideline)	$m=10^5$, $M=5\times10^5$, $n=5$, $c=2$

n, the number of sample units; m, the threshold value for the number of bacteria (satisfactory if not exceeded); M, the maximum value for the number of bacteria (unsatisfactory if exceeded); c, the number of sample units where the bacterial count may be between m and M. (For further explanation see p. 3.)

Milk

Untreated milk

Raw milk may contain pathogens derived from the cow (or other milk animal) such as *Campylobacter* spp., *Salmonella* spp., *Cryptosporidium*, *E. coli* O157, *S. aureus* and *L. monocytogenes*. Raw milk is a recognized vehicle for food poisoning.

The methylene blue dye reduction test, as a statutory test for cows' milk for drinking, was replaced in the Milk (Special Designation) Regulations 1989 [17] by a colony count and coliform test. Directive 92/46/EEC [12] allows a colony count of up to 5×10^4 cfu/mL for cows' milk for drinking purposes and does not cover raw milk from other sources. However, the UK legislation, enacting the EC Directive, the Dairy Products (Hygiene) Regulations (1995) [13] retains the more stringent specification of up to 2×10^4 cfu/mL for raw cows' milk sold directly to the consumer, as found in the 1989 regulations, and applies them to milk from ewes, goats and buffaloes as well. The EC Directive also specifies an examination for *S. aureus* and *Salmonella* spp., and requires that pathogenic microorganisms and their toxins shall not be present in quantities that might affect the health of consumers. In the UK legislation the requirements on *Salmonella* spp. and *S. aureus* apply only to milk for export to a Member State.

The EC Directive and the UK legislation also contain specifications for raw milk intended for the production of milk-based products or pasteurized milk. These vary according to the proposed use of the milk and the animal source.

Test	Section/method
◆ *Salmonella* spp.	6.12
◆ *Staphylococcus aureus*	6.14
◆ Colony count (30°C)	7.2, method 1
◆ Coliforms (30°C)	7.1, method 2
▲ *Campylobacter* spp.	6.4
▲ *Escherichia coli*	6.6
■ *Brucella* spp.	6.3
■ *Listeria monocytogenes*	6.10
■ *Yersinia* spp.	6.18
■ *Cryptosporidium* spp.	Appendix C

◆ Dairy Products (Hygiene) Regulations (1995) [13]

Microbiological criteria for untreated milk for drinking

Dairy Products (Hygiene) Regulations (1995) [13]

Milk sold directly to the consumer (cow, goat, ewe, buffalo):
Pathogenic microorganisms and their toxins shall not be present in quantities that may affect the health of the consumer.

Colony count (30°C)	$\leq 2 \times 10^4$/mL
Coliforms (30°C)	< 100/mL

Cows' milk for export to another Member State:

Colony count (30°C)*	$\leq 5 \times 10^4$/mL
Staphylococcus aureus/mL	$m = 10^2$, $M = 5 \times 10^2$, $n = 5$, $c = 2$
Salmonella spp.	Absent in 25 mL, $n = 5$, $c = 0$

---

*Colony count taken as the geometric average over a period of 2 months with a minimum of two samples per month.

n, the number of sample units; m, the threshold value for the number of bacteria (satisfactory if not exceeded); M, the maximum value for the number of bacteria (unsatisfactory if exceeded); c, the number of sample units where the bacterial count may be between m and M. (For further explanation see p. 3.)

Microbiological criteria for raw milk intended for the manufacture of dairy products which will have no further heat treatment

Dairy Products (Hygiene) Regulations (1995) [13]

Cows' milk:

Colony count (30°C)	$< 1 \times 10^5$/mL
Staphylococcus aureus/mL	$m = 500$, $M = 2000$, $n = 5$, $c = 2$

Goats', ewes' or buffaloes' milk:

Colony count (30°C)	$< 1.5 \times 10^6$/mL
Staphylococcus aureus/mL	$m = 500$, $M = 2000$, $n = 5$, $c = 2$

---

n, the number of sample units; m, the threshold value for the number of bacteria (satisfactory if not exceeded); M, the maximum value for the number of bacteria (unsatisfactory if exceeded); c, the number of sample units where the bacterial count may be between m and M. (For further explanation see p. 3.)

Pasteurized milk

The phosphatase enzyme present in raw milk is destroyed by pasteurization and a test for residual phosphatase activity should be used to check that effective heat treatment has been achieved. The Milk and Milk-based Products Directive 92/46/EEC [12] also stipulates a peroxidase test, which is used to indicate whether overheating (greater than 75°C) of pasteurized milk has taken place.

The Dairy Products (Hygiene) Regulations 1995 [13] require pasteurized cows' milk sampled at the heat treatment premises to satisfy a pre-incubated colony count, coliform test and phosphatase test and to give a positive reaction in the peroxidase test. Procedures for the collection and transport of samples and the test methods are specified in Commission Decision 91/180/EEC [18], and guidelines have been produced for enforcement purposes [19,20]. It is no longer a statutory requirement to perform the methylene blue test on pasteurized milk. The EC Directive does not stipulate a colony count, nor do the UK regulations incorporating the directive into national law (Dairy Products [Hygiene] Regulations 1995 [13]). There is also a requirement for the absence of pathogens and toxins in quantities that may be harmful to the consumer, but the Commission Decision [18] states that if the specified tests are satisfactory testing for pathogens is only necessary in instances where food poisoning is suspected. The Dairy Products (Hygiene) Regulations apply to pasteurized milk not only from cows but also from ewes, goats and buffaloes.

Test	Section/method
◆ *Listeria monocytogenes*	6.10
◆ *Salmonella* spp.	6.12
◆ Pre-incubated colony count (21°C)*	7.1, method 1
◆ Coliforms (30°C)	7.1, method 2
◆ Phosphatase test	7.1, method 3
◆ Peroxidase test	7.1, method 4
■ *Campylobacter* spp.	6.4
■ *Yersinia* spp.	6.18

◆ Dairy Products (Hygiene) Regulations (1995) [13]
*After pre-incubation at 6°C for 5 days.

Microbiological criteria for pasteurized drinking milk (all milks)

Dairy Products (Hygiene) Regulations (1995) [13]

Pathogenic microorganisms	Absent in 25 g; $n=5$, $c=0$
Pre-incubated colony count/mL	$m=5\times10^4$, $M=5\times10^5$, $n=5$, $c=1$
Coliforms/mL	$m=0$, $M=5$, $n=5$, $c=1$

n, the number of sample units; m, the threshold value for the number of bacteria (satisfactory if not exceeded); M, the maximum value for the number of bacteria (unsatisfactory if exceeded); c, the number of sample units where the bacterial count may be between m and M. (For further explanation see p. 3.)

Sterilized and ultra heat treated milk

The designation 'sterilized' is used for milk that is heated in its final container to a temperature of at least 100°C for several minutes (usually in the range 105–120°C for 10–30 min). The heating process should result in complete denaturation of the soluble milk proteins and destruction of viable organisms. The completeness of protein denaturation used to be monitored by the turbidity test, which detects any undenatured whey protein; however, this test is not included in either Directive 92/46/EEC [12] or the UK regulations (the Dairy Products (Hygiene) Regulations 1995 [13]).

The designation 'UHT' (ultra heat treated) is used for milk that has been treated by the ultra high temperature method, that is, heated to a temperature of 135–150°C for a sufficient length of time to produce a satisfactory level of commercial sterility (usually 138–142°C for 2–5 s). Thus all residual spoilage microorganisms and their spores are destroyed with minimal chemical, physical and organoleptic changes to the milk. The UHT milk is then put into containers under aseptic conditions.

Both sterilized milk and UHT milk are required to satisfy a statutory colony count test after pre-incubation at 30°C for 15 days (or 55°C for 7 days if heat resistant spores are likely to cause a problem) if collected at the processing plant [12,13].

Test	Section/method
Sterilized and UHT milk:	
◆ Colony count (30°C)*	7.3, method 1

◆ Dairy Products (Hygiene) Regulations (1995) [13]
*After incubation of the milk at 30°C for 15 days or 55°C for 7 days.

Microbiological criteria for sterilized and UHT milk

Dairy Products (Hygiene) Regulations (1995) [13]

Colony count (30°C)*	≤100/mL

*After incubation of the milk at 30°C for 15 days or 55°C for 7 days.

Semi-skimmed and skimmed milk

Both semi-skimmed (fat content 1.5–1.8%) and skimmed (fat content not more than 0.3%) milk are required to be subject to a heat treatment process (pasteurization, sterilization or UHT method). The test schedules applicable to these milks are as given for whole milk under the appropriate heat treatment heading.

Other milk-based products

Milk-based drinks

Milk-based drinks may be prepared for retail sale by the addition of flavourings to pasteurized, sterilized or UHT milk. No specific reference is made to milk-based drinks in Directive 92/46/EEC [12], or the UK legislation [13] but they should be considered as liquid milk-based products and the appropriate tests applied. The directive and UK legislation (Dairy Products [Hygiene] Regulations, 1995 [13]) specify that colony counts on UHT or sterilized milk-based products are performed after incubation of the intact container at 30°C for 15 days. There is a general requirement for absence of pathogens and their toxins as well as specific standard and guideline criteria.

Test	Section/method
Pasteurized milk-based drinks:	
◆ *Listeria monocytogenes*	6.10
◆ *Salmonella* spp.	6.12
◆ Coliforms (30°C) (guideline)	7.4, method 1
■ *Yersinia* spp.	6.18
■ Phosphatase test	7.1, method 3b
■ Colony count	7.4, method 8
Sterilized or UHT milk-based drinks:	
◆ Colony count	7.3, method 1

◆ Dairy Products (Hygiene) Regulations (1995) [13]

Microbiological criteria for milk-based drinks

Dairy Products (Hygiene) Regulations (1995) [13]

For liquid milk-based products on removal from the processing plant:

◆ *Listeria monocytogenes*	Absent in 1 g, $n=5$, $c=0$
◆ *Salmonella* spp.	Absent in 25 g, $n=5$, $c=0$
◆ Coliforms (30°C)/mL (guideline)	$m=0$, $M=5$, $n=5$, $c=0$

Milk-based products that are UHT or sterilized and intended for conservation at room temperature:

◆ Colony count (30°C)*	≤100 cfu/mL milk

---

*After incubation of the milk at 30°C for 15 days.

n, the number of sample units; m, the threshold value for the number of bacteria (satisfactory if not exceeded); M, the maximum value for the number of bacteria (unsatisfactory if exceeded); c, the number of sample units where the bacterial count may be between m and M. (For further explanation see p. 3.)

Dried milk

Liquid milk to be used for the production of dried milk is required to be stored under conditions that do not allow multiplication of potential pathogens. *S. aureus* in particular must be prevented from multiplying and producing enterotoxin to a concentration that would be a hazard in the dried product.

The microflora of dried milk is determined by a number of factors, notably the temperature to which the milk is raised before drying and the drying process employed. Milk may be spray dried or roller dried. The temperature achieved in roller drying is higher than that for spray drying and consequently roller-dried milk contains fewer organisms than spray-dried milk. Organisms may be introduced during processing and packing. The low water content of dried milk will result in a decrease in the number of viable organisms during storage and spore-forming organisms will usually predominate.

When dried milk is reconstituted surviving organisms will be able to multiply, so reconstituted milk should be treated with the same care as fresh milk.

Occasionally, salmonellae have been detected in dried milk and have been responsible for outbreaks of food poisoning. The level of *Salmonella* contamination may be extremely low and so it may be necessary to examine a large number of samples of greater quantity in order to detect the presence of the organism. In an outbreak associated with *Salmonella* Ealing in a dried formula for infants the level of contamination was shown to be less than two salmonellae/450 g pack of baby milk.

A pre-enrichment step is also important to allow recovery of cells damaged by the heat treatment applied during the drying process.

Test	Section/method
◆ *Listeria monocytogenes*	6.10
◆ *Salmonella* spp.	6.12
◆ *Staphylococcus aureus*	6.14
◆ Coliforms (30°C) (guideline)	7.4, method 1
▲ Colony count	5.3–5.6; 7.4, method 8
▲ *Bacillus* spp.	6.2
▲ *Escherichia coli*	7.4, method 1; 6.6

◆ Dairy Products (Hygiene) Regulations (1995) [13]

Yoghurt

Yoghurt is mostly made by first heating milk, usually to 85°C for 30 min or 90–95°C for 5–10 min. This is followed by cooling, inoculation with *Lactobacillus bulgaricus* and *Streptococcus thermophilus* and incubation at 40–42°C. The starter organisms produce acid, lowering the pH and giving the product its characteristic flavour. Yoghurt is frequently flavoured and sweetened; fruit is a common addition. Pathogenic organisms that may be introduced with fruit or other flavourings will not multiply at the low pH of the product. Yeasts and moulds are little affected by the low pH and may cause spoilage.

In the Dairy Products (Hygiene) Regulations (1995) [13], fermented products such as yoghurt would be required to meet the criteria listed for milk-based products.

Test	Section/method
◆ *Listeria monocytogenes*	6.10
◆ *Salmonella* spp.	6.12
◆ Coliforms (30°C) (guideline)	7.4, method 1
▲ pH	4.5
▲ *Escherichia coli*	7.7, method 1; 6.6
■ *Staphylococcus aureus*	6.14
■ Shelf-life tests to determine the behaviour of contaminating organisms, e.g. yeasts, coliforms	Incubate sample at 4°C for 10 days/20°C for 3 days before testing

---

◆ Dairy Products (Hygiene) Regulations (1995) [13]

3.11   Dried foods

This heading refers to dried foods in general, although some specific foods are mentioned briefly. Animal feeds, baby foods, cereals and rice, coconut, milk, eggs and gelatin, all in the dried form, are considered under separate headings elsewhere in this section.

Microorganisms vary in their minimum requirements for water and the amount of available water influences their ability to grow. Some foods are sufficiently dry when harvested to prevent microbial growth; others are preserved by the removal of water, that is, by a drying process. A dried food can be expected to contain spore-bearing bacteria and moulds that are difficult to remove by the heat applied in the drying process. Foods of plant origin such as cereals, grains, herbs and spices are particularly likely to contain sporing bacilli, a major source of the contamination being the soil and environment in which the plants grow. Grain is naturally contaminated by soil and dust and also by rodent and bird faeces. Contamination levels may be increased during transportation and handling of the produce. Dried food stored under humid conditions will absorb water at its surface, it can then support the growth of moulds and, if more water is absorbed, eventually yeasts and then bacteria. Food stored in a sealed polythene bag, which prevents the escape of water vapour from the atmosphere surrounding it, collects moisture on its surface and becomes more liable to spoilage. Dried food may be a source of contamination to other food, which may in turn provide suitable conditions for growth. Organisms present in the original food may be damaged during the drying processing, therefore, a resuscitation step is necessary in the microbiological examination of the product.

Dried foods that are likely to require examination, in addition to those covered under separate headings elsewhere in this section, include cake mixes, cornflour, herbs, spices, instant desserts, soups, vegetables and dehydrated meats.

Mycotoxins, of which aflatoxins are the most important, have been detected in a variety of dried foods including soya beans, ground spices, rice, maize and spaghetti. Nuts such as peanuts are susceptible to mould contamination, growth and mycotoxin production. Damaged nuts, particularly those stored under hot, humid conditions, may become heavily contaminated and associated with poisoning. Aflatoxins may not be destroyed by the heat employed in the process of cooking. The significance to human health of the small amounts of such toxins that are present in a number of dried foods has not been established.

Test	Section/method
▲ Colony count	Section 5, e.g. 5.3–5.6
▲ *Bacillus* spp.	6.2
▲ Clostridia	6.5
▲ Coliforms/*Escherichia coli*	6.6
▲ Enterobacteriaceae	6.7
▲ *Salmonella* spp.	6.12
▲ *Staphylococcus aureus*	6.14
▲ Yeasts and moulds	6.17
■ Mycotoxins	Appendix C

3.12 Eggs

Eggs are used in catering in a variety of forms; for example, in small quantities as separated albumen and yolk from shell eggs broken out by hand, or in larger quantities, as homogenized pasteurized liquid egg, egg powder, egg albumen, crystalline or powdered egg albumen in commercial kitchens. All of these products may be contaminated with a variety of organisms including salmonellae and *Bacillus cereus* and each requires a different examination, depending on the nature of the investigation being undertaken. The test schedules for a number of egg products (shell eggs, raw bulk liquid egg, pasteurized bulk liquid egg, liquid egg albumen, crystalline egg albumen, powdered egg and other preserved eggs) follow under separate subheadings. Further details on methods are given in Section 8 of this manual.

Shell eggs

Shell eggs may be contaminated with various *Salmonella* spp. during their passage down the oviduct of the laying bird. The organism is then usually present in the egg contents in small numbers, but in pure culture, and may be present as a microcolony lying in the albumen near to the yolk. Levels of *Salmonella* usually remain relatively low for up to 2 weeks, but if the eggs are stored at ambient temperature for prolonged periods very high levels may be reached without apparent physical changes. The shell may also be contaminated during the passage of the egg down the oviduct or from the environment after laying. On the shell,

Salmonella spp. may be mixed with other organisms including coliform bacilli, *Pseudomonas* spp., *Bacillus* spp., staphylococci and faecal streptococci.

Shell eggs are normally examined just for the presence of *Salmonella* spp. Each method involves some compromise owing to the practical difficulty of separating shell, albumen and yolk. There are several methods available and the choice of method will be determined by the purpose of the examination.

The most sensitive technique is the examination of individual eggs without disinfection of the shells, but there is a risk of contamination of the contents by the dirty shell. This therefore needs to be taken into account on interpretation of the results. Similar considerations apply when eggs are examined by bulking batches of three or six without shell disinfection. Batch examination may result in some loss of sensitivity, particularly if the incubation of the enrichment culture is not sufficiently prolonged. Shell disinfection removes the risk of contamination of the contents but swabbing of the shells is likely to result in a reduced sensitivity.

Eggs may also be examined by separating the albumen and yolk, but this is complicated by the unavoidable contamination of one component by another, since the yolk and shell are always coated with albumen. For research purposes, a most probable number (MPN) technique can be applied to determine the number of salmonellae present, but the low isolation rate, small quantity of material available and viscous nature of egg present particular problems.

The most useful information may be obtained by the examination of eggs from the following sources:
- The homes of cases of salmonellosis.
- The producer of the eggs consumed by the cases of salmonellosis (retail outlet and/or farm).
- The retail outlet from which eggs were purchased by cases.
- Travelling salesmen of eggs in the same geographical area as cases.
- The oviduct of laying hens at post-mortem.
- Retail outlets, packing stations, etc. as part of a survey.

There is a statutory requirement under the Zoonoses Order 1989 to report the isolation of *Salmonella* spp. from eggs that can be identified with certainty as coming from a particular flock [21].

Test	Section/method
Salmonella spp., individual eggs:	
▲ Without shell disinfection	8.1, method 1
▲ With shell disinfection	8.1, method 2
Salmonella spp., batched eggs:	
▲ Without shell disinfection	8.1, method 3
▲ With shell disinfection	8.1, method 4

Raw bulk liquid egg

Unpasteurized (raw) bulk liquid egg is commonly heavily contaminated with a wide variety of different organisms. This, in combination with its extremely adhesive characteristics, makes it pernicious material to have in the laboratory. It should therefore be treated with the extra care applied to highly infected clinical material. Examination is normally made for the presence of salmonellae. Several serotypes may be present in one sample and multiple samples will give differing results if the product is not homogeneous. The sensitivity of the isolation procedure is increased by the use of an MPN technique with dilution of the sample.

Examinations for colony count, coliforms and *Escherichia coli* and other organisms may also be made where necessary.

Test	Section/method
■ Colony count	5.3–5.6
■ Coliforms/*Escherichia coli*	6.6
■ Enterobacteriaceae	6.7
▲ *Salmonella* spp.	8.2, method 1

Pasteurized bulk liquid egg

Egg products were a major source of human salmonellosis before statutory pasteurization of liquid egg was introduced in 1964. It is important to monitor the effectiveness of pasteurization. The alpha-amylase test is based on inactivation of the enzyme naturally present in egg by the pasteurization process and is widely used. However, some effective pasteurization processes do not completely inactivate the enzyme. A colony count can be used instead of the alpha-amylase test. It has been demonstrated that post-pasteurization contamination with salmonellae does occur. It is recommended that all egg products be examined routinely for salmonellae. A Statutory Instrument, The Egg Products Regulations 1993 [22] implements an EC directive on egg products (89/437/EEC) [23a] which contains microbiological standards for *Salmonella* spp., Enterobacteriaceae, *Staphylococcus aureus* and colony counts in the product from the treatment establishment.

Test	Section/method
◆ Colony count (30°C)	5.3–5.6
◆ Enterobacteriaceae	6.7
◆ *Salmonella* spp.	6.12
◆ *Staphylococcus aureus*	6.14
◆ Alpha-amylase	8.2, method 3
▲ *Bacillus* spp.	6.2

◆ The Egg Products Regulations (1993) [22]

Microbiological criteria for egg products

The Egg Products Regulations (1993) [22]. EC Directive 89/437/EEC [23a]

Colony count (30°C)	$m=10^5$/g or mL
Enterobacteriaceae	$m=10^2$/g or mL
Staphylococci	Absent in 1 g or mL
Salmonella spp.	Absent in 25 g or 25 mL

Liquid egg albumen

Liquid egg albumen cannot be pasteurized at the temperatures that are used for homogenized whole liquid egg as the heating damages the functional qualities of the product (whipping, emulsifying, coagulation, etc.). The use of lower temperatures increases the chance of survival of salmonellae. Liquid egg albumen should therefore be examined for the presence of *Salmonella* spp. and for other organisms as required (e.g. according to current legislation).

It should be noted that egg albumen contains antibacterial substances that should be diluted out in the pre-enrichment culture for salmonellae.

Test	Section/method
◆ Colony count (30°C)	5.3–5.6
◆ Enterobacteriaceae	6.7
◆ *Salmonella* spp.	6.12
◆ *Staphylococcus aureus*	6.14
▲ *Bacillus* spp.	6.2

◆ The Egg Products Regulations (1993) [22]

Microbiological criteria for liquid egg albumen

As for pasteurized bulk liquid egg

Crystalline egg albumen

Chinese crystalline egg albumen was contaminated in the 1960s with *Salmonella* Paratyphi B. Culture methods therefore should be selected that will allow this organism to grow. Selenite cystine or a tetrathionate broth should be included in the enrichment procedure if this organism is suspected.

Test	Section/method
◆ Colony count (30°C)	5.3–5.6
◆ Enterobacteriaceae	6.7
◆ *Salmonella* spp.	6.12, method 1
◆ *Staphylococcus aureus*	6.14
■ *Bacillus* spp.	6.2
■ *Escherichia coli*	6.6

◆ The Egg Products Regulations (1993) [22]

Microbiological criteria for crystalline egg albumen

As for pasteurized bulk liquid egg.

Powdered egg

Drying kills most of the bacteria initially present in the egg. Once dried the microbial flora is stabilized, and further decline is slow over prolonged storage. The predominant organisms are the most resistant members of the original flora, enterococci and aerobic sporing bacilli. Salmonellae will be reduced in num-bers but some may survive. Thus powdered egg products, including whole egg, egg yolk and albumen, should be examined for the presence of salmonellae. Tests for colony counts and other organisms such as Enterobacteriaceae, *E. coli* and *B. cereus* may be included where necessary.

Test	Section/method
◆ Colony count (30°C)	5.3–5.6
◆ Enterobacteriaceae	6.7
◆ *Salmonella* spp.	6.12
◆ *Staphylococcus aureus*	6.14
■ *Bacillus* spp.	6.2
■ *Escherichia coli*	6.6

◆ The Egg Products Regulations (1993) [22]

Microbiological criteria for powdered egg

As for pasteurized bulk liquid egg

Eggs preserved by other methods

Eggs preserved by the addition of a salt or sugar, coating with clay or by fermentation should all be examined for the presence of salmonellae. Other tests should be selected depending on the purpose of the examination.

Test	Section/method
▲ *Salmonella* spp.	6.12, method 1

3.13 Fish, crustaceans and molluscan shellfish [23]

Fish

Unless caught in polluted waters, fresh fish are unlikely to be a source of human pathogens. The only organisms of public health significance that are normally associated with fish are *Vibrio parahaemolyticus*, which is mainly found in fish from sea water, and *Clostridium botulinum*. In some countries outbreaks of botulism have been associated with the consumption of raw, preserved fish, mostly caused by *C. botulinum* type E [24]. The microbial flora of fish is predominantly psychrotrophic and, in marine fish, halophilic.

Contamination usually occurs during processing and storage. Gutting of the catch on board ship can spread intestinal flora over the surface of the fish, and ice used for chilling in the holds of the ships often becomes heavily contaminated by potential spoilage organisms. Poor temperature control of the fish after landing encourages bacterial growth. The flesh of fish is more perishable than that of animals. The loss of bright surface colours, changes in the smell, and the presence of surface slime are the best indicators of spoilage, which in ice-stored fish is mainly due to pseudomonads. Colony counts of uncooked fish are of little value, but investigation for potential pathogens may be useful for monitoring both the product and the aquatic environment.

Conventional cooking should kill vegetative bacteria and freshly cooked fish is unlikely to cause bacterial food poisoning. However, spores may survive and, on subsequent poor storage, germinate and multiply to levels that can cause food poisoning. Incidents of both *Clostridium perfringens* and *Bacillus cereus* food poisoning have been reported from the consumption of cooked fish held at inappropriate temperatures after cooking. Post-cooking contamination can also occur. Fish products such as fish cakes and fish sticks may be contaminated during production and staphylococci may be introduced during handling. Faults in canning have given rise to occasional outbreaks of botulism due to *C. botulinum* type E [25].

Scombrotoxic fish poisoning is associated with the consumption of fish of the families *Scomberesocidae* and *Scombridae*, which include tuna, bonito and mackerel. These fish naturally contain large amounts of histidine. Toxicity is associated with bacterial spoilage where bacteria break down the histidine to histamine and possibly other toxic end products. Poisoning is prevented by ensuring that the fish is properly refrigerated from the time of catching until consumption. Estimation of the number of spoilage organisms present is not a reliable indicator of possible toxicity. The toxic substance(s) are not destroyed by cooking or curing the fish. Non-scombroid fish, such as sprat and pilchards, have been incriminated in several incidents. The heat stability of the toxin(s) means that commercially canned fish may cause poisoning. Introduction of the appropriate organisms into cooked fish, e.g. in restaurants and sandwich bars, followed by inadequate storage has resulted in proliferation of the organisms, production of toxin and subsequent scombrotoxic fish poisoning

Ciguatera toxin poisoning is common in certain parts of the world and follows the consumption of some species of carnivorous fish found in the tropics (e.g. sea bass and barracuda). The ciguatoxin is acquired from toxic dinoflagellates, which are part of the food chain of the fish. The toxin is heat stable and is not destroyed by ordinary cooking methods. Large adult fish are most likely to contain high levels of toxin.

Test	Section/method
Raw fish:	
▲ *Pseudomonas* spp.	6.11
▲ *Salmonella* spp.	6.12
▲ *Vibrio parahaemolyticus* and other *Vibrio* spp.	6.15
■ *Aeromonas* spp.	6.1

continued

■ Scombrotoxin	Appendix C
■ Ciguatera toxin	Appendix C

Cooked fish:

▲ Colony count	5.3–5.6
▲ *Escherichia coli*	6.6
▲ Enterobacteriaceae	6.7
▲ *Salmonella* spp.	6.12
▲ *Staphylococcus aureus*	6.14
▲ *Vibrio* spp.	6.15
■ *Bacillus cereus* and *Bacillus* spp.	6.2
■ Clostridia	6.5
■ *Listeria monocytogenes*	6.10
■ *Pseudomonas* spp.	6.11
■ *Shigella* spp.	6.13
■ Scombrotoxin	Appendix C
■ Ciguatera toxin	Appendix C

Crustaceans

Crustaceans include shrimps, prawns, crabs, crayfish, lobster and scampi. When freshly caught they are highly perishable due to the activities of spoilage bacteria and natural enzymes. Shrimps and crabs should be either frozen or boiled as soon as possible after they are caught, but storage in ice is also common. Lobsters may be kept alive in water until they are required for cooking. Crustaceans taken from polluted waters may be contaminated by organisms from untreated sewage. *Vibrio parahaemolyticus* and other *Vibrio* spp. are found in shallow coastal waters and are common contaminants. *Yersinia enterocolitica* has also been isolated from raw crustaceans, but the strains found are considered to be non-pathogenic to humans. A major hazard from raw crustaceans is cross-contamination to processed foods.

Ready-to-eat, cooked frozen peeled prawns and shrimps are exported from many countries, especially those in the Far East. *Vibrio parahaemolyticus* has been isolated from these products on many occasions, and occasionally salmonellae. Guidelines for the microbiological quality of this product were introduced in the UK in 1975 [26]. Application of these guidelines resulted in rejection of many batches of prawns and shrimps, often on the basis of the colony count alone [27].

Specifications were extended to the rest of the EU by Commission Decision 93/51/EEC [28] which lays down microbiological criteria applicable to the production of cooked crustaceans and molluscan shellfish. These criteria have not been published as UK legislation.

Test	Section/method
Raw crustaceans:	
▲ *Aeromonas* spp.	6.1
▲ *Salmonella* spp.	6.12
▲ *Vibrio* spp.	6.15
Cooked crustaceans:	
◆ Colony count (30°C)	5.3–5.6
◆ Thermotolerant coliforms/*Escherichia coli*	6.6
◆ *Salmonella* spp.	6.12
◆ *Staphylococcus aureus*	6.14
■ *Shigella* spp.	6.13
■ *Vibrio* spp.	6.15

◆ Commission Decision 93/51/EEC [28]

Microbiological criteria for crustaceans

Commission Decision 93/51/EEC (cooked crustaceans and molluscan shellfish) includes the following [28]:

Pathogens:

Salmonella spp.	Absent in 25 g, $n=5$, $c=0$

Organisms indicating poor hygiene (shelled or shucked products):

Staphylococcus aureus	$m=10^2$, $M=10^3$, $n=5$, $c=2$
Thermotolerant coliforms or *Escherichia coli*	$m=10$, $M=10^2$, $n=5$, $c=2$

Indicator organisms (guidelines). Colony count (30°C):

Whole products	$m=10^4$, $M=10^5$, $n=5$, $c=2$
Shelled or shucked products (except crab meat)	$m=5 \times 10^4$, $M=5 \times 10^5$, $n=5$, $c=2$
Crab meat	$m=10^5$, $M=10^6$, $n=5$, $c=2$

---

n, the number of sample units; m, the threshold value for the number of bacteria (satisfactory if not exceeded); M, the maximum value for the number of bacteria (unsatisfactory if exceeded); c, the number of sample units where the bacterial count may be between m and M. (For further explanation see p. 3.)

Molluscan shellfish

Molluscs are estuarine animals and are liable to gross faecal contamination from sewage pollution of the waters in which they live. They can be subdivided into the bivalves (oysters, clams, mussels, cockles and escallops) and gastropods (whelks and periwinkles). Bivalve molluscs are self-cleaning 'filter feeders' and if placed in water of good microbiological quality, will eliminate any faecal bacteria from their bodies (depuration). Unfortunately, this process may not remove viruses, and the presence or absence of faecal bacteria used for monitoring the safety of this product is not a reliable test for excluding viral contamination. A search for enteroviruses, which can be detected by tissue culture, may not reliably indicate contamination by hepatitis A virus or viruses causing gastroenteritis such as the Norwalk-like virus (NLV) group. Satisfactory tests for these viruses need to be developed.

Oysters, which are eaten raw, are particularly hazardous [29]. Other molluscs are boiled for retail sale, but this cooking may not be properly controlled and may be inadequate. Several members of the genus *Vibrio* are pathogenic in humans and have caused illness following the ingestion of undercooked or raw seafood. *Vibrio parahaemolyticus* is the most common [30], but *V. vulnificus*, which can produce a severe septicaemic illness, may be associated with the consumption of raw oysters. Outbreaks of cholera have also been attributed to the consumption of molluscan shellfish. Filter-feeding molluscs may be toxic to humans following the accumulation of toxin derived from marine dinoflagellates (e.g. paralytic, diarrhetic and amnesic shellfish poisoning) [31]. These organisms are widely distributed, but poisoning only occurs when there are relatively large numbers present in the water. Natural loss of toxin from molluscs may take several weeks.

Shellfish production in the UK is controlled and includes rearing in approved areas or cleansing by approved plants. The presence of *E. coli* is usually accepted as an indication of less than optimal hygienic conditions of cultivation or of insufficient heat treatment. The EUC Directive on shellfish hygiene [32] stipulates standards for molluscan shellfish and includes both microbiological limits and limits for certain toxins such as paralytic shellfish poison. Shellfish rearing areas are classified on the basis of faecal coliform or *E. coli* levels and the produce from these areas will be processed according to these levels. The standards have been incorporated into UK legislation [33,34] (see Section 9).

Test	Section/method
Raw molluscan shellfish:	
◆ *Salmonella* spp.	6.12
◆ *Escherichia coli*	Section 9, method 1
◆ Dinoflagellate toxins (PSP, DSP, ASP)	Appendix C
■ *Staphylococcus aureus*	6.14
■ *Vibrio* spp.	6.15
■ Viruses	Appendix C

◆ The Food Safety (Fishery Products and Live Shellfish) (Hygiene) Regulations (1998) and Amendment Regulations (1999) [33,34]
ASP, amnesic shellfish poison; DSP, diarrhetic shellfish poison; PSP, paralytic shellfish poison.

continued

Cooked molluscan shellfish:

- ◆ Colony count   5.3–5.6
- ◆ Thermotolerant coliforms/*Escherichia coli*   6.6 (plate method)
- ◆ *Salmonella* spp.   6.12
- ◆ *Staphylococcus aureus*   6.14
- ▲ *Vibrio* spp.   6.15

- ◆ Commission Decision 93/51/EEC [28]

Microbiological criteria for raw molluscan shellfish

The Food Safety (Fishery Products and Live Shellfish) (Hygiene) Regulations (1998) and Amendment Regulations (1999) [33,34], EC Directive 91/492/EEC [32]

Live bivalve molluscs and other shellfish intended for immediate consumption:

Faecal coliforms, or	<300/100 g
Escherichia coli	<230/100 g
Salmonella spp.	Absent in 25 g
Paralytic shellfish poison (PSP)	≤80 µg/100 g
Diarrhetic shellfish poison (DSP)	Must not give a positive result with biological testing method
Amnesic shellfish poison (ASP)	≤20 µg/g

The microbiological criteria for the classification of shellfish harvesting areas is found in Section 9. The EC microbiological criteria for cooked molluscan shellfish are found in Commission Decision 93/51/EEC and are the same as those for cooked crustaceans [28].

Some shellfish, e.g. cockles, lose their acceptability to the customer unless cooking is limited to retain taste and flavour. Special cooking procedures for these shellfish have been devised [35].

Preserved seafoods

Curing, smoking or pickling is used for the preservation of freshwater foods and seafoods. Salting prevents the growth of many spoilage organisms, particularly pseudomonads. Many food poisoning organisms are inhibited at a salt concentration of 10% or less but *V. parahaemolyticus* and some toxigenic staphylococci have a greater salt tolerance (up to 18% for some strains of *S. aureus*). Salting may be undertaken prior to smoking. Fish may be either cold or hot smoked, the former being the more common treatment for smoked salmon. Cold smoking imparts flavour to the food, but produces only relatively minor changes in the microbial flora of the product. Liquid smokes, into which the fish are dipped, have also been developed.

Numbers of bacteria on fully cured foods should be low unless there has been extensive surface contamination. Lightly smoked products or those brined only to improve flavour are only slightly more stable than the raw products. The temperatures achieved during hot smoking should destroy vegetative cells. The salt concentration plays an important part in preservation, e.g. in smoked salmon where the inhibition of *Clostridium botulinum* is essential. The acidity of vinegar (pH 4.5 or lower) should suppress the growth of bacteria and the only test considered necessary for pickled products is a pH determination.

Test	Section/method
▲ Colony count	5.3–5.6
▲ *Escherichia coli*	6.6
▲ Enterobacteriaceae	6.7
▲ *Listeria monocytogenes*	6.10
▲ *Salmonella* spp.	6.12
▲ *Staphylococcus aureus*	6.14
▲ *Vibrio* spp.	6.15
■ pH (pickled in vinegar)	4.5
■ Clostridia	6.5
■ *Pseudomonas* spp.	6.11
■ Yeasts and moulds	6.17
■ Ciguatera toxin	Appendix C
■ Dinoflagellate toxins (PSP, DSP, ASP)	Appendix C
■ Scombrotoxin	Appendix C

ASP, amnesic shellfish poison; DSP, diarrhetic shellfish poison; PSP, paralytic shellfish poison.

3.14 Frozen lollies

The following products come under this heading:
(a) **Ice-water lollies** which consist of frozen mixtures of water, sugar, flavouring and citric acid. The pH of the mixture should be 4.5 or less.
(b) **Ice-cream lollies** [36] which consist of ice-water lolly mixture on the outside, with a centre of ice-cream. The ice-water mixture should be examined separately from the ice-cream.
(c) **Ice-milk lollies** which are similar to ice-cream but contain less milk fat and sugar but more non-milk fat solids than ice-cream. If both (b) and (c) contain dairy ice-cream they are frozen milk-based products and should be governed by the microbiological parameters laid down in the Milk and Milk-based Products Directive 92/46/EEC [12], which are incorporated into the Dairy Products (Hygiene) Regulations (1995) [13].

Test	Section/method
(a) Ice-water lolly mixture	
▲ pH	4.5
(b) Ice-cream and (c) ice-milk	
◆ *Listeria monocytogenes*	6.10
◆ *Salmonella* spp.	6.12
◆ *Staphylococcus aureus*	6.13
◆ Coliforms (30°C) (guideline)	7.4, method 1
◆ Colony count (30°C) (guideline)	7.4, method 8
■ *Escherichia coli*	6.6

◆ Dairy Products (Hygiene) Regulations (1995) [13]

3.15 Fruit juice, beverages and slush

Beverages with a low pH or containing a chemical preservative are unlikely to be a hazard to health, although salmonellae have been found to survive in low pH cider and apple juice. Apple cider (the US equivalent of apple juice) was implicated in an outbreak of salmonellosis in 1974 and of *E. coli* O157 infection in 1993. Spoilage of products with a pH of 4.5 or less may be caused by acid-tolerant organisms such as yeasts, moulds, and the lactic acid bacteria; normally only these groups of organisms need be sought in these products. Spore-forming bacteria have also occasionally caused spoilage.

Slush drinks, made from a neutral base and ice, have not been associated with outbreaks of illness and extensive routine bacteriological examination is not considered necessary. The water supply used for dilution of the base should be of potable quality and the dispensing machines should be cleaned regularly.

Fruit juices should be concentrated prior to testing. Centrifuge a known volume at 3000 rev/min for 15 min and examine the deposit produced. Membrane filtration techniques have also been used.

Carbonated soft drinks may be concentrated by membrane filtration, the method of choice for these products.

Test	Section/method
Fruit juice:	
▲ pH	4.5
■ Colony count	5.3–5.6
■ *Bacillus* spp.	6.2
■ Clostridia	6.5

continued

Coliforms/*Escherichia coli*	6.6
Lactobacilli and other lactic acid bacteria	6.9
Salmonella spp.	6.12
Yeasts and moulds	6.17

Carbonated soft drinks:

| ▲ pH | 4.5 |

pH greater than 4.5:

■ Colony count	5.3–5.6
■ Coliforms/*Escherichia coli*	6.6
■ *Salmonella* spp.	6.12
■ *Staphylococcus aureus*	6.14
■ Yeasts and moulds	6.17

Slush drinks — diluted base:

| ▲ pH | 4.5 |

pH greater than 4.5:

| ▲ Colony count | 5.3–5.6 |

3.16 Gelatin

Gelatin is a dried meat protein marketed in powder or leaf form [37]. The extraction, drying and blanching processes involved in its production all have a bactericidal effect. The residual flora consists mainly of spore-forming bacteria, micrococci and faecal streptococci. Salmonellae and clostridia may be introduced by contamination from meat, and *Staphylococcus aureus* and *Bacillus cereus* during processing. Multiplication of the bacteria in the product is prevented while the gelatin is kept dry, but once it is rehydrated contaminating bacteria may grow. Further contamination may be introduced if other ingredients are added to the reconstituted gelatin during manipulation by the food handler or from contact with dirty utensils and equipment. Since gelatin is a dried product, resuscitation techniques should be used to aid the recovery of thermally injured organisms.

Test	Section/method
▲ Colony count	5.3–5.6
▲ *Bacillus* spp.	6.2
▲ Clostridia	6.5
▲ *Salmonella* spp.	6.12
▲ *Staphylococcus aureus*	6.14
■ Enterobacteriaceae, or	6.7
■ Coliforms/*Escherichia coli*	6.6

3.17 Mayonnaise and sauces

These products [38,39], which may contain eggs, milk or cream, can be a source of salmonellae, particularly when made in catering or domestic premises and using unpasteurized ingredients. In addition other organisms, such as *Bacillus cereus* and *Staphylococcus aureus*, may be introduced during preparation.

Many of these products, which are basically emulsions of oil and water with starch as stabilizer, are made with vinegar (acetic acid) or lemon juice (citric acid) and should have a pH of less than 4.5. The low pH will prevent multiplication of food poisoning bacteria, but may allow growth of yeasts and moulds. Where the pH is 4.5 or above, there is a greatly increased chance of multiplication of bacteria if the storage temperature is not properly controlled.

Most bottled sauces and mayonnaise contain preservatives and gas production due to yeast growth is the most frequent cause of spoilage. Owing to the wide variety of potential ingredients and methods of production of these products as much information as possible should be gathered on the food item before it is tested. It is most important to determine whether it is produced locally in a kitchen or mass-produced in a factory.

The use of fresh shell eggs in the production of mayonnaise and other sauces such as Hollandaise and Béarnaise in catering has resulted in outbreaks of salmonellosis. Examination of eggs from the same supplier is important in tracing outbreaks. Pasteurized egg should be used in the preparation of these products.

Test	Section/method
▲ pH	4.5
▲ Colony count	5.3–5.6
■ *Bacillus* spp.	6.2
■ Clostridia	6.5
■ Enterobacteriaceae	6.7
■ Coliforms/*Escherichia coli*	6.6
■ *Salmonella* spp.	6.12
■ *Staphylococcus aureus*	6.14
■ Yeasts and moulds	6.17

3.18 Meat

This food heading is subdivided as follows:
- Raw meat and poultry.
- Cooked meat and poultry.
- Cooked meat pies.
- Cured and processed meats.

Raw meat and poultry

The importance of veterinary sources of food-borne illness was reviewed by Johnston [40]. Intensive rearing of livestock increases considerably the spread of organisms from animal to animal and, in slaughter and processing, from carcass to carcass. Animals may excrete salmonellae or campylobacters without showing symptoms. The prevalence of salmonellae on raw red meats is variable and will differ depending on the type of meat animal and method of rearing.

Chickens and other poultry are most often infected and a high proportion of retail carcasses may be contaminated [41,42]. Infections caused by *Salmonella enteritidis* phage type 4 increased in the 1980s and this organism may infect eggs during their formation in the oviduct (see Section 3.12). Commercial breeding flocks, laying flocks and hatcheries must be registered and tested for salmonellae. Those positive for *S*. Enteritidis or *S*. Typhimurium were slaughtered under regulations introduced in 1989, although early in 1991 the requirement to slaughter flocks harbouring *S*. Typhimurium was discontinued. Vaccination of flocks against these salmonellae has been introduced and the effects of this programme are reflected in the decrease in human cases of salmonellosis reported to the Public Health Laboratory Service (PHLS) in the late 1990s [43].

Chickens, particularly those retailed fresh, are heavily contaminated with campylobacters [44,45]. The incidence in red meats at the point of sale is lower [46]; however, offal is more likely to be contaminated [47–49].

Chickens frequently harbour *Listeria monocytogenes* [50,51] and *Yersinia enterocolitica* [52] and aeromonads have also been reported in raw meats. Contaminated pork may be an important source of sporadic *Yersinia* infections [53]. Refrigeration temperatures may not be low enough to stop the growth of these bacteria. *Escherichia coli* and *Clostridium perfringens* can be expected on carcasses, but their numbers are low where meat is produced with good hygienic practices. In some countries ground beef, in particular undercooked beefburgers, may be an important source of verocytotoxigenic *E. coli* infections [54]. Lamb products have also been reported as a source of *E. coli* O157 [55]. The major outbreak in Scotland in 1996 [56] led to recommendations [57] in relation to practices and hygiene in butchers premises. A study undertaken in 1997 [58] of some 1400 manufacturing butchers' premises showed that the majority of these premises selling raw and cooked/ready-to-eat meat products did have appropriate control measures in place to minimize risk of cross-contamination. However there were still some practices that required attention.

Most spoilage bacteria are aerobes and grow on the surface of the meat. These may be distributed unevenly throughout the product by mincing or chopping. The flora of raw meat packed in non-permeable wrappings will change as carbon dioxide gradually replaces oxygen and the aerobes are suppressed.

Test	Section/method
■ Colony count	5.3–5.6
■ *Campylobacter* spp.	6.4
■ Verotoxigenic *Escherichia coli*	6.6
■ Lactobacilli and other lactic acid bacteria	6.9
■ *Listeria monocytogenes*	6.10
■ *Pseudomonas* spp.	6.11
■ *Salmonella* spp.	6.12
■ *Staphylococcus aureus*	6.14
■ *Yersinia enterocolitica*	6.18

Cooked meat and poultry

The temperatures achieved during cooking should be sufficient to kill vegetative cells, but spores such as those of *C. perfringens* may survive and germinate if foods are not cooled and refrigerated rapidly after cooking. Any cooking process will drive off oxygen from the tissues and produce an environment that favours the growth of anaerobic bacteria. The centre temperature achieved during the cooking of large joints of meat may not even be sufficient to kill vegetative bacteria [59]. Cooked meat may also be recontaminated from surfaces and equipment and during packaging and handling. Many types of meat are sold ready-sliced and cross-contamination from slicing machines has been identified as an important hazard. Cross-contamination from raw to cooked meats is a major problem. The growth of food poisoning bacteria introduced in this way is not restricted by the competing organisms normally found in the raw product. Strict separation of raw and cooked meats is therefore essential, together with storage at appropriate temperatures and attention to personal hygiene to reduce the risk of transmission by and growth of food poisoning bacteria in these products [60,61]. A hazard analysis approach (hazard analysis critical control point, HACCP) should be adopted during the production, storage and distribution of meat products. A study of cold ready-to-eat sliced meats from catering establishments [62] showed that, while 74% of almost 3500 samples were of acceptable quality, 26% were unsatisfactory, mainly due to high aerobic colony counts, and <1% were unacceptable, due to the presence of high levels of *E. coli*, *S. aureus*, *Listeria* spp. and/or *C. perfringens*. The quality of the samples were judged according to the guidelines produced by the PHLS in 1996, the most recent guidelines (Table 2.1, Section 2, p. 17) would not judge some of the samples 'unacceptable' on the basis of the levels of *E. coli*.

Test	Section/method
▲ Colony count (aerobic)	5.3–5.6
▲ *Bacillus* spp.	6.2
▲ Clostridia	6.5
▲ Coliforms/*Escherichia coli*	6.6
▲ Enterobacteriaceae	6.7
▲ *Listeria monocytogenes*	6.10
▲ *Salmonella* spp.	6.12
▲ *Staphylococcus aureus*	6.14
■ *Campylobacter* spp.	6.4
■ Enterococci	6.8
■ Lactobacilli and other lactic acid bacteria	6.9
■ *Pseudomonas* spp.	6.11
■ *Shigella* spp.	6.13
■ Yeasts and moulds	6.17

The guidelines for ready-to-eat foods at the point of sale (Table 2.1, Section 2, p. 17) could be applied to these products.

Cooked meat pies

These may be eaten either hot, such as steak or chicken pies, or cold, such as pork pies or sausage rolls. For those eaten hot the meat filling is pre-cooked, added to the pastry case, and the pie cooked again. Pies eaten cold usually contain cured meats. During baking the temperatures achieved should kill vegetative cells and thus any subsequent bacterial growth will arise from the germination of surviving spores of *Bacillus* and *Clostridium* species. Jelly, which is made from gelatin, spices, flavouring and water is added after baking to some pies eaten cold, e.g. pork pies. To prevent the survival of vegetative cells, the jelly should be adequately heated (boiled for 5 min) and kept at a high temperature (not less than 77°C) until it reaches the pie. Any gelatin or stock remaining after the filling process must be discarded and not retained for incorporation into the next batch of product. The reservoir and injection apparatus should be emptied, dismantled and cleaned each day as a routine procedure. A separate microbiological examination of the meat and the surrounding jelly can prove useful.

Test	Section/method
▲ Colony count (aerobic)	5.3–5.6
▲ Bacillus spp.	6.2
▲ Clostridia	6.5
▲ Coliforms/Escherichia coli	6.6
▲ Enterobacteriaceae	6.7
▲ Enterococci	6.8
▲ Salmonella spp.	6.12
▲ Staphylococcus aureus	6.14
■ Listeria monocytogenes	6.10
■ Shigella spp.	6.13
■ Yeasts and moulds	6.17

The guidelines for ready-to-eat foods (Table 2.1, p. 17) could be applied to these products.

Cured and processed meats

The test schedules for these products are given below under the following headings:
• Canned and sliced cured meats. This heading includes shelf-stable cured canned meats, perishable cured canned meats and sliced cured meats.
• Cured fermented sausages.
• Processed non-cured meats and meat products.

Canned and sliced cured meats

Curing processes usually involve injecting the meat with a pickle containing sodium chloride, sodium or potassium nitrate and sodium nitrite followed by immersion in a brine solution for 7–14 days (see Section 3.6). Some canned cured meat, notably ham and mixtures containing ham, are only given a minimal heat treatment. Also, in response to consumer preference, there has been a trend towards decreased concentration of curing salts and shorter immersion times, and this has resulted in a product that is more perishable. The salt concentration is not by itself sufficient to prevent growth of spoilage and some food poisoning organisms and so, in addition, adequate refrigeration of this product is required. Sliced cured meats may be sold raw (bacon) or cooked (ham).

The test schedule for canned foods is given in Section 3.7 and procedures for the preliminary examination of cans are given in Section 4.4.

Cured fermented sausages

The initial stage in the production of these meats involves a simultaneous process of curing in brine and fermentation in which multiplication of lactic acid bacteria, present in the meat, takes place and is accompanied by a decrease in the number of Gram-negative bacteria. Starter cultures are often added at the commencement of curing. After curing and fermentation the product may be dried and is usually smoked. Finally, the sausages are 'ripened' or 'mellowed' for up to 4 weeks.

Outbreaks of staphylococcal food poisoning from cured fermented sausages have been reported and occasionally also salmonellae infections [63]. Multiplication of *S. aureus* can be limited by holding the meat at refrigeration temperatures during initial fermentation. If refrigeration is not used, the addition of starter culture and/or a chemical acidulant will promote rapid acidification and consequent inhibition of growth of *S. aureus*. The temperature, relative humidity and time for these stages vary according to the product. Cured sausages are classified as dry, with a moisture content of less than 40%, e.g. salami, pepperoni; or semi-dry, with a moisture content of 40–45%, e.g. Cervelat, Thuringer. Cured sausages are usually consumed without cooking.

Many cured or processed meats are sliced before sale and contamination from the slicing machine can be important. They are also sold in vacuum or modified atmosphere packs that help maintain the freshness of the product. The permeability of the packaging to water vapour and to certain gases is important in controlling microbial spoilage. Cured meats are packed in oxygen-impermeable film because oxidation causes fading of the meat colour [64].

Test	Section/method
Cured fermented sausages and products to be consumed without further cooking:	
▲ *Salmonella* spp.	6.12
■ pH	4.5
■ Water activity (a_w)	4.7
■ Colony count	5.3–5.6
■ Clostridia	6.5
■ Coliforms/*Escherichia coli*	6.6
■ Enterobacteriaceae	6.7
■ Enterococci	6.8
■ Lactobacilli and other lactic acid bacteria	6.9
■ *Listeria monocytogenes*	6.10
■ *Pseudomonas* spp.	6.11
■ *Staphylococcus aureus*	6.14
■ Yeasts and moulds	6.17
Products to be cooked before consumption:	
▲ *Salmonella* spp.	6.12

Processed non-cured meats and meat products

A number of non-cured meats and meat products are retailed from delicatessen counters. The safety of these products depends on the hygiene of handling and especially on maintenance of low temperatures in chilled display counters. *Listeria* spp. can become a problem with this type of product due to their ubiquity and persistence of survival in the environment and their ability to grow at chill temperatures. These organisms can grow in 10% sodium chloride and survive drying, freezing and thawing. Problems have been encountered with *L. monocytogenes* in pâté [65] and refrigerated sliced meats [66], often present in large numbers. Improved production practices and temperature control relating to these products has reduced both the frequency of occurrence and numbers of *L. monocytogenes* present.

Test	Section/method
▲ Colony count	5.3–5.6
▲ Clostridia	6.5
▲ Coliforms/*Escherichia coli*	6.6
▲ Enterobacteriaceae	6.7
▲ *Listeria monocytogenes* and other *Listeria* spp.	6.10
▲ *Salmonella* spp.	6.12
▲ *Staphylococcus aureus*	6.14
■ Lactobacilli and other lactic acid bacteria	6.9
■ *Pseudomonas* spp.	6.11
■ Shigella	6.13
■ Yeasts and moulds	6.17

3.19 Pre-prepared foods — chilled and frozen

Ready-to-eat foods

Low temperature storage has been used for many years as a means of preserving food [67]. Refrigeration, provided that it is adequately controlled, prevents the growth of many organisms including the food-borne pathogens. Notable exceptions include *Clostridium botulinum* type E, *Yersinia enterocolitica* and *Listeria monocytogenes*, all of which can grow slowly at these temperatures. Numerous studies have reported the presence of *L. monocytogenes* in chilled foods [68]. Psychrophilic bacteria and many moulds are also able to grow and cause spoilage. The Food Safety (Temperature Control) Regulations 1995 identified maximum storage temperatures for certain chilled foods as at or below 8°C [69].

Freezer cabinets are usually maintained at −18°C to −20°C. At these temperatures all microbial growth is suppressed. Low-temperature spoilage due to the action of naturally occurring enzymes in foods can take place during prolonged storage or if the freezer temperature is not adequately controlled. In the microbiological examination of frozen foods, omission of a resuscitation step for cold-shocked organisms can lead to artificially low counts or failure to isolate a particular pathogen.

There are many types of chilled or frozen pre-cooked convenience foods. A hygiene failure during bulk production could expose large numbers of people to the risk of infection. Hot foods should be chilled quickly, preferably in pre-cooling units. The practice of cooling cooked food in chill rooms can be dangerous as large quantities of hot food take many hours to cool. During this time bacterial multiplication may occur and the presence of bulks of hot food may result in a significant rise in the temperature of the chill room. Measures to prevent post-cooking contamination are essential, particularly as competing organisms will have been destroyed during cooking.

Prepared salads may contain large numbers of bacteria. Adequate washing of ingredients and proper temperature control during storage are important. In restaurants salads may be kept at ambient temperatures for long periods for customers to serve themselves. Ready-to-eat desserts may contain cream or custard and *S. aureus* is an added risk.

Test	Section/method
▲ Colony count	5.3–5.6
▲ *Bacillus* spp.	6.2
▲ Clostridia	6.5
▲ Coliforms/*Escherichia coli*	6.6
▲ Enterobacteriaceae	6.7
▲ *Listeria monocytogenes* and other *Listeria* spp.	6.10
▲ *Salmonella* spp.	6.12
▲ *Staphylococcus aureus*	6.14
■ Lactobacilli and other lactic acid bacteria	6.9
■ *Pseudomonas* spp.	6.11
■ *Shigella* spp.	6.13
■ Yeasts and moulds	6.17

Microbiological criteria for ready-to-eat foods

PHLS guidelines for ready-to-eat foods at retail sale: applicable across a wide range of foods in Section 3 of this manual, are summarized in Table 2.1, Section 2, p. 17.

continued

	Sandwiches/rolls					
	With salad (cfu/g)			Without salad (cfu/g)		
	Target	Acceptable	Reject	Target	Acceptable	Reject
Colony count (30°C)	$<10^5$	10^5	$>10^6$	$<10^4$	10^4	$>10^5$
Coliforms (37°C)	$<10^3$	10^3	$>10^4$	$<10^2$	10^2	$>10^3$
Escherichia coli	<10	10	$>10^2$	<10	10	$>10^2$
Staphylococcus aureus	<10	10	$>10^2$	<10	10	$>10^2$
Salmonella spp.	Absent in 25 g	Absent in 25 g	Present in 25 g	Absent in 25 g	Absent in 25 g	Present in 25 g
Listeria spp. (presence in the product must be investigated)	Absent in 25 g	Absent in 25 g	Present in 25 g	Absent in 25 g	Absent in 25 g	Present in 25 g

Airline Catering Technical Coordinating Committee code of practice (see Section 2.7

Lists microbiological guidelines for seven categories of airline catering food items based on the degree of manipulation and cooking the food receives

Cook–chill and cook–freeze meals

These types of ready meals are popular at retail and are also used extensively in catering particularly if on a large scale. There are detailed guidelines for the times and temperatures for preparation, cooking, chilling and freezing during the production of cook–chill and cook–freeze meals in catering systems [70]. Both systems are popular in hospitals and in other forms of institutional catering as they give better and more controlled use of labour and resources. The systems are based on the cooking of food followed by fast chilling or freezing and subsequent storage in controlled temperature conditions, above freezing point (0–3°C) for cook–chill foods or deep frozen (−18°C) for cook–freeze foods. Provided that there is adherence to certain basic principles cook–chill foods should not present either public health or spoilage problems. All raw materials should be of good microbiological quality. The principles set out by the Department of Health can be summarized as follows:

- The food should be subjected to an initial cooking treatment which will ensure destruction of vegetative stages of any pathogenic microorganisms present.

Cook–chill process:

- After completion of the cooking and portioning process, and in any event within 30 min of the food leaving the cooker, the chilling process should commence. The food should be chilled to between 0°C and 3°C within 1.5 h. Most pathogenic organisms will not grow below 7°C. The temperature of 3°C is required to reduce growth of spoilage organisms. Slow growth of spoilage organisms will still occur so storage life cannot be more than 5 days.

- Once chilled the food should be stored at a controlled temperature between 0°C and 3°C.
- The chilled food should be distributed under controlled conditions to minimize temperature changes during distribution.
- For both safety and palatability, the food should be reheated immediately upon removal from chill conditions to a temperature of at least 70°C.
- A temperature of 10°C should be regarded as the critical safety limit for chilled food. Should the temperature of the food rise above this limit during storage or distribution, the food must be discarded.
- Once reheated, the food should be consumed as soon as possible and all unconsumed food must be discarded.

Cook–freeze process:
- After completion of the cooking and portioning process, and in any event within 30 min of the food leaving the cooker, the freezing process should commence. The food should reach a centre temperature of −5°C or colder within 1.5 h of entering the freezer and subsequently should reach a storage temperature of −18°C.
- The frozen food should be stored at a temperature of −18°C or colder.
- Food that has thawed either partially or completely should not be refrozen.
- The shelf-life of the food will vary according to the type of food but in general it may be stored for up to 8 weeks without significant loss of nutrients or palatability.
- Some frozen foods may require thawing before reheating. Thawed food should be held at below 3°C and never above 10°C until reheated. The food should be reheated to at least 70°C.
- Once reheated, the food should be consumed as soon as possible and all unconsumed food must be discarded.

A procedure related to cook–chill is *sous-vide* in which foods are slow cooked under vacuum at low temperatures (60–65°C). This system gives a long shelf-life under refrigerated conditions.

Good manufacturing practices and quality control programmes are essential for pre-cooked food systems. A HACCP approach should be applied at all stages of the process [60,61]. Microbiological surveillance is required when a new cook–chill or cook–freeze system is established or when material alterations are made to an existing system. Once established, only periodic checks on finished products are required. Process control is the best way of achieving a good quality, safe product.

Test	Section/method
▲ Colony count	5.3–5.6
▲ Clostridia	6.5
▲ Coliforms/*Escherichia coli*	6.6
▲ Enterobacteriaceae	6.7
▲ *Listeria monocytogenes*	6.10
▲ *Salmonella* spp.	6.12
▲ *Staphylococcus aureus*	6.14

Microbiological criteria for cook–chill and cook–freeze meals in catering systems examined immediately before reheating

Department of Health guidelines (1989) [70].

	cfu/g
Colony count	$<10^5$
Clostridium perfringens	$<10^2$
Escherichia coli	<10
Staphylococcus aureus	$<10^2$
Listeria monocytogenes	Not detected in 25 g
Salmonella spp.	Not detected in 25 g

3.20   Surfaces and containers

There are three main reasons for collecting environmental samples:
• As part of an investigation of a suspected food poisoning outbreak where surfaces are thought to be the likely vehicles of cross-contamination.
• To trace the route of contamination from dirty to clean situations.
• As part of an educational programme designed to test the standard of hygiene and efficiency of cleaning procedures in catering premises.

In many ways environmental sampling complements food examination and may provide additional useful information to Environmental Health Officers during inspections of high-risk food premises [71]. Tests used may be quantitative or qualitative. Since no method will pick up all bacteria on a surface, quantitative methods should be used only as a guide to contamination levels.

Hands

Where hands are suspected as the source of contamination of foods, agar impressions of the thumb and fingertips can be collected. Impressions can be made on a non-selective medium which, after a short period of incubation, can be replicated on selective media to look for potential pathogens. In some instances a finger-rinse technique may be better. Samples are collected from finger-tips by rubbing each finger against the bottom of a jar containing a small volume of suitable diluent or by massaging the hand inside a plastic bag containing diluent. Colony counts may be performed on the diluent and, if required, potential pathogens may be sought. Larger volumes of diluent can be processed by membrane filtration.

Staphylococcus aureus may be transferred from raw foods, from various normal carriage sites on the human body, or from infected lesions. Staphylococci survive for long periods on the skin and in the nose. Food handlers are often shown to play a major role in *S. aureus* food poisoning.

Both salmonellae and *E. coli* are susceptible to drying and normally survive for relatively short periods on human skin. They are loosely adherent and may be transferred to foods and to surfaces. The presence of these organisms on the hands may indicate direct faecal contamination, or contamination acquired by handling raw foods. Food handlers excreting salmonellae are unlikely to spread the salmonellae to foods provided that they have good personal hygiene and no symptoms of gastroenteritis, i.e. they have formed stools [72].

Test	Section/method
▲ Colony count:	
Surface contact *or*	5.8 and 5.9
Rinse in known volume of diluent	5.11
▲ *Escherichia coli*	6.6
▲ *Salmonella* spp.	6.12
▲ *Staphylococcus aureus*	6.14

Food surfaces and equipment

Comparison of bacterial contamination on surfaces before and after cleaning provides a useful guide to cleaning efficiency. Sampling during use will give very variable results, but high counts on surfaces used for cooked foods could serve as a warning. Various factors determine the number of bacteria on surfaces. A damp, porous wooden surface can be expected to carry many more bacteria than one of clean, dry metal. The interval between use and sampling will influence the numbers of bacteria recovered. Some organisms will die on the surface during drying. The choice of sampling method will depend on the situation. Agar-contact plates or slides are convenient and particularly suitable for relatively clean areas. After a short period of incubation, the plate can be replicated on to another medium that is more selective. This facilitates the detection of specific bacteria and also helps the recovery of damaged organisms. Dip slides coated with cystine lactose electrolyte deficient agar (CLED) or violet red bile glucose agar (VRBGA) or plate count agar (PCA) can be used for this recovery technique as the medium supports the growth of most of the aerobic pathogens. CLED dip slides can be returned to their original containers that can then be filled with the relevant enrichment medium.

Dirty areas may be better examined by swabbing. The resulting bacterial suspension may be diluted before counting. A confluent growth on a contact plate, however, usually provides sufficient information. Swabbing may be used to test surfaces that cannot be sampled with contact plates, e.g. nail brushes or the insides of containers. Where specific bacteria are sought a large area may be swabbed and the swab placed in enrichment medium. Several swabs may be placed in the same enrichment broth. Alternatively the suspension obtained with a surface swab for enumeration of organisms may be added to enrichment media specific to the organisms sought. Dip slides can also be placed in enrichment medium, but unless multiple impressions are taken the area sampled is small.

Contact plates can be used to demonstrate cleaning efficiency to staff. The incubated plates should be sprayed with domestic hair spray to minimize aerosols and to lessen the risk of infection. However, this procedure does not completely eliminate the risk. Cultures should be returned to the laboratory for disposal.

A rapid method for the determination of surface contamination is by the assessment of the concentration of microbial adenosine triphosphate (ATP) per surface area by bioluminometry. The results should be interpreted with care because part of the measured ATP levels can originate from plant or animal tissues. The method is widely used for 'real time' and 'on site' inspection of the food environment.

Test	Section/method
▲ Colony count	Section 5, methods 8–10
▲ Listeria monocytogenes	6.10
▲ Salmonella spp.	6.12
▲ Staphylococcus aureus	6.14
■ Campylobacter spp.	6.4
■ Clostridia	6.5
■ Coliforms/Escherichia coli	6.6
■ Enterobacteriaceae	6.7
■ Enterococci	6.8
■ Yersinia spp.	6.18

Cloths

Reusable wiping cloths are important cross-contamination hazards. In many catering premises raw and cooked food areas are still cleaned with a single cloth. Many cloths are disinfected infrequently and are often heavily contaminated with bacteria [73,74]. Paper is much less likely to spread contamination, but is generally unpopular in commercial kitchens [75]. Fabric cloths that are used throughout the day and then discarded may be heavily contaminated, particularly if used in different food areas. Cloths colour-coded for specific areas, while theoretically should reduce the risk of cross-contamination, rarely do as they do not remain in their designated areas. Cloths may be examined by contact impressions or by immersing the whole or a known area into a diluent. Both qualitative and quantitative tests may be performed.

Test	Section/method
▲ Colony count	5.8 or any method in Section 5 appropriate to the suspension obtained by immersion
■ *Escherichia coli*	6.6
■ Enterobacteriaceae	6.7
■ Enterococci	6.8
■ *Listeria* spp.	6.10
■ *Salmonella* spp.	6.12
■ *Staphylococcus aureus*	6.14

Containers

The internal surfaces of some containers may be sampled with swabs. If the container can be sealed a rinse technique similar to that used for milk bottles is suitable. With small containers the rinse fluid may be added in the laboratory. Where containers are very large the fluid may be added on site and then transferred to a sterile bottle and sent to the laboratory for examination. For milk and soft-drink bottles, less than 200 cfu/bottle is regarded as satisfactory [76,77]. In general, counts should be <1/mL of capacity of the container, i.e. for 1 L capacity the count should be <1000.

Test	Section/method
▲ Colony count:	
Swabs *or*	5.9
Bottle rinse	5.12

Microbiological criteria

Guidelines for the bacteriological cleanliness of milk bottles (Ministry of Agriculture and Fisheries technique No. B743/T.P.B.) [76] (see also Section 5.12)

<200 cfu/bottle	Satisfactory
200–600 cfu/bottle	Acceptable
>600 cfu/bottle	Unsatisfactory

3.21 Vegetables and fruit

Fresh fruit and vegetables [78,79] carry a surface flora of microorganisms consisting mainly of soil saprophytes, air-borne fungal spores and, possibly, plant parasites. Fungi are mainly responsible for spoilage of fruit, but bacterial spoilage is important in vegetables. Washing, unless controlled, will distribute organisms particularly if the wash water is recirculated. Vegetables are frequently presented for sale in supermarkets in a washed, peeled or chopped state. These further manipulations often serve to spread surface organisms throughout the product and the juices released provide an improved environment for microbial growth.

Some vegetables are blanched, particularly before freezing. Blanching is used primarily to inactivate degradative enzymes in the plant tissue, but the process is also sufficient to kill vegetative cells of pathogenic organisms present on the plant surface. The final bacteriological content of blanched products is largely determined by the hygiene employed in handling and packaging after blanching.

In some countries salad and root crops may be contaminated with faecal pathogens following fertilization/irrigation with raw or partially treated sewage. Watercress may also become contaminated if grown in polluted water. Consumption of uncooked fresh vegetables and fruit has occasionally been reported to cause disease in humans. Infections reported include salmonellosis, bacillary and amoebic dysentery, cholera, leptospirosis, viral hepatitis [80], viral gastroenteritis and fascioliasis. The infectious agent was usually present as a surface contaminant. Examination for *E. coli* may be used to monitor contamination of the plant surface. Criteria for *E. coli* colony counts on green vegetables are available only for watercress [81].

Listeria spp. are common environmental organisms and may often be found on plant material. *L. monocytogenes* has been isolated from a variety of salad vegetables. Isolation is more frequent with chopped, prepared salads that contain a mixture of many vegetables and sometimes fruit ingredients [82]. The addition of mayonnaise to mixed salads will reduce the pH and help to control the growth of organisms, but to be effective the pH needs to be less than 4.5. Mixed salads are often available from salad bars in restaurants where they may be left for long periods at ambient temperatures for customers to serve themselves. Bacterial levels in these salads can therefore be high. An ever increasing range of sandwiches, often containing salad ingredients, are available from many retail outlets, some of which have inadequately controlled or no low-temperature display units. Sandwiches from such sources often have high colony counts and may contain potential pathogens.

Sprouting seeds such as bean sprouts and alfalfa may be a problem owing to the conditions of high temperature and humidity in which they are grown. High total counts are not uncommon and pathogens may also proliferate if there is not strict hygienic control of production. An outbreak of *Salmonella* infection was traced to the consumption of raw mung bean sprouts; the source of the salmonellae was the original dried bean. Alfalfa sprouts have been incriminated in incidents of *Salmonella*, *L. monocytogenes* and *E. coli* O157 infection. A major outbreak of *E. coli* O157 infection occurred in Japan in the late 1990s involving more than 6000 people; it was associated with the consumption of white radish sprouts. *Bacillus cereus* intoxication has also been associated with similar sprouting beans. A code of practice for the manufacture, distribution and retail sale of sprouting seeds (especially mung beans) produced by the Campden Food and Drink Research Association (see Section 2.7, p. 22) includes microbiological criteria for guidance, but not as a basis for acceptance/rejection. Guidance is also given on sampling.

Dried vegetables and fruits, while they may occasionally be contaminated with salmonellae, are infrequently involved in food-borne illness. If properly rehydrated and heated any vegetative cells of pathogenic bacteria present in the product will be eliminated. However, if added to a dish at the end of cooking for additional flavouring, e.g. with herbs and spices, the organisms may survive.

A few vegetables contain naturally occurring toxins that may cause illness if eaten raw. For example red kidney beans contain a haemagglutinin which is denatured if the beans are boiled thoroughly before cooking, but which can cause illness if the beans are eaten raw or undercooked.

Test	Section/method
Green vegetables:	
▲ Escherichia coli	5.11
Other fresh fruit and vegetables:	
▲ Colony count	5.3–5.6
▲ Escherichia coli	6.6
▲ Escherichia coli O157	6.6
▲ Salmonella spp.	6.12
■ Aeromonas spp.	6.1
■ Listeria monocytogenes	6.10
■ Shigella spp.	6.13
■ Vibrio spp.	6.14
Blanched and frozen:	
▲ Colony count	5.3–5.6
▲ Escherichia coli	6.6

Microbiological criteria

Campden Food and Drink Research Association guidelines for sprouting seeds (for mung beans especially) (see Section 2.7, p. 22).

Category 1 (recommended tests for final product)

Salmonella spp.	Absent in 25 g
Escherichia coli	<10/g of dried beans
	<10^3/g of final product*
	Absent in 100 mL water (coliforms <3/100 mL)
Listeria monocytogenes	Absent in 25 g of final product*

Category 2 (recommended additional tests)

Colony count	10^5/g of dried beans
	<10^7/g of final product
Coliforms	10^3/g of dried beans
	<10^6/g of final product*

PHLS guidance for watercress [81]

Escherichia coli:	≤5/g	Satisfactory
	>5/g	Unsatisfactory

---

*Immediately after packing.

3.22 Water

Potable water

In England and Wales, the Water Supply (Water Quality) Regulations 2000 [83] amend, for a limited period, the Water Supply (Water Quality) Regulations 1989 [84] and on 1 January 2004, revoke and replace those Regulations. They are primarily concerned with the quality of water supplied, in England and Wales, for drinking, washing, cooking and food preparation for domestic purposes and for food production, and also with arrangements for the publication of information about water quality. They are directed at the achievement of the objective set out in Council Directive 98/83/EC [85] to protect human health from the adverse effects of any contamination of water intended for human consumption by ensuring that it is wholesome and clean. Parts of the Regulations come into force before 1 January 2004 such as those, for example, specifically relating to *Cryptosporidium* (Regulations 27–29) and prescribing new standards of wholesomeness (Regulation 4). The Private Water Supplies Regulations 1991 [86] apply to water from private supplies, used for drinking, washing, cooking or for food production purposes. More specific requirements on the supply and use of potable water for food production purposes can be found in the Food Safety (General Food Hygiene) Regulations 1995 [87]. The Ministry of Agriculture,

Fisheries and Food (MAFF) Animal Health Circular 92/86 gives guidance on water testing procedures in EC approved fresh meat premises [88].

The Water Quality Regulations 2000 provide a legal definition of the term 'wholesomeness' and include a number of chemical and microbiological parameters. Provision is made in the Regulations for the water undertaker to monitor the water supplied for Regulation 4 purposes to a specified level of sampling. Local authorities are charged with (a) making such arrangements with relevant water undertakers as will secure that the authority is notified as soon as may be after the occurrence of any event which gives rise to or is likely to give rise to a significant risk to health, and (b) the taking of such samples that they may reasonably require and arranging for their analysis.

Ordinary potable water, supplied in containers (bottles), as well as spring water and natural mineral waters are subject to the Natural Mineral Water, Spring Water and Bottled Drinking Water Regulations 1999 [89] which incorporate the requirements of the EC Directives on natural mineral water [90] and bottled drinking water [91].

Owing to the possible presence of water-borne pathogens, in small numbers and intermittently, and the technically demanding methods used for their detection, potable water is examined instead for the presence of organisms indicative of faecal pollution, usually total and (especially) faecal coliforms or *E. coli*. These are relatively easy to isolate and enumerate and, if found, imply that pathogens may also be present. If an outbreak of water-borne infection is suspected, it may then be worth attempting to isolate the particular pathogen such as *Cryptosporidium* spp. or *Campylobacter* spp. To ensure the continuing safety of a water supply it is necessary to examine the water regularly and frequently; the examination of a single sample will provide information on the condition of the water only at a particular time and place.

As well as providing evidence of possible faecal contamination in a water supply, colony counts can also give an indication of the overall microbiological quality of the water. Enumerations of organisms are made after 24 h or 48 h incubation at 37°C, and after 72 h incubation at 22°C. The count obtained after 37°C incubation will give an indication of the content of organisms that are more likely to include those of extraneous origin. The count obtained at 22°C incubation will give an indication of the 'normal water flora'. Each water supply, depending on its source, level of nutrients and degree of treatment, will tend to have colony counts that are fairly constant although there may be seasonal variations.

Any significant increase in the expected level of organisms, particularly at 37°C, may indicate a supply problem with possible contamination and a need for further investigation. However, it is not possible to give any numerical guidance on what may constitute a significant increase. This can only be judged with knowledge of what the usual variations of a particular supply may be.

The Water Quality Regulations 2000 require that samples should be taken by the water undertakers from consumers' taps selected at random and also from other supply points. There may be marked changes in the quality of the water beyond this point of entry into a building, especially in large buildings or complexes, such as hospitals and tower blocks with water storage tanks, long and complex pipelines and 'dead legs', particularly at raised ambient temperatures. Inappropriate plumbing materials, water softeners and filters may contribute to bacterial overgrowth with the formation of biofilms, some of which may contain coliforms and pseudomonads. Examination of samples from various points along the supply lines may give an indication of the location of the problem. Similar considerations apply to water supplied to ships, trains and aircraft.

The regulations give details of the tests required and frequencies of sampling. The essential tests specified in the directive are an examination for enterococci and faecal coliforms. UK legislation also requires total coliforms as an essential test and specifies *E. coli* in place of faecal coliforms. Schedule 2 of the Directive deals with indicator parameters and specifies *Clostridium perfringens* and total coliforms together with colony counts at 37°C and 22°C. The frequency of testing depends upon the population supplied, increasing *pro rata*. The organisms specified should not be detected in a sample of 100 mL water. No figures are specified for colony counts, but no abnormal change should be detected. In certain circumstances examination for enterococci and *C. perfringens* may be required. Technical details of the required methods are given in The Microbiology of Drinking Water (2002) [92] and are prescribed in the legislation [83,84]. A procedure for the detection of *Cryptosporidium* oocysts is detailed in the methods document prepared by the Drinking Water Inspectorate [93].

Test	Section/method
Potable water (including that used in food production)	
◆ Colony count at 37°C and 22°C	See [92]
◆ Total coliforms in 100 mL	See [92]
◆ Faecal coliforms/*E. coli* in 100 mL	See [92]
◆ *Clostridium perfringens* in 100 mL	See [92]
◆ Enterococci in 100 mL	See [92]
■ *Cryptosporidia in water*	See [93]

Microbiological criteria for potable water

Water Supply (Water Quality) Regulations 2000 [83]

Table A of Schedule 1 and Schedule 2.

Item	Parameter	Concentration	Point of compliance
Directive requirements (Schedule 1 Table A, part I):			
1	Enterococci	0/100 mL	Consumers' taps
2	*Escherichia coli*	0/100 mL	Consumers' taps
National requirements (Schedule 1 Table A, part II):			
1	Coliform bacteria	0/100 mL	Service reservoirs* and water treatment works
2	*Escherichia coli*	0/100 mL	Service reservoirs* and water treatment works
Indicator parameters (Schedule 2):			
1	*Clostridium perfringens*	0/100 mL	Supply point†
2	Coliform bacteria	0/100 mL	Consumers' taps
3	Colony counts (22°C)	No abnormal change (per mL)	Consumers' taps, service reservoirs and treatment works
4	Colony counts (37°C)	No abnormal change (per mL)	Consumers' taps, service reservoirs and treatment works

*Compliance required as to 95% of samples from each service reservoir (Regulation 4(6)).
†May be monitored from samples of water leaving treatment works or other supply point, as no significant change in distribution.

Natural mineral water and other water in containers

Natural mineral water is defined as microbiologically wholesome water originating in an underground water table or deposit and emerging from a spring tapped at one or more natural or bore exits. It differs from ordinary drinking water in its mineral content, its trace elements or other constituents and (where appropriate) certain effects; it is also different in its original state. Any form of disinfection is prohibited although carbon dioxide may be introduced (or reintroduced). The source must be protected from all pollution risks, both microbiological and chemical. An outbreak of cholera in Portugal was attributed to bottled mineral water [94,95] but there is no other evidence of ill-health.

If any type of water is to be used for bottling or putting into another container type all organisms specified should be sought in 250 mL [89].

Test	Section/method
Natural mineral water	
◆ Plate count at 37°C and 22°C	See [89,91,92]
◆ Total coliforms/*Escherichia coli* in 250 mL	See [89,91,92]
◆ Faecal streptococci in 250 mL	See [89,91,92]
◆ Sulphite reducing sporulated anaerobes in 50 mL	See [89,91,92]
◆ *Pseudomonas aeruginosa* in 250 mL	See [89,91,92]

◆ The Natural Mineral Water, Spring Water and Bottled Drinking Water Regulations (1999) [89]

Microbiological criteria for natural mineral water

The Natural Mineral Water, Spring Water and Bottled Drinking Water Regulations 1999 [89], EC Directive 80/777/EEC [91]

Colony count:

At source	Shall conform to the normal viable colony count of that water
For the period of 12 h following bottling while kept at 4 ± 1°C	<100/mL after 72 h incubation at 20–22°C <20/mL after 24 h incubation at 37°C

Other organisms:

At source and during its marketing:

Coliforms	Absent in any 250 mL sample
Escherichia coli	Absent in any 250 mL sample
Faecal streptocci	Absent in any 250 mL sample
Pseudomonas aeruginosa	Absent in any 250 mL sample
Sulphite reducing sporulated anaerobes	Absent in any 50 mL sample

---

The colony count must not exceed that which results from the normal increase in the bacterial content at source (which may not be known to the examiner).
A mineral water must also be free from parasites and pathogenic microorganisms (no tests specified).

Test	Section/method
Spring water and drinking water (bottled)	
◆ Colony count at 37°C and 22°C*	See [91,92]
◆ Coliforms†	See [91,92]
◆ Faecal coliforms	See [91,92]
◆ Faecal streptococci	See [91,92]
◆ Sulphite reducing sporulated anaerobes in 20 mL	See [91,92]

*The colony counts should be measured within 12 h of bottling with the sample water being kept at a constant temperature during that 12-h period.
†By multiple tube method.

Microbiological criteria for spring water and bottled drinking water

The Natural Mineral Water, Spring Water and Bottled Drinking Water Regulations (1999) [89]

Total coliforms	0/100 mL
Faecal coliforms	0/100 mL
Faecal streptococci	0/100 mL
Sulphite reducing clostridia	≤1/20 mL
Colony counts:	
At 22°C	100/mL
At 37°C	20/mL

Any increase in the colony count of the water between 12 h after bottling and the time of sale shall not be greater than that normally expected.

Water in vending machines

Water is a major ingredient in drinks from beverage vending machines. The water supplied to the machines must be of potable quality and satisfy the parameters above. Once the water has entered the machine it is regarded as a food and so the Food Safety Regulations apply [87]. The testing of water from vending machines assesses the quality and safety of the vended product and the adequacy of cleaning of the machines. Guidance on good hygiene practice has been introduced by the industry [96]. It is recognized that bacterial growth will occur in the vending machine and that colony counts of 10^5/mL are not uncommon, particularly if usage is infrequent. However total coliform counts exceeding 10^3/100 mL or presence of *E. coli* in 100 mL indicate the need for sanitization of the machine.

3.23 References

1   Great Britain. *The Animal By-Products Order 1999*. Statutory Instrument No. 646. London: HMSO, 1999.

2   Anderton A, Howard JP, Scott DW. Microbiological control in enteral feeding. *Human Nutr: Appl Nutr* 1986; **404**: 163–7.

3   Anderton A, Howard JP, Scott DW. *Microbiological Control in Enteral Feeding. A Guidance Document. Parenteral and Enteral Nutrition Group*. London: British Dietetic Association, 1986.

4   Nazarowec-White M, Farber JM. *Enterobacter sakazaki*: a review. *Int J Fd Microbiol* 1997; **34**: 103–13.

5   Food and Agriculture Organization (FAO)/World Health Organization (WHO). *Microbiological Specifications for Foods. Report of the Second Joint FAO/WHO Expert Consultation 1977*. Rome: FAO, 1977.

6   Mossel DAA, Corry JEL, Struijk CB, Baird JM. *Essentials of the Microbiology of Foods*. Chichester: John Wiley & Sons, 1995: 388–9.

7   Craven PC, Mackel DC, Baine WB, *et al*. International oubreak of *Salmonella eastbourne* infection traced to contaminated chocolate. *Lancet* 1975; **i**: 788–93.

8   Gill ON, Sockett PN, Bartlett CLR, *et al*. Outbreak of *Salmonella napoli* infection caused by contaminated chocolate bars. *Lancet* 1983; **i**: 574–7.

9   Gardner GA. Microbiological examination of curing brines. In: Board RG, Lovelock DW, eds. *Sampling—Microbiological Monitoring of Environments. Society for Applied Bacteriology Technical Series No. 7*. London: Academic Press, 1973: 21–7.

10 International Commission on Microbiological Specifications for Foods. *Microorganisms in Foods. 2. Sampling for Microbiological Analysis. Principles and Specific Applications*, 2nd edn. Oxford: Blackwell Scientific, 1986.

11 International Commission on Microbiological Specifications for Foods. Chapter 8: Cereals and cereal products. In: *Microbial Ecology of Foods. Vol 2. Food Commodities*. London: Blackie Academic and Professional, 1998: 313–55.

12 Council of the European Communities. Directive No. 92/46/EEC. Laying down the health rules for the production and placing on the market of raw milk, heat treated milk and milk-based products. *Official J Eur Communities* 1992; **L268**: 1–32.

13 Great Britain. *The Dairy Products (Hygiene) Regulations 1995*. Statutory Instrument No. *1086*. London: HMSO, 1995.

14 British Standards Institution (BSI). BS 4285. *Microbiological Examination for Dairy Purposes. Parts 0–3*. London: BSI, 1986–93.

15 Great Britain. *The Ice-Cream (Heat Treatment, Etc.) Regulations 1959*. Statutory Instrument No. *734*. London: HMSO, 1959.

16 Great Britain. *The Ice-Cream (Heat Treatment, Etc.) (Amendment) Regulations 1963*. Statutory Instrument No. *1083*. London: HMSO, 1963.

17 Great Britain. *The Milk (Special Designation) Regulations 1989*. Statutory Instrument No. *2383*. London: HMSO, 1989.

18 European Commission. 91/180/ EEC. Commission decision laying down certain methods of analysis and testing of raw milk and heat treated milk. *Official J Eur Communities* 1991; **L93/1**: 1–48.

19 Food Safety Act 1990. *Code of Practice No. 18: Enforcement of the Dairy Products (Hygiene) Regulations 1995 and the Dairy Products (Hygiene) (Scotland) Regulations 1995 ('the Regulations')*. London: HMSO, 1995.

20   Ministry of Agriculture, Fisheries and Food, Department of Health, Scottish Office, Welsh Office. *Dairy Products (Hygiene) Regulations 1995—Guidance Notes*. London: MAFF, 1995.

21   Great Britain. *The Zoonoses Order 1989. Statutory Instrument No. 285*. London: HMSO, 1989.

22   Great Britain. *The Egg Products Regulations 1993. Statutory Instrument No. 1520*. London: HMSO, 1993.

23a   Council of the European Communities. Directive No. 98/437/EEC. Hygiene and health problems affecting the production and placing on the market of egg products. *Off J Eur Communities* 1989; **L212**: 87–100.

23   International Commission on Microbiological Specifications for Foods. Chapter 3: Fish and fish products. In: *Microbial Ecology of Foods. Vol 2. Food Commodities*. London: Blackie Academic and Professional, 1998: 130–89.

24   Johnson EA, Goodnough MC. Botulism. In: Collier L, Balows A, Sussman M, eds. *Topley and Wilson's Microbiology and Microbial Infections*, 9th edn, vol. 3. *Bacterial Infections*. London: Arnold, 1998: 723.

25   Ball AP, Hopkinson RB, Farrell ID, *et al*. Human botulism caused by *Clostridium botulinum* type E. The Birmingham outbreak. *Q J Med* 1979; **48**: 473–91.

26   Editorial. Guidelines on microbiological quality for imported frozen cooked prawns. *Environ Hlth* 1975; **83**: 367.

27   Gilbert RJ. The microbiology of some foods imported into England through the Port of London and Heathrow (London) Airport. In: Kurata H, Hesseltine CW, eds. *Control of Microbial Contamination of Foods and Feeds in International Trade: Microbial Standards and Specifications*. Tokyo: Saikon Publishing, 1982: 105–19.

28   Council of the European Communities. Commission Decision No. 93/51/EEC on the microbiological criteria applicable to the production of cooked crustaceans and molluscan shellfish. *Official J Eur Communities* 1993, **L13**: 11–13.

29   Editorial. Shuck your oysters with care. *Lancet* 1990; **ii**: 215–16.

30   Doyle MP. Pathogenic *Escherichia coli*, *Yersinia enterocolitica* and *Vibrio parahaemolyticus*. *Lancet* 1990; **i**: 1111–15.

31   Scoging A. Illness associated with seafood. *PHLS Commun Dis Rep* 1991; **1 Review No 11**: R117–22.

32   Council of the European Communities. Directive No. 91/492/EEC on shellfish hygiene: classification and monitoring of shellfish harvesting water. *Official J Eur Communities* 1991; **L268**: 1–14.

33   Great Britain. *The Food Safety (Fishery Products and Live Shellfish) (Hygiene) Regulations 1998. Statutory Instrument No. 994*. London: HMSO, 1998.

34   Great Britain. *The Food Safety (Fishery Products and Live Shellfish) (Hygiene) Amendment Regulations 1999. Statutory Instrument No. 399*. London: HMSO, 1999.

35   Early JC, Nicholson FJ. *Specification for a Model Cockle Processing Plant*. MAFF, Torry Research Station 1988; Report No. TD 2106 amended 1990; Report No. 2401.

36   International Commission on Microbiological Specifications for Foods. Chapter 16: Milk and dairy products. In: *Microbial Ecology of Foods. Vol 2. Food Commodities*. London: Blackie Academic and Professional, 1998: 521–76.

37   International Commission on Microbiological Specifications for Foods. Chapter 1: Meat and meat products. In: *Microbial Ecology of Foods. Vol 2. Food Commodities*. London: Blackie Academic and Professional, 1998; 1–74.

38   Smittle RB. Microbiology of mayonnaise and salad dressing: a review. *J Food Protect* 1977; **40**: 415–22.

39   International Commission on Microbiological Specificaions for Foods. Chapter 11: Oil and fat based foods. In: *Microbial Ecology of Foods. Vol 2. Food Commodities.* London: Blackie Academic and Professional, 1998: 390–417.

40   Johnson AM. Veterinary sources of food-borne illness. *Lancet* 1990; **ii**: 856–8.

41   Humphrey TJ, Mead GC, Rowe B. Poultry meat as a source of human salmonellosis in England and Wales. *Epidem Infect* 1988; **100**: 175–84.

42   Department of Health Ministry of Agriculture Fisheries and Food. *Surveillance of Salmonella in UK Produced Raw Chicken on Retail Sale. No. 2 in a Joint Series.* London: Department of Health, 1996.

43   Public Health Laboratory Service. Facts and figures—*Salmonella* in humans 1981–2000. 16 March 2001.
      http://www.phls.co.uk/facts/Gastro/Salmonella/salmHumAnn.htm

44   Hood AM, Pearson AD, Shahamat M. The extent of surface contamination of retailed chickens with *Campylobacter jejuni* serogroups. *Epidem Infect* 1988; **100**: 17–25.

45   Lammerding AM, Garcia MM, Mann ED, *et al*. Prevalence of *Salmonella* and thermophilic *Campylobacter* in fresh pork, beef, veal, and poultry in Canada. *J Fd Prot* 1998; **51**: 47–52.

46   Turnbull PCB, Rose P. *Campylobacter jejuni* and salmonella in raw red meats. *J Hyg* 1982; **88**: 29–37.

47   Bolton FJ, Dawkins HC, Hutchinson DN. Biotypes and serotypes of thermophilic campylobacters isolated from cattle, sheep and pig offal and other red meats. *J Hyg* 1985; **95**: 1–6.

48   Kramer JM, Frost JA, Bolton FJ, Wareing DRA. *Campylobacter* contamination of raw meat and poultry at retail sale: Identification of multiple types and comparison with isolates from human infection. *J Fd Prot* 2000; **63**: 1654–9.

49   Fricker CR, Park RWA. A 2-year study of the distribution of 'thermophilic' campylobacters in human, environmental and food samples from the Reading area with particular reference to toxin production and heat stable serotype. *J Appl Bact* 1989; **66**: 477–90.

50   Pini PN, Gilbert RJ. The occurrence in the UK of *Listeria* spp. in raw chickens and soft cheeses. *Int J Fd Microbiol* 1988; **6**: 317–26.

51   Miettinen MK, Palmu L, Bjorkroth KJ, Korkeala H. Prevalence of *Listeria monocytogenes* in broilers at the abattoir, processing plant, and retail level. *J Fd Prot* 2001; **64**: 994–9.

52   Brewer RA, Corbel MJ. Characterization of *Yersinia enterocolitica* strains isolated from cattle, sheep and pigs in the United Kingdom. *J Hyg* 1983; **90**: 325–33.

53   Tauxe RV, Vandepitte J, Wauters G, *et al*. *Yersinia enterocolitica* infections and pork: the missing link. *Lancet* 1987; **i**: 1129–32.

54   Doyle MP, Schoeni JL. Isolation of *Escherichia coli* O157: H7 from retail fresh meats and poultry. *Appl Environ Microbiol* 1987; **53**: 2394–6.

55   Chapman PA, Siddons CA, Cerdan Malo AT, Harkin MA. A 1-year study of *Escherichia coli* O157 in raw beef and lamb products. *Epidem Infect* 2000; **124**: 207–13.

56   Cowden JM. Scottish outbreak of *Escherichia coli* O157 November–December 1996. *Eurosurveillance* 1997; **2**: 1–2.

57   The Pennington Group. *Report on the Circumstances Leading to the Outbreak of Infection with Escherichia coli O157 in Central Scotland, the Implications for Food Safety and the Lessons to be Learned.* Edinburgh: The Stationery Office, 1997.

58   Little CL, de Louvois J. The microbiological examination of butchery products and butchers' premises in the United Kingdom. *J Appl Microbiol* 1998; **85**: 177–86.

59   Sutton RGA, Kendall M, Hobbs BC. The effect of two methods of cooking and cooling on *Clostridium welchii* and other bacteria in meat. *J Hyg* 1972; **70**: 415–24.

60   Campden and Chorleywood Food and Drink Research Association. *HACCP: A Practical Guide*, 2nd edn. *Technical Manual No. 38*. Chipping Campden: Campden and Chorleywood Food and Drink Research Association, 1997.

61   International Commission on Microbiological Specifications for Foods. *Microorganisms in Foods. 4. Application of the Hazard Analysis Critical Control Point (HACCP) System to Ensure Microbiological Safety and Quality*. Oxford: Blackwell Scientific, 1988.

62   Gillespie I, Little CL, Mitchell R. Microbiological examination of cold ready-to-eat meats from catering establishments in the United Kingdom. *J Appl Microbiol* 2000; **88**: 467–74.

63   Cowden JM, O'Mahony M, Bartlett CLR, *et al.* A national outbreak of *Salmonella typhimurium* DT 124 caused by contaminated salami sticks. *Epidem Inf* 1989; **103**: 219–25.

64   Hayes PR. *Food Microbiology and Hygiene*, 2nd edn. London: Elsevier Applied Science, 1992: 121–5.

65   Morris IJ, Ribeiro CD. *Listeria monocytogenes* and pâté. *Lancet* 1989; **ii**: 1285–6.

66   Velani S, Gilbert RJ. *Listeria monocytogenes* in pre-packed ready-to-eat sliced meats. *PHLS Microbiol Dig* 1990; **7**: 56–7.

67   Frazier WC, Westhoff DC. *Food Microbiology*, 4th edn. New York: McGraw-Hill, 1988: 121–33.

68   Gilbert RJ, Hall SM, Taylor AG. Listeriosis update. *PHIS Microbiol Dig* 1989; **6**: 33–7.

69   United Kingdom. *Food Safety (Temperature Control) Regulations 1995*. Statutory Instrument No. 2200. London: HMSO.

70a British Sandwich Association (BSA). Code of practice and minimum standards for sandwich manufacturers (producers), revised 2001. Ardington: BSA.

70   Department of Health. *Chilled and Frozen. Guidelines on Cook-Chill and Cook-Freeze Systems*. London: HMSO, 1989.

71   Tebbutt GM. Assessment of hygiene risks in premises selling take-away foods. *Environ Health* 1991; **99**: 97–100.

72   Cruickshank JG, Humphrey TJ. The carrier food handler and non-typhoid salmonellosis. *Epidemiol Infect* 1987; **98**: 223–30.

73   Davis JG, Blake JR, Woodall CM. A survey of the hygienic condition of domestic dishcloths and tea-towels. *Med Officer* 1968; **120**: 29–32.

74   Gilbert RJ. Cross-contamination of cooked-meat slicing machines and cleaning cloths. *J Hyg* 1969; **67**: 249–54.

75   Tebbutt GM, Southwell JM. Comparative study of visual inspections and microbiological sampling in premises manufacturing and selling high-risk foods. *Epidem Infect* 1989; **103**: 175–86.

76   Ministry of Agriculture and Fisheries. National Milk Testing and Advisory Scheme. *The rinse method for the examination of washed milk bottles. A provisional technique*. 1947. Technique No. B743/T.P.B. London: MAFF.

77   British Standards Institution (BSI). BS 4285. *Microbiological Examination for Dairy Purposes. Part 4. Methods for Assessment of Hygienic Conditions*. London: BSI, 1991.

78   International Commission on Microbiological Specifications for Foods. Chapter 5: Vegetables and vegetable products; Chapter 6: Fruit and fruit products. In: *Microbial*

Ecology of Food Commodities. London: Blackie Academic and Professional, 1998: 215–73.

79 Swaminathan B, Sparling PH. The bacteriology of foods excluding dairy products. In: Collier L, Balows A, Sussman M, eds. *Topley and Wilson's Microbiology and Microbial Infection*, 9th edn, vol. 2. *Systematic Bacteriology*. London: Arnold, 1998: 395–416.

80 Reid TMS, Robinson HG. Frozen raspberries and hepatitis A. *J Hyg* 1987; **98**: 109–12.

81 Tee GH. Bacteriological examination of watercress. *Mon Bull Min Health PHLS* 1962; **21**: 73–8.

82 Velani SK, Roberts D. *Listeria monocytogenes* and other *Listeria* spp. in pre-packed mixed salads and individual salad ingredients. *PHLS Microbiol Dig* 1991; **8**: 21–2.

83 England and Wales. *The Water Supply (Water Quality) Regulations 2000. Statutory Instrument No. 3184*. London: HMSO, 2000.

84 Great Britain. *The Water Supply (Water Quality) Regulations 1989. Statutory Instrument No. 1147*. London: HMSO, 1989.

85 Council of the European Union. Council Directive 98/83/EC on the quality of water for human consumption. *Official J Eur Communities* 1998; **L330**: 32–54.

86 Great Britain. *The Private Water Supplies Regulations 1991. Statutory Instrument No. 2790*. London: HMSO, 1991.

87 Great Britain. *The Food Safety (General Food Hygiene) Regulations 1995. Statutory Instrument No. 1763*. London: HMSO, 1995.

88 Ministry of Agriculture Fisheries and Food, Department of Agriculture and Fisheries for Scotland, Welsh Office Agriculture Department. *Animal Health Circular* 1992: **92/86**.

89 England and Wales. *The Natural Mineral Water, Spring Water and Bottled Drinking Water Regulations 1999. Statutory Instrument No. 1540*. London: HMSO, 1999.

90 Council of the European Communities. Directive 80/777/EEC of 15 July 1980 on the approximation of the laws of the Member States relating to the exploitation and marketing of natural mineral waters. *Official J Eur Communities* 1980; **L229**: 1–10.

91 Council of the European Communities. Directive No. 80/778/EEC relating to the quality of water intended for human consumption in relation to other drinking water which is bottled or sold in a bottle (as defined in regulation 2). *Official J Eur Communities* 1980; **L229**, 11.

92 Standing Committee of Analysts. *Methods for the Examination of Waters and Associated Materials. The Microbiology of Drinking Water (2002)—Part I—Water Quality and Public Health*. Environment Agency, 2002.

93 Drinking Water Inspectorate. Standard operating protocols for laboratory and analytical procedures and for performing risk assessment for the monitoring of *Cryptosporidium* oocysts in treated water supplies to satisfy Water Supply (Water Quality) (Amendment) Regulations 1999, SI 1524. Part 2. Laboratory and analytical procedures. http://www.dwi.gov.uk/regs/crypto/index.htm.

94 Blake PA, Rosenberg ML, Costa JB, Ferreira PS, Guimaraes CL, Gangarosa EJ. Cholera in Portugal, 1974. I. Modes of transmission. *Am J Epidemiol* 1977; **105**: 337–43.

95 Blake PA, Rosenberg ML, Florencia J, Costa JB, Quintino LDP, Gangarosa EJ. Cholera in Portugal, 1974. II. Transmission by bottled mineral water. *Am J Epidemiol* 1977; **105**: 344–8.

96 The Automatic Vending Association. *Industry Guide to Good Hygiene Practice: Vending and Dispensing Guide Supplement (to the Catering Guide)*. London: Chadwick House Group Ltd, 2000.

4 Preparation of samples

4.1   Receipt and storage

Food samples collected under the Food Safety Act 1990 that may be the subject of legal proceedings need to be handled according to Code of Practice No. 7, 'Sampling for Analysis or Examination' (revised October 2000) [1] and the associated 'Guidance on Food Sampling for Microbiological Examination' [2]. The guidelines laid down in these documents are applicable also to all samples of food taken for microbiological examination. In the context of the code 'examination' means microbiological examination by a food examiner (microbiologist). A copy of this code should be available in every laboratory. The provisions of Part III, 'Samples for Examination', of the Code of Practice and the Guidance are summarized below.

Size and nature of sample for examination

The quantity of sample submitted should normally be at least 100 g. The sample may consist of a single unit or a number of units. This will depend on the purpose of the examination, for example whether a particular pathogen is being sought. Existing national sampling protocols should be taken into consideration. In any case of doubt the food examiner should be consulted.

Handling for examination

Officers should ensure that, as far as possible, samples for examination reach the laboratory in a condition microbiologically unchanged from that existing at the time of sampling. Contamination of the sample and microbial growth or death during sampling, transport and storage should be avoided. Aseptic handling techniques should be used throughout the sampling process.

Containers

All samples should be placed in containers before submission to the food examiner. The owner of the food, if present, should be given the opportunity to observe the sampling procedure.

Sampling instruments and containers that come into direct contact with food should be sterile. Samples taken from unpacked or opened cans or packets of foods should first be placed in clean, dry, sterile leakproof containers such as wide-mouth glass or food-quality plastic jars or sterile plastic bags with closures. Jars and bottles should be closed with suitable caps with insoluble, non-absorbent cap-liners. If the sample is already contained within unopened packaging, in the vendor's wrapping or if the container is securely closed, for example a leak-proof screw top jar, disposable food grade plastic bags may be used to further contain them. Plastic bags should be sealed securely so that they cannot leak or become contaminated during normal handling.

The contained sample should be secured with a tamper-evident seal and labelled. Information recorded on the label should include the name of the food, the names of the sampling officer and the authority, the place, date and time of sampling and a unique tagging identification number. If the label is likely to become damaged during transport the sample should be placed in a second container, such as a plastic bag, and sealed to prevent tampering. The label should remain visible.

Transportation and storage

Samples should be transported and stored under conditions that inhibit changes in microbial numbers, i.e.:

- Frozen foods need to be kept frozen as far as possible.
- Chilled/refrigerated foods and other perishable foods need to be kept in a surrounding air temperature at or below 8°C and preferably between 0°C and 4°C [3], but not frozen.
- Hot or warm samples should be kept separate from other food samples and cooled down as quickly as possible to a temperature of 8°C or below.
- Dried foods, unblown cans and other shelf-stable items need not be cooled but should be stored and transported at a temperature less than 40°C.

Refrigerated insulated containers or insulated containers cooled by means of frozen ice or gel packs should be used to hold and transport chilled or frozen samples. If frozen packs are used their volume should form at least 10% of the volume of the insulated container.

Samples should be delivered to the laboratory as soon as possible, preferably within 4h. If there is likely to be a delay the samples must be stored under conditions that will minimize microbial change.

The air temperature of the cool box should be recorded on arrival in the laboratory.

Request for examination

All relevant information should accompany a food sample to ensure that it is subjected to the most appropriate examination and to enable the food examiner to interpret the results:

- Name and authority of sampling officer.
- Sample identification number.
- Date, time and place of sampling.
- The temperature and storage conditions at the place of sampling.
- Description of sample including batch/lot number, canning code, etc. and durability date (use by, best before, etc.).
- Reason(s) for sampling and whether legal action may result.
- Name of owner, manufacturer, importer, seller, buyer, as appropriate.
- The process and date of cooking (if known) of cooked foods.
- Country of origin, conditions and duration of transport (if known).
- Other relevant storage factors, e.g. condition of packages, humidity, sanitation.
- Method of sampling (random throughout lot, random throughout accessible units, otherwise).
- Clinical and epidemiological details (in cases of suspected food poisoning).
- Storage and transport conditions since the sample was taken.
- The time of delivery to the laboratory.

Standard request forms for examination of formal samples are available from the Public Health Laboratory Service (PHLS). If legal action is likely to result from the examination, samples taken in accordance with the Food Safety (Sampling and Qualifications) Regulations 1990 [4] and the requirements of Code of Practice No. 7 should be submitted to a laboratory accredited for the purpose of examination and which appears on the list of official control laboratories (published on the Food Standards Agency website: www.foodstandards.gov.uk).

Receipt and description at the laboratory

Food samples may be received at the laboratory in containers of various types and aseptic techniques need to be used to open them. The container should be disinfected if necessary to avoid contamination of the sample. Other batches of a similar product can provide useful background information and should be tested together with any suspect sample in case of complaint or consignment defect. The following details should be recorded on the report form:

- **Type of packaging**—this may have an effect on the condition of the contents and should be recorded to aid interpretation of the results. For example, the environment within vacuum packages is anaerobic whilst meats sliced at a delicatessen counter are in an aerobic atmosphere and will have a much shorter overall shelf life. The gas mixtures used for modified atmosphere packaging will also influence the microbiology of a food. Defects such as dents and imperfect seals should also be noted.

- **Appearance**—describe the food sample in general terms, e.g. '70 g of machine-sliced, paper-wrapped, pink-coloured, cooked ham'. Signs of deterioration, abnormal colour and mould should also be recorded.
- **Texture**—bacterial deterioration can cause products to become soft or semi-liquid; this applies particularly to meat products.
- **Smell**—this is an indication of spoilage or contamination. A full organoleptic test includes taste, but this should not be undertaken in the laboratory.

Storage before and after examination

The bacterial and fungal content of food that is not shelf stable may increase greatly between the time of collection and the time of examination if simple precautions are not taken. On arrival in the laboratory the samples should be transferred to a refrigerator at 0–4°C [5] while the clerical work is completed. If the tests cannot be commenced on the day of receipt, perishable samples should be stored at 0–4°C and examined preferably within 24 h of sampling. If received frozen the sample should be kept at below –18°C until the day of the test. Generally frozen samples should be thawed in a refrigerator at 0–4°C (bulky samples may require overnight thawing) and kept there until the examination is about to take place. Alternatively the frozen sample may be placed at ambient temperature in the laboratory for 2–3 h (meat products) [6] or 1 h (fish products) [7] immediately before examination.

After the examination the remainder of the sample should be stored at 0–4°C or below –18°C, as appropriate, and discarded only when proper authority has been obtained.

4.2 Preparation of sample suspension

The diluent recommended for general use is a peptone saline solution of composition 0.1% peptone and 0.85% sodium chloride in distilled water [5]. This solution is referred to as 'maximum recovery diluent' (MRD). Certain food products such as some dairy and fish products require the use of specific diluents other than MRD. Information about specific diluents can be found in ISO 6887, parts 2–4 [6,7,8], in ISO 8261 [9] and in Sections 7 and 9. These diluents are required for acid foods, highly salted foods, products with a high fat content, etc., and are used to achieve a uniform aqueous suspension of approximately isotonic concentration.

The sample suspension may be prepared in either a stomacher (peristaltic homogeniser), a rotary food blender or a pulsifier as described below. For most products a 1/10 (10^{-1}) sample suspension is prepared by mixing one part of sample with nine parts of diluent. For some dehydrated products with high absorbency it will be necessary to prepare a more dilute homogenate such as 1/20 in order to obtain some free liquid.

Stomacher* (peristaltic homogeniser)

Solid foods have to be rendered into a suspension in liquid in order to apply the counting and culturing techniques described in Sections 5–9. The stomacher provides a suitable means of doing this. It blends the food by means of paddles that pound against a sterile plastic bag containing the food plus diluent. A weighed sample of food (25 g) is homogenized in a measured volume of diluent (225 mL) to give a 10^{-1} homogenate. Less than 25 g of sample is not recommended unless the quantity of sample submitted is insufficient to allow use of this amount. Aseptic techniques need to be used throughout all sampling and handling procedures to avoid the introduction of microorganisms into the sample from the operator, equipment or environment.

The stomacher may be used for most foods but is not suitable for products which may puncture the stomacher bag or for products of tough texture such as salami-type sausage.

Procedure

(a) Place the sample and the diluent in the appropriately sized stomacher bag taking care not to touch the inside of the bag with the hands when opening. Do not include sharp objects such as bone in the sample as these may puncture the bag.

(b) Open the door of the stomacher by lifting the handle and place the bag between the door and the paddles allowing about 7 cm of the open end of the bag to project above the top of the door.

(c) Close the door by pulling the handle forwards, thus clamping the bag in place.

(d) Switch on the machine and operate it for 1 min. Longer periods may be required to produce a homogeneous food suspension.

(e) Switch off the machine. Hold the open end of the bag and open the door to release the bag.

(f) Pour the contents of the bag into a suitable sterile container.

(g) Use this 10^{-1} homogenate, or a decimal dilution of this homogenate, for counting and culturing techniques as described in Sections 5–9.

Rotary blender

If a stomacher is not available or is not suitable, a rotary blender may be used to produce a food suspension. This consists of a sterilizable glass or metal jar fitted with a mixing blade at the base and a close fitting lid. The blender should have a rotational speed of between 8000 and 45 000 rev/min.

*Stomacher® is a registered trade mark of Seward Medical Ltd, 98 Great North Road, London N2 0GN. Tel: 0208 3654100; Fax: 0208 3653999.

Procedure

(a) Place the weighed sample (25 g) and all or a portion of the diluent (225 mL) into a sterile blender jar. Seal the jar with a sterile lid. The volume of diluent required will depend on the size of the blender jar. For safety reasons, i.e. to prevent aerosols, it is advisable to add only a portion of the diluent before blending.

(b) Operate the blender to achieve 15 000–20 000 revolutions of the mixing blade within 2.5 min. Operation of the blending apparatus for longer periods will generate heat.

(c) Transfer the homogenate to a suitable sterile container and add the remainder of the diluent. Mix well.

(d) Use this 10^{-1} homogenate, or a decimal dilution of it, for counting and culturing techniques as described in Sections 5–9.

Pulsifier*

This equipment is used in a similar way to a stomacher but the pulsifier uses a metal ring to beat the outside of the sample bag at high frequency (3500 rev/min). The beating action produces a combination of shock waves and intense mixing which releases the organisms into suspension. Unlike the other methods of homogenate preparation, the food pieces remain relatively intact and the suspensions remain clear. This reduces the likelihood of bag punctures and facilitates pipetting as well as reducing interference due to sample debris.

4.3 Preparation of decimal dilutions

Use the 10^{-1} sample homogenate to prepare further decimal dilutions as required by adding one part of the 10^{-1} homogenate to nine parts of MRD to form the 10^{-2} dilution. Do not introduce the pipette more than 1 cm into the sample homogenate and avoid contact between the pipette containing the inoculum and the sterile diluent. Use a vortex mixer to mix the dilution thoroughly before preparation of a further dilution. Repeat this procedure to prepare further dilutions by adding one part of each dilution to nine parts of MRD until sufficient dilutions have been made to achieve a density of colonies that is countable. Always use MRD as the diluent for further dilutions regardless of the diluent used to prepare the 10^{-1} dilution, unless xerophilic or osmophilic organisms are sought (see Section 6.17, method 2).

If a more dilute sample homogenate was prepared because of the nature of the food product, compensate for this when preparing the 10^{-2} dilution by adding two parts of sample homogenate to eight parts of MRD if the initial suspension was 1/20, three parts of sample homogenate to seven parts of MRD if a 1/30 was used, etc.

*The pulsifier is available from Microgen Bioproducts Ltd, 1 Admiralty Way, Camberley, Surrey GU15 3DT. Tel: 01276 600081; Fax: 01276 600151.

Do not allow more than 30 min to elapse between preparation of the sample homogenate and preparation of further dilutions, or more than 45 min to elapse between preparation of the sample homogenate and contact with the culture medium [5].

4.4 Preliminary examination of cans and flexible long-life packs [10–12]

Pre-examination incubation of shelf-stable foods

(a) Examine up to six abnormal packs and at least two normal packs as soon as possible after receipt.
(b) Incubate 12–24 normal packs at 30°C for 7–14 days. Examine any that develop into blown packs as soon as possible. Examine six of the remaining normal packs at the end of the incubation period.

Preparation and external examination

(a) Maintain canned meats at a temperature of 4°C for several hours after pre-examination incubation to allow any gelatin to set; this will aid removal of the sample from the can.
(b) Examine the can for rust and leakage as follows (Fig. 4.1a). Examine the outer surface of the label for signs of underlying rust. Note where the edges of the label overlap and secure the position of the label at this point with short strips of adhesive tape over the seam. With a sharp knife cut the label vertically, opposite the overlap as illustrated and part it carefully from the can to locate any rust spots or staining of the label due to leakage from body or seam. If any rust spots on the label are uniform and light in colour, leakage is unlikely, but if a rust spot has a darker inner area then the can may be perforated. Probe the dark area with a fine needle to check if there is a pinhole.
(c) Examine the appearance of the seam as follows (Fig. 4.1b). Remove the label and examine the seam visually for any signs of product leakage or irregularity. Any physical defect, for example a 'spur' as shown in the illustration, could be a point of leakage. View the seam along a line nearly parallel to the can body, and examine the line of contact between the can seam and the can body for any lack of tightness as shown. Check that both seams look alike and look tight. In the case of a slack seam, there is a more obvious gap at the point marked 'x'.
(d) Examine the metal of the ends for fracture by deep impression coding or damage to the score or rivet area of any ring-pull feature and for metal fracture of the body at the extremities of deep dents or at score lines. If the contents are solid, examine for plate fracture, which may be present without obvious product leakage.

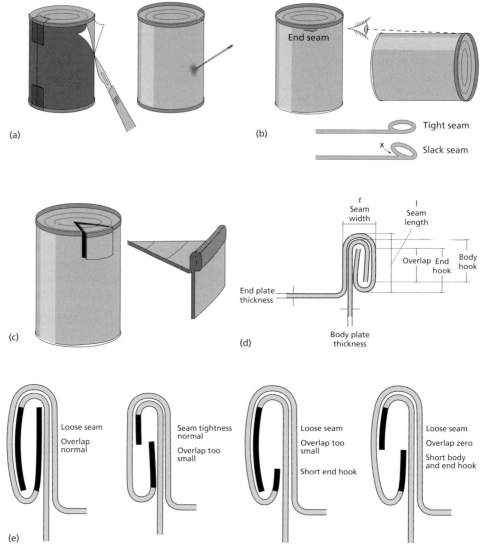

(a)

(b)

Tight seam

x — Slack seam

t
Seam
width

I
Seam
length

Overlap End — Body
hook — hook

End plate
thickness

Body plate
thickness

(c)

(d)

(e)

Loose seam

Overlap
normal

Seam tightness
normal

Overlap too
small

Loose seam

Overlap too
small

Short end hook

Loose seam

Overlap zero

Short body
and end hook

End seam

Fig. 4.1 Preliminary examination of cans: (a) rust and leakage; (b) seam appearance; (c) cut section of seam; (d) seam section; (e) seam dimensions (black shading indicates seam overlap).

(e) Attach can labels to the worksheet.
(f) Clean the outside of the can with soap and cold water to remove dust and grease.
(g) Record observations of the external appearance of the can.

Opening

Procedure

(a) Immerse the non-coded end of the can in a solution containing 100–300 p.p.m. available chlorine for at least 10 min Remove the excess liquid by draining, then wipe the top of the can with 70% alcohol and allow to evaporate.*

(b) Keep the disinfected top covered with a sterile dish.

(c) Check the vacuum/pressure within the can if possible.

(d) Open the non-coded end of the can or a small area of that end with a sterile opener. Avoid cutting the rim and damaging any code mark. Remove the can contents. Large cans need to be opened around the side walls.

(e) Cut a section of the seam and measure its dimensions t and l (Fig. 4.1c,d). Use a micrometer or a small rule having slots of various widths that serve as 'go'–'no-go' gauges† to make the measurements. Examine the cut seam under a hand lens for possible defects. Examine the side seam for tightness, continuous welded joint and any defects at either end. The integrity of a seam is very dependent on the way in which the folds of metal interlock and the tightness of the interlock (Fig. 4.1e). Interpretation of the results needs experience, but major defects can usually be located.‡

For metal cans, dimensional measurements should be carried out to check both the seam length and seam thickness at four points 90° apart round the can end seam (away from the body side seam). These should be compared with the customer's seam specification data. Any discrepancies may suggest irregularities (such as those illustrated in Fig. 4.1e) that may have led to leaker spoilage after processing. Many types of ends are produced for metal cans with a wide variety of seam dimensions. These may differ significantly for the same can diameter. In Europe these have been classified by Secretariat of the European Federation of Light Metal Packaging Manufacturers (SEFEL)§ and the current guideline publication is available from them.

---

*Other methods of disinfection are also used. These include spraying the can with peracetic acid plus surfactant. Good ventilation and a safety cabinet are essential for this procedure.

†Gauges for seam measurement are available from: Blackpole Jig & Tool Ltd, Worcester Trading Estate, Blackpole Road, Worcester WR3 8H.

‡Specialist facilities are available for can examination; see Appendix C.

§SEFEL, Agoria, Biamant Building, 80 Boulevard A Reyers, 1030 Brussels, Belgium. Tel: 00 322706 7958.

Sampling

Solid foods

Procedure

(a) Take scrapings with a sterile spatula from the exposed surfaces of the food. Take a separate central core sample using a suitable sterile instrument such as a core borer or a spoon. Remove the food from the can, take scrapings from the remaining surfaces and add to the first scrapings sample.

(b) Swab the upper rim seam of the can with a sterile cotton wool swab. Swab the body seam and the lower rim seam with a second swab.

Semi-liquid foods

> **Procedure**
> (a) Take a representative 100 g sample with a sterile implement.
> (b) Record the internal condition of the can, i.e. presence/absence of lacquer, rusting, blackening, and corrosion.

4.5   pH measurement

It is important to determine the pH of the food sample before undertaking microbiological examination as this can influence the range of examinations applied and organisms sought. In general, in foods with a pH below 4.5 pathogens would not be expected to survive; the organisms present would be limited to yeasts, moulds and a few acid tolerant bacteria. Foods with a pH above 4.5 require full microbiological examination.

> **Procedure**
> (a) Remove a portion from the sample for pH measurement to avoid contamination of the bulk of the food.
> (b) Calibrate a pH meter and measure the pH directly at the surface of the food using a surface probe.

4.6   Direct microscopic examination

Examination for organisms — Gram stain

It may be helpful to perform a Gram stain on the sample homogenate before further examination if the sample has been submitted as a spoilage complaint or as the cause of possible toxigenic food-borne illness. In these cases the samples will contain high levels ($>10^6$ colony forming units (cfu)/g) of the causative organisms at some point, although culture may not recover them due to heat treatment or die off.

> **Procedure**
> (a) Smear the surface of a slide thinly with the food material or a small drop of the 10^{-1} homogenate.
> (b) Fix the preparation by heat and defat if necessary with xylenol.
> (c) Stain by Gram's method (see Section 10.6)
> (d) Examine the stained dry slide by optical microscopy at high magnification (oil immersion objective) for Gram positive or Gram negative bacteria.
>
> **continued**

(e) Record the levels of the different types of bacteria seen, e.g. large, moderate or scanty numbers of Gram positive cocci or Gram negative bacilli.

In some instances the product may interfere with the Gram stain and it may be more practical to examine the 10^{-1} homogenate under direct illumination as a wet preparation (without any staining). Viable motile spoilage bacteria can then be observed more easily as may bacterial spores. Gram staining can also be performed at a later stage on culture isolates recovered from broth or agar plate media.

Examination for fungi — wet preparation

Procedure
(a) Using a clean glass microscope slide scrape the surface of the food where fungal growth is seen or suspected.
(b) Emulsify the material in distilled water on another slide and cover with a cover slip.
(c) Add one drop of lactophenol cotton blue stain to the edge of the cover slip.
(d) Examine the slide by optical microscopy at low magnification for fungal elements.

4.7 Water activity

The water activity (a_w) of a food is a measure of availability of water for the metabolic activity and growth of microorganisms. This available or 'free' water is expressed as a ratio of the water vapour pressure of the food to that of pure water at the same temperature, and depends on the nature and quantity of the particles dissolved in the aqueous phase of the product. Values range from 0.0 for a completely anhydrous sample to 1.0 for pure, salt-free water.

Measurement of a_w is usually performed using an electric hygrometer, which consists of a potentiometer, a sample/sensor holder and a sensor. The sample holder needs to be vapour-tight and sufficiently large to accommodate a representative sample. The sensors vary according to manufacturer but usually contain an immobilized electrolyte. When the sample and airspace within the sample holder are at equilibrium changes in the equilibrium relative humidity (ERH) are reflected in changes in the conductance of an electric current through the sensor and across the electrolyte. This is detected electrically by the equipment and can be converted to water activity using a simple equation [13,14].

The equipment should be calibrated before use with standards consisting of solutions of saturated salts prepared in deionized distilled water. Precise control of temperature is very important when taking measurements and the equipment should be calibrated at the same temperature as that used for the samples. The material to be measured should be uniform in nature and placed in the sample holder quickly to minimize moisture exchange with ambient air. Further information is given in the instruction manual accompanying the equipment.

Different species of microorganisms have different minimum levels of water activity that permit growth. The water activity of a food product can therefore be used to predict microbial growth and to determine the microbiological stability of a food product. This can be a useful measurement to perform on canned foods that yield growth on enrichment culture in order to determine the likelihood of outgrowth during storage. As a general guide, the growth of most bacteria and fungi occurs only at a_w values above 0.90; if the a_w is below 0.8 the only organisms likely to grow are xerophilic moulds and osmophilic yeasts.

4.8 Good laboratory practice

Good laboratory practice is essential to ensure that:
1 The organisms isolated from a food sample originated from that sample.
2 The organisms in the food do not contaminate the environment or other samples.
3 The organism counts obtained truly reflect the organism levels in the food.
4 The techniques used in the laboratory are reproducible between operators in the same laboratory and repeatable in other laboratories.
   In order to achieve this:
(a) Environmental contamination should be minimized. This may require a filter ventilation system for incoming air or the use of a clean-air laminar flow cabinet.
(b) A strict regime for cleaning and disinfection of surfaces and equipment should be in operation.
(c) Staff should be well trained in aseptic technique.
(d) Equipment should meet the specifications shown below [3,5,15]:
   • Balances for weighing samples should be capable of weighing to 0.1 g or less.
   • Accuracy for addition of diluent to the sample during preparation of the homogenate should be ±5% of the target volume or weight.
   • Accuracy of volumes for dilution fluid used for preparation of decimal dilutions should be ±2% of the target volume.
   • Accuracy of sample volumes used in preparation of decimal dilutions and inoculation of media should be ±5% of the target volume. In order to achieve this accuracy the use of fixed volume calibrated displacement pipettors and sterile disposable tips should be considered.
   • pH meters should be capable of measuring to an accuracy of ±0.1 pH units with a minimum measurement threshold of 0.01 pH units.
   • Incubators and water baths should be capable of maintaining a stable temperature which is evenly distributed to within ±1°C for incubators and within ±0.5°C for water baths.
   • The accuracy of temperature measurement should be four times greater than the requested accuracy; for example for a requested accuracy of ±2°C, the measurement accuracy should be ±0.5°C.

- Loading of incubators should ensure adequate air circulation. Plates, tubes and bottles should not be in contact with the sides of the incubator. Bottles, tubes and stacks of plates should not be in contact with one another and plates should not be stacked more than six high.

4.9 Laboratory accreditation

One of the essential criteria for many laboratories is accreditation by an external body to a recognized standard. This may be to an internationally recognized standard such as ISO 17025 [16] or to an industry-based standard. In order to achieve accreditation the laboratory must demonstrate that it is working to the requirements of a documented quality system. A key element of accreditation is the demonstration of full traceability of results, which is also a prerequisite for samples that are likely to proceed to legal action. Testing should only be undertaken by appropriately trained staff or under their direct supervision, and full training records are necessary. In order to demonstrate competency the laboratory will need to undertake a programme of internal quality assurance testing and participate in an external scheme for proficiency testing. Such a scheme is available from the PHLS.

Food external quality assurance (EQA) schemes run by the PHLS are:
- **The Standard Scheme** — suitable for European official laboratories and all other laboratories offering examination for pathogens and microbial enumerations.
- **The Extended Scheme** — suitable for public health and other laboratories offering a wide range of examinations.
- **The Shellfish Scheme** — suitable for laboratories offering examination of raw bivalve molluscs for end product testing or classification of shellfish harvesting beds.
- **The Dairy Scheme** — suitable for all laboratories offering examination of dairy products (pathogen-free option available).
- **The Non-Pathogen Scheme** — suitable for all laboratories offering tests for aerobic colony counts, indicator and spoilage organisms that prefer not to introduce pathogens onto their premises.
- **The Flexible Schedule** — suitable for laboratories that require a limited number of samples which may be chosen from more than one of the above EQA schemes.

Further information is available from: PHLS Food EQA Schemes, Food Safety Microbiology Laboratory, PHLS Central Public Health Laboratory, 61 Colindale Avenue, London NW9 5HT. Tel: 0208 200 4400; Fax: 0208 200 8264; E-mail: foodeqa@phls.nhs.uk.

4.10 References

1 Food Standards Agency. *Food Safety Act 1990. Code of Practice No. 7: Sampling for Analysis or Examination*. London: Food Standards Agency, 2000.

2   Local Authorities Coordinating Body on Food and Trading Standards (LACOTS). *Guidance on Food Sampling for Microbiological Examination*. London: LACOTS, 2002.

3   ISO 7218 (BS 5763 Part 0). Microbiology of Food and Animal Feeding Stuffs—General Rules for Microbiological Examinations. Geneva: International Organization for Standardization (ISO), 1996.

4   Great Britain. *Statutory Instrument No. 2463. The Food Safety (Sampling and Qualifications) Regulations 1990*. London: HMSO, 1990.

5   BS EN ISO 6887-1. Microbiology of Food and Animal Feeding Stuffs—Preparation of Test Samples, Initial Suspension and Decimal Dilutions for Microbiological Examination. Part 1: General Rules for the Preparation of the Initial Suspension and Decimal Dilutions. Geneva: International Organization for Standardization (ISO), 1999.

6   ISO/CD 6887-2. Part 2. Specific rules for the preparation of the initial suspension and decimal dilutions of meat and meat products. In preparation.

7   ISO/CD 6887-3. Part 3. Specific rules for the preparation of the initial suspension and decimal dilutions of fish products. In preparation.

8   ISO/CD 6887-4. Part 4. Specific rules for the preparation of the initial suspension and decimal dilutions of products other than milk and milk products, meat and meat products, fish products. . In preparation.

9   ISO 8261. Milk and Milk Products—Preparation of Test Samples and Dilutions for Microbiological Examination. Geneva: International Organization for Standardization (ISO), 2001.

10 Department of Health. *Guidelines for the Safe Production of Heat Preserved Foods*. London: HMSO, 1994.

11 Rees JAG, Bettison J, eds. *Processing and Packaging of Heat Preserved Foods*. London: Blackie and Son Ltd, 1990.

12 Footitt RJ, Lewis AS. *The Canning of Fish and Meat*. Glasgow: Blackie Academic and Professional, 1994.

13 ISO 13369. Microbiology of food and animal feeding-stuffs—Horizontal method for the determination of water activity. Geneva: International Organization for Standardization (ISO), 2000.

14 Troller JA, Scott VN. Measurement of water activity (a_w) and acidity. In: Vanderzant C, Splittstoesser DF, eds. *Compendium of Methods for the Microbiological Examination of Foods*, 3rd edn. Washington, D.C.: American Public Health Association, 1992.

15 Peterz MEG. Temperature in agar plates and its influence on the results of quantitative microbiological food analyses. *Int J Food Microbiol* 1991; **14**: 59–66.

16 ISO/IEC 17025. General Requirements for the Competence of Testing and Calibration Laboratories. Geneva: International Organization for Standardization (ISO), 1999.

5   Enumeration of microorganisms

Choice of method

A range of methods is available for the enumeration of microorganisms in food. The choice of method will depend on a number of factors.

- Type of sample.
- Characteristics, including the physiological state, of specific organisms sought.
- Characteristics of specific media.
- Lower limit of enumeration required.
- Purpose of the examination.
- Time available.

Legislation sometimes prescribes a specific counting method for the enumeration of microorganisms in a particular product, for example the pour plate method is specified in European Union (EU) milk legislation. For environmental samples such as surfaces, utensils and equipment a surface contact technique may be the most useful method to choose.

Any of a number of methods given in this section may be selected for enumeration of microorganisms in food. Whilst the pour plate method using plate count agar is regarded as the standard international method of enumeration for a total aerobic colony count, it is common for laboratories to use surface methods such as the surface drop and spiral plate. Apart from the obvious convenience of using pre-poured plates, these surface methods have the advantages that they eliminate possible heat stress to the organisms from the molten agar, provide fully aerobic conditions of growth and facilitate identification of the organism types present.

Pour plate methods require the use of a clear growth medium to allow counting of colonies that have grown below the surface of the medium. This also applies to counts performed by automated colony counters using transmitted light.

In most instances surface methods are preferable when selective media are used for enumeration of specific groups of organisms because they allow full manifestation of colonial properties such as morphology, pigmentation, haemolysis, haloes of precipitation around the colonies or changes in colour around the surrounding medium. However, some organisms with particular atmospheric requirements, such as anaerobes, may be best enumerated by a pour plate method where the depth of medium helps maintain an anaerobic environment.

The use of a liquid method such as a multiple tube method for enumeration of organisms that are highly stressed, due to drying or high salt content for example, may allow better recovery and growth of the target organism and thus result in a more accurate assessment of the level of the target organism in the food sample. Multiple tube methods are also useful for enumeration of low numbers of organisms (below 100/g) but are less suitable when high numbers are expected.

If an enumeration is performed in order to determine compliance with limits set in microbiological standards, guidelines or specifications the choice of enumeration method may also be affected by the required lower limit of detection. Pour plate methods, membrane filtration and multiple tube methods are capable of detecting lower counts than surface methods of enumeration because a larger quantity of the sample can be examined.

Where large numbers of similar samples are to be checked for a microbial load within a defined range, such as in production runs within a factory, increasing use is being made of sophisticated equipment that detects bacterial growth electronically by impedance or conductance within the growth medium. For any given product it is first necessary to produce a calibration curve for growth in a defined medium under carefully controlled test conditions. The advantage of such methods is that batch rejection can be triggered as soon as a predefined point on the calibration curve is reached and means that the samples with the highest bacterial count will be detected in the minimum period of time, sometimes within 6 h. These methods are not included in this manual because of the diversity of foods which most non-industrial laboratories are required to examine.

Factors affecting the results [1]

The successful performance of the pour plate technique depends heavily on adequate and appropriate tempering of the molten agar. Bottles of molten agar should be placed in a water bath set at 44–47°C. The length of time required for tempering to that temperature will depend on the volume of agar in each bottle and should be determined on an individual basis. The number of bottles placed in the water bath will also affect the rate of cooling. Extended storage of the molten agar will reduce the gelling properties. Molten agar should be used within 8 h of melting and preferably within 3 h, and should not be remelted once it has set. For some particularly sensitive media such as agars containing bile, the duration of holding in the molten state should not exceed 3 h. Even if adequate tempering of the molten agar has been ensured, heat stress of organisms may still occur, particularly in chilled and frozen foods.

Many of the organisms found in foods are obligate aerobes, for example some species of *Pseudomonas* and *Bacillus*. The relatively anaerobic conditions found in the depths of the agar in a pour plate may result in under-recovery of these organisms. Use of surface methods utilizing pre-poured plates will remove these variables and may result in a more accurate determination of the levels of these organisms. Pre-poured plates usually require some drying before use, so that the inoculum used in the test is absorbed within 15 min of application. Over-drying must be avoided as this can result in concentration of inhibitory components at the surface of the plate with subsequent inhibition of growth.

Inoculated plates should be placed in the incubator as soon as possible after the agar has set or the inoculum absorbed. International standards recommend that plates should be stacked no more than three high to ensure good heat penetration. This may be difficult to achieve in practice and studies have shown that plates stacked six high are not subject to significant variation in heat penetration [1].

At the end of the incubation period it is not always possible to perform the colony counting, for example due to lack of time or work of a higher priority. In most cases it is acceptable to refrigerate the plates until counting can be performed. ISO 7218 [2] permits refrigerated storage of plates for up to 24 h after the incubation period unless otherwise specified in the method. For media containing pH indicators such as violet red bile agars the plates must be allowed to regain ambient temperature before attempting to count the colonies to ensure accurate identification of suspect colonies.

It is good practice to monitor the microbial contamination of the laboratory environment, and this should be performed at regular intervals determined by the level of activity in the laboratory. Settle plates may be used to monitor the level of aerial environmental contamination in areas of sample processing by exposing the agar surface for a defined length of time, e.g. 15 min. The number of organisms are then counted after incubation. An action level should be established above which remedial action should be taken, for example thorough cleaning of the laboratory. Surface swabs may also be taken to monitor general levels of hygiene and to ensure the absence of pathogens.

Preparation of dilutions [3]

In order to enumerate fully the number of organisms in a food sample it may be necessary to prepare dilutions of the food homogenate. Commonly serial decimal dilutions in peptone saline solution (maximum recovery diluent, MRD) are prepared from the sample homogenate by adding 1 mL of sample homogenate to 9 mL of diluent etc. to the required endpoint. The accuracy of the volumes of diluent used should be ±2% and the accuracy of the sample volume dispensed should be ±5%. The use of automatic pipettors and associated sterile tips is advocated to help ensure accuracy when preparing dilutions. Precision of ±1% is achievable with automatic pipettors compared with ±5% with volumetric graduated pipettes. All automatic pipettors should be checked regularly to ensure that the desired volume is being delivered. For dispensing volumes of 0.1 mL or more, the pipettor should be used in total delivery mode, that is the plunger is depressed only to the first stop when drawing up the liquid, but fully depressed when discharging the liquid. If the volume to be dispensed is less than 0.1 mL, the reverse pipetting technique should be used whereby the plunger is fully depressed when aspirating the liquid but only depressed to the first stop when discharging. In all cases care must be taken to prevent jump back of the liquid inoculum that may result in contamination of the pipettor, as this may also result in contamination of the sample inocula; regular sanitizing of the pipettor is recommended.

If total delivery volumetric pipettes are used, correct delivery is ensured by touching the tip of the pipette on an inside wall of the container when emptying.

Quality control of media

Solid and liquid media used for the enumeration of microorganisms in foods should be subjected to quality control tests using reference cultures. Details of cultures for use in relation to media specific for particular organisms or groups of organisms are given in Section 6. The organisms listed in Table 5.1 are recommended for testing media used for enumeration of 'total' microbial content and other non-selective procedures.

Table 5.1 Control organisms for testing enumeration and non-selective media.

Control strain		Media for control
NCTC 6571	Staphylococcus aureus	Blood agar base, tryptone soya
NCTC 662	Lactococcus lactis	agar, tryptone soya broth
NCTC 662	Lactococcus lactis	
NCTC 775	Enterococcus faecalis	Plate count agar, yeast extract agar, milk plate count agar
NCTC 10418/9001	Escherichia coli	
NCTC 662	Lactococcus lactis	
NCTC 10418/9001	Escherichia coli	Nutrient agar
NCTC 10418/9001	Escherichia coli	
NCTC 11994	Listeria monocytogenes	Dilution fluid, e.g. MRD
NCTC 662	Lactococcus lactis	
NCTC 4840	Salmonella poona	
NCTC 11994	Listeria monocytogenes	Buffered peptone water

MRD, maximum recovery diluent; NCTC, National Collection of Type Cultures.

Uncertainty of measurement [4]

Uncertainty of measurement is a quantity associated with the result of a test measurement that characterizes the dispersion of values that could reasonably be attributed to that measurement (such as a count per g). Each laboratory should evaluate the uncertainty associated with test methods used by that laboratory.

- The *standard uncertainty* of a test method is defined as one standard deviation.
- The *combined standard uncertainty* is the result of the combination of all the standard uncertainty components associated with that test method.
- The *expanded uncertainty* is obtained by multiplying the combined standard uncertainty by a coverage factor (see below).
- *Type A evaluations of uncertainty* are done by calculations from a series of re-peated observations, using statistical methods.
- *Type B evaluations of uncertainty* are derived from other sources, e.g. calibration data.

Likely sources of uncertainty are shown in Table 5.2.

In microbiological testing the greatest sources of uncertainty arise from sampling and the non-homogeneous distribution of microorganisms in the sample. In order to evaluate uncertainty it has to be assumed that the organisms are distributed randomly. When performing a microbiological test, type B un-certainties usually form part of a type A evaluation and so may not need to be considered separately. In addition, they usually represent such a small contribu-

Table 5.2 Factors contributing to uncertainty of measurement in microbiology.

Sample stability
Representative nature of subsampling in the laboratory
Uncertainty associated with weighing balance
Uncertainty associated with diluting equipment (dispensers, pipettors)
Uncertainty associated with inoculum volume (pipettes, pipettors)
Integrity of filtration membrane (quality, pore size)
Uncertainty of temperature measurement (thermometers)
Stability of incubation conditions
Penetration of heat during incubation
Achievement of designated incubation duration
Performance of the isolation medium (yield)
Uncertainty associated with counting:
   particle statistical variation
   crowding effect
   between operator variation
   accuracy of colony counter
   personal interpretation of the target
Uncertainty associated with confirmatory tests:
   number of colonies selected

tion to the combined standard uncertainty that they do not make a significant contribution. Thus for microbiological testing purposes, the type A evaluation is the dominant component and is not significantly different from the standard uncertainty. Generally, the type B components can therefore be ignored for microbiological tests.

Duplicate results from tests performed by different operators as part of internal or external quality control samples can be used to calculate uncertainty of measurement using the analysis of variance to obtain the repeatability standard deviation. This is equivalent to the standard uncertainty. In order to obtain a level of confidence of approximately 95% the standard uncertainty (standard deviation) is multiplied by a coverage factor of two. The value obtained is known as the expanded uncertainty of the test.

This analysis should be repeated on a regular basis to maintain an estimate that is relevant to the laboratory in its current situation. Results from all staff should be included, to provide a result for the laboratory as a whole.

Interpretation of counts [4]

If a numerical limit is specified in a standard, guideline or specification and a statement of compliance is required but no reference is made to taking uncertainty into account, the following approach is recommended [4].

- Expand the count obtained in the test by the uncertainty interval at a level of confidence of 95% before comparison with the numerical standard. For microbiological tests, maximum values are usually specified.
- Compliance is achieved if the standard lies above the upper limit of the uncertainty interval.
- If the standard is exceeded even when the measured count is decreased by half the uncertainty interval, a statement of non-compliance can be made.
- If the lower limit of the uncertainty interval does not exceed the standard it is not possible to confirm compliance or non-compliance. The test result and expanded uncertainty should be reported together with a statement that compliance was not demonstrated.

EXAMPLE

The uncertainty for a test at a 95% confidence level is ±0.21 (expressed as a logarithmic value).
The standard to be met is 1.0×10^5/g (or $\log_{10} 5.0000$).
The measured count for the test is 1.3×10^5/g (or $\log_{10} 5.1139$).
The measured count expanded by the uncertainty is:

$\log_{10} 4.9039 - \log_{10} 5.3239$ or $8.0 \times 10^4 - 2.1 \times 10^5$.

Because the measured count lowered by half the uncertainty interval (8.0×10^4) is less than the standard it is not possible to confirm compliance or non-compliance.

ENUMERATION METHODS

5.1 | Dip slide culture

Dip slides may be used for estimating numbers of bacteria in liquid food products and in food homogenates prepared as described in Section 4.2. The use of dip slides for surface contact methods is described in method 3 of Section 5.8. There is a wide choice of dip slides available and the selection of a particular type will depend on the following:

- The organism or group of organisms sought (and therefore the agar medium used).
- The potential use of the dip slide (the same medium or different media can be used to coat the two sides of the slide).
- The surface area of the slide.
- The availability and storage life.
- Cost.

Procedure

(a) Remove the dip slide from its container and immerse the agar-covered area in the sample.

(b) Remove the dip slide and drain.

(c) Replace the dip slide in its container and incubate as appropriate for the organisms sought (see Section 6 for guidance).

After incubation

Estimate the number of microorganisms/mL of sample from diagrams supplied by the manufacturer of the slide or count the number of colonies on each side of the slide.

Calculation

For watery liquids only:

$$\frac{\text{Total colonies on slide}}{\text{Agar surface area (cm}^2)} \times 1000 = \text{colony forming units (cfu)/mL}.$$

Calibration is necessary for other types of liquids, e.g. oil–water emulsions, milk or milk products.

5.2 | Membrane filtration [5]

This method is suitable for water, beverages and liquid food products. Any measured volume of sample that is compatible with the equipment available may be used, so this method is particularly useful for examining larger sample sizes such as 100 mL or 1 L. If the sample is likely to contain high numbers of organisms, the use of a small volume or preparation of serial decimal dilutions is recommended.

Procedure

(a) Filter a measured volume of the sample or dilution using sterile membrane filtration equipment and a membrane with pore size 0.45 μm. For sample volumes of less than 10 mL, aseptically pour 20 mL of sterile diluent into the filtration funnel before addition of the measured volume of sample. Vacuum filtration is recommended.

(b) After filtration, remove the filter membrane with sterile forceps and place it on a culture pad previously soaked in appropriate culture medium or on the surface of a suitable agar medium (see Section 6 for guidance).

(c) Incubate the culture pad or agar plus filter membrane as appropriate for the organisms sought (see Section 6 for guidance).

After incubation

Count the number of colonies on the membrane and relate the number of colonies to the volume (and dilution) of sample filtered to obtain a count per mL.

5.3   Pour plate [6]

This method is suitable for liquid food products or food homogenates. Serial decimal dilutions of the sample should be made using peptone saline solution (MRD) as diluent. As a guide, with 'clean' products dilution to 10^{-3} may be sufficient whereas heavily contaminated products may require dilution to 10^{-6}.

Procedure

(a) Place 1 mL of the dilution into each of two sterile Petri dishes.

(b) Add about 15 mL of molten clear agar, tempered to 44–47°C, to each plate (e.g. plate count agar for a total colony count).

(c) Mix each plate well by moving it five times in a vertical, clockwise, horizontal and anticlockwise direction as shown, then allow the plates to set.

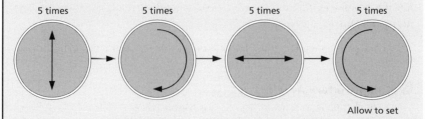

| 5 times | 5 times | 5 times | 5 times |

Allow to set

(d) Incubate all plates as appropriate for the organisms sought (see Section 6 for guidance). For a total mesophilic aerobic colony count using plate count agar, incubate for 72±3 h at 30°C.

continued

Calculation

Use the plates containing fewer than 300 colonies at two consecutive dilutions to calculate the results from a weighted mean. The number (N) of cfu/g or mL of test sample is calculated as follows:

$$N = C/v \, (n_1 + 0.1\,n_2)\, d$$

where: C is the sum of colonies on all plates counted
v is the volume applied to each plate
n_1 is the number of plates counted at the first dilution
n_2 is the number of plates counted at the second dilution
d is the dilution from which the first count was obtained.

Round the result to two significant figures and express it as a number between 1.0 and 9.9 multiplied by 10^x where x is the appropriate power of 10.

EXAMPLE

Number of colonies at first dilution (10^{-3}) = 171 and 194.
Number of colonies at second dilution (10^{-4}) = 14 and 20.
Volume added to each plate = 1 mL.

$$N = (171 + 194 + 14 + 20)/1 \times (2 + [0.1 \times 2]) \times 10^{-3}$$
$$= 399/0.0022 = 181\,363.$$

When rounded to two significant figures this becomes 180 000 or 1.8×10^5 cfu/g or mL.

Note: all counts from plates of the selected dilutions should be used, including any plate with no colonies if the corresponding plate at that dilution contains colonies, unless the count exceeds 300 or is overgrown.

If a differential or selective medium (such as violet red bile glucose agar [VRBGA]) is used for the pour plate method, plates containing no more than 150 colonies should be selected for counting.

If plates at only one dilution contain countable colonies, calculate the count using the formula $N = C/2 \, v \, d$.

If only one plate contains countable colonies, calculate the count using the formula $N = C/v \, d$.

Confidence intervals

In certain circumstances, plates with colony counts falling within the count limits expanded by the 95% confidence interval (CI) may be used for counting (Tables 5.3 and 5.4).

continued

Table 5.3 Enumeration of total colony count (e.g. aerobic plate count) using non-selective medium.

Count

First dilution (d_1)	Second dilution (d_2)	Expression
$n \geq 15$ and ≤ 300	Any	Weighted mean
$n \geq 15$ and ≤ 300	None	Arithmetic mean
$n < 15$	None	Arithmetic mean
$n = 0$	None	Less than $1/d_1$
$n > 300$ and ≤ 324	~<15	Weighted mean
$n > 324$	$n \geq 10$	Arithmetic mean d_2
$n > 324$	$n < 10$	Not acceptable
$n > 300$	$n > 300$	More than $300 \times 1/d_2$
$n > 300$	$n < 300$	Arithmetic mean d_2

d, dilution (10^{-1}, 10^{-2}, etc.); n, total number of colonies.

Table 5.4 Enumeration of characteristic colonies on selective media.

Count

First dilution (d_1)	Second dilution (d_2)	Expression
$n \geq 15$ and ≤ 150 with cc	Any with cc	Weighted mean
$n \geq 15$ and ≤ 150 with cc	No cc	Arithmetic mean d_1
$n < 15$ with cc	No cc	Arithmetic mean d_1
$n = 0$	No cc	Less than $1/d_1$
$n \geq 150$ with cc	$n \leq 150$ no cc	Less than $1/d_2$ and more than $1/d_1$
$n \geq 150$ no cc	$n \leq 150$ no cc	Less than $1/d_1$
$n > 150$ and ≤ 167 with cc	$n < 15$ with cc	Weighted mean
$n > 167$ with cc	$n < 15$ with cc	Arithmetic mean d_2
$n > 150$ with cc	$n > 150$ with cc	More than $150 \times 1/d_2$
$n > 150$ with cc	$n \leq 150$ with cc	Arithmetic mean d_2

cc, characteristic colonies; d, dilution (10^{-1}, 10^{-2}, etc.); n, total number of colonies.

For a 95% probability, the CI can be calculated from the following equation:

$$CI = [C/B + 1.92/B \pm 1.96 \sqrt{C/B}]\,1/d$$

where $B = v(n_1 + 0.1n_2)$.

The limits of the CI can then be expressed as a percentage. An example of this is shown below for the extreme counts of 15 and 300.

continued

No. colonies counted			
Dilution d	Dilution $d+1$	Weighted mean	CI
300	30		278–324
300	30	300	From −7% to +8%
15	1		10–20
15	1	14	From −29% to +43%

The CI for counts derived from plates containing less than 15 colonies at the lowest dilution are wide. Values may be found in tables contained in ISO 7218 [2]. For example, for a microorganism count of 10 derived from two Petri dishes, for a 95%CI the range is 6–15, the per cent error for the lower limit is −39% and for the upper limit is +54%. If only one plate is used, the range is 5–18 with per cent errors of −52% and +84%. Plates containing less than 10 colonies that are not part of a weighted mean count should only be used if they contain the lowest dilution used.

Full details of rules for counts by the pour plate method outlined above can be found in ISO 4833 [6].

5.4 Spiral plate

This method is suitable for liquid food products or food homogenates, but it is necessary to allow all food particles to settle before proceeding with the test. The spiral plater is a dispenser which distributes a set volume of liquid on to the surface of a rotating agar plate. The dispensing arm moves from near the centre of the plate towards the outside edge, depositing the sample in an Archimedes' spiral. A cam-activated syringe dispenses a continually decreasing volume of sample, resulting in a concentration range of up to $10\,000:1$ on a single plate. The volume of sample on any particular segment of a plate is known and is constant.

Procedure
(a) Prepare a clear agar plate with a flat surface (e.g. plate count agar, lysed blood agar). Always use plates with the same volume of agar.
(b) If required dilute the sample or food homogenate prepared as described in Section 4.2 and allow particles to settle to avoid blockage of the stylus.

continued

(c) Disinfect the dispensing stylus of the spiral plater with 2–5% sodium hypochlorite solution and rinse with sterile distilled water.

(d) Take up the liquid in the dispensing stylus and distribute the set volume (usually 0.05 mL but may be up to 0.4 mL) on to the agar plate located on the rotating table of the apparatus.

(e) Incubate the agar plate as appropriate for the organisms sought (see Section 6 for guidance). For a mesophilic aerobic colony count, incubation is normally carried out at 30°C for 48±2 h.

(f) Repeat step (c) after each sample or between each dilution if higher than the previous dilution.

After incubation

Count the colonies on the agar plate. This can be done manually with a viewing grid or with a laser colony counter or other automated counter/image analyser. For manual counting, select any segment and count the colonies from the outer edge into the centre until 20 colonies have been counted; continue to count the remaining colonies in the subdivision of the segment containing the 20th colony. Record this count together with the number assigned to the subdivision of the segment. Count the colonies in the same area on the opposite side of the plate and record the count. Add the counts together to obtain the number of colonies in that designated subdivision. If the whole plate contains fewer than 160 colonies count the colonies on the whole plate.

Calculation

To calculate the count, divide the total count obtained by the volume constant for the subdivision counted, then multiply by the appropriate dilution factor. Alternatively, use the tables supplied by the manufacturer. If a 0.05-mL volume has been used the countable range of cfu/mL of test dilution is $20–10^5$.

5.5 Surface drop [7]

This method is suitable for liquid food products or food homogenates. Serial decimal dilutions should be made using MRD as diluent. As a guide, with clean products dilutions to 10^{-3} may be sufficient whereas heavily contaminated products may require dilution to 10^{-6} or higher.

Procedure

(a) Start with the highest dilution of the sample (e.g. 10^{-6}).

(b) Mix well, preferably using a vortex mixer.

(c) Using the reverse pipetting technique, draw up a known volume of the liquid, e.g. 20 μL using an automatic pipettor and sterile tip.

(d) Dispense the aspirated volume as a drop onto one sector of at least two agar plates (e.g. plate count agar).

continued

(e) Repeat steps (b)–(d) for the remaining dilutions to produce two or more sectored plates. The number of sectors will equal the number of dilutions, to a maximum of six sectors per plate.

(f) Incubate the plates as appropriate to the organisms sought (see Section 6 for guidance).

After incubation

Count the colonies on all sectors containing 30 or fewer colonies per drop.

Calculation

Determine the mean number of colonies per drop for the dilutions counted, C/x. Calculate the number of cfu/g or mL of sample (N) as follows:

$$N = C/x \ v \ d$$

where: C is the sum of the colonies

d is the sample dilution used

x is the number of drops used at that dilution

v is the volume of sample dilution used per drop.

If there are countable colonies at more than one dilution, use a weighted mean, i.e. $N = C/x \ (1.1 \ v) \ d$, where d is the dilution from which the first counts were obtained.

5.6 Surface spread plate [7]

This method is suitable for liquid food products or food homogenates. Serial decimal dilutions should be made using MRD as diluent. As a guide, with 'clean' products dilutions to 10^{-3} may be sufficient whereas heavily contaminated products may require dilution to 10^{-6}.

Procedure

(a) Prepare at least two agar plates (e.g. plate count agar) for each dilution to be tested.

(b) Starting with the highest dilution, use an automatic pipettor and sterile disposable tip to transfer 0.1 mL of each test dilution to the surface of the appropriately labelled dried agar plates.

> If greater sensitivity is required, a volume of up to 0.5 mL of the 10^{-1} homogenate may be applied to the agar plates, giving a lower detection limit of 10 cfu/g or mL.

(c) Spread the inoculum evenly over the entire surface of the plates using a sterile bent spreader (glass or plastic). Avoid touching the sides of the plate.

continued

(d) Incubate all plates as appropriate for the organisms sought (see Section 6 for guidance). For a total mesophilic aerobic colony count, incubation is normally performed at $30\pm1°C$ for 48 ± 2 h or 72 ± 3 h.

After incubation

Count all colonies on plates containing 300 or fewer colonies per plate or, if the medium is selective, 150 colonies or fewer per plate.

Calculation

Use the plates containing not more than 300 colonies (or 150 for selective media) at two consecutive dilutions to calculate the results. Calculate the number (N) of cfu/g or mL of test sample as follows:

$$N = C/v\,(n_1 + 0.1n_2)\,d.$$

For the key to symbols and an example of calculation see Section 5.3. In this instance, the volume added per plate, v, is 0.1 mL (or 0.5 mL).

5.7 Multiple tube (most probable number) methods

Multiple tube methods, also known as most probable number (MPN) methods, are suitable for liquid food products or food homogenates. The methods are based on the probability of finding bacterial growth after culture of successive dilutions of the food sample in a liquid medium. They are used for enumeration of specific organisms or groups of organisms such as *Escherichia coli* and coliforms, and not for 'total' microbial counts on a product. The most commonly used procedures are based on the use of three serial decimal dilutions of the sample (methods 3 and 4) using three or five aliquots of each dilution; further dilutions can be made if necessary. The degree of dilution necessary and the number of tubes at each dilution used depends on the initial bacterial load. For a sample that is unlikely to contain many organisms to be counted, culture of 6×18 mL aliquots of a single dilution (method 1) would give a counting range of 1–10 organisms/100 mL of the dilution used. For a wider count range, 10×1 mL aliquots of a single dilution will allow counting of 10–230 organisms/100 mL of the dilution used (method 2). Higher number of organisms can be counted and greater accuracy achieved with the methods utilizing three serial dilutions.

Method 1 Six tube (six by 18 mL or 18 g) test

Procedure

(a) If the sample is liquid, add 18 mL volumes to each of six 180 mL volumes of the chosen liquid medium (e.g. buffered peptone water (BPW) or selective enrichment medium). If the sample is solid, prepare six homogenates using 18 g of sample with 180 mL of chosen liquid medium.

continued

(b) Incubate overnight at the temperature appropriate for the organism sought (see Section 6 for guidance).

After incubation

Test all six tubes for the characteristic reactions of the organisms sought by subculture from each tube to a suitable selective agar or liquid medium. If the medium used has no characteristic reactions, subculture all the tubes. Incubate the plates or broths and record the number of tubes that contain the target bacteria. Obtain the MPN of bacteria/g or mL of the food sample from Table 5.5, taking into account any dilution factor of the original sample.

Table 5.5 Most probable number (MPN)/100 mL or 100 g using six 18 mL or 18 g aliquots.

Number positive	MPN/100 mL or 100 g
1	1
2	2
3	4
4	6
5	10
6	>10

Method 2 Ten tube (10 by 1 mL or 1 g) test

Procedure

(a) For liquid samples add 1 mL volumes to 10 tubes of chosen liquid medium (e.g. buffered peptone water or selective enrichment medium). For solid samples add 10 mL of the 10^{-1} homogenate (equivalent to 1 g) to either 10 mL of double strength medium or 90 mL of single strength medium.

(b) Incubate overnight at the temperature appropriate for the organism sought (see Section 6 for guidance).

After incubation

Test all 10 tubes for the characteristic reactions of the organisms sought by subculture from each tube to a suitable selective agar or liquid medium. If the medium has no characteristic reactions subculture all tubes. Incubate the plates or broths and record the number of original tubes that contain the target bacteria. Obtain the MPN of bacteria/g or mL of the food sample from Table 5.6.

Table 5.6 Most probable number (MPN)/100 mL or 100 g using 10×1 mL or 1 g aliquots.

Number positive	MPN/100 mL or 100 g	95% confidence limits
0	0	<0–37
1	10	0.25–59
2	22	3–81
3	36	7–106
4	51	13–134
5	69	21–168
6	92	30–211
7	120	43–270
8	160	59–368
9	230	81–600
10	>230	118–>600

Method 3 Nine tube (3,3,3 tube) test [8,9]

Procedure
(a) Make serial decimal dilutions of the liquid food sample, or 10^{-1} food homogenate prepared as described in Section 4.3, using MRD as diluent.
(b) Prepare nine tubes, each containing 10 mL of single strength growth medium appropriate for the organisms sought (e.g. BPW or a selective enrichment broth).
(c) Add 1 mL of the liquid food sample or food homogenate to each of three tubes containing growth medium.
(d) Repeat step (c) for each of two subsequent decimal dilutions.
(e) Incubate all nine tubes as appropriate for the organisms sought (see Section 6 for guidance).

> If greater sensitivity is required, also prepare three tubes containing 10 mL of double strength medium and add 10 mL of liquid sample or 10^{-1} food homogenate to each tube. If high numbers of target organisms are expected, prepare three tubes of single strength growth medium for each additional decimal dilution to be used and inoculate each of them with 1 mL of the additional dilution.

After incubation
Test those tubes showing the characteristic reactions of the organisms sought by subculture from each tube to a suitable confirmatory agar or liquid medium. If the medium has no characteristic reactions subculture all the tubes. Incubate the plates or broths and record the number of original tubes at each dilution that contain the target bacteria.

Selection of dilutions [2,8,9]
Select three consecutive dilutions to obtain the MPN of bacteria/g or mL of the food sample from Table 5.7. Select the highest dilution (i.e. that having the lowest sample

continued on p. 122

Table 5.7 Most probable number (MPN): three tubes at each dilution.

10⁻¹	10⁻²	10⁻³	MPN/g or mL	Category when the number of tests is 1	95%CI
0	0	0	<3		0.0–9.4
0	0	1	3	3	0.1–9.5
0	1	0	3	2	0.1–10.0
0	1	1	6	0	1.2–17.0
0	2	0	6	3	1.2–17.0
0	3	0	9	0	3.5–35.0
1	0	0	4	1	0.2–17.0
1	0	1	7	2	1.2–17.0
1	0	2	11	0	4.0–35.0
1	1	0	7	1	1.2–20.0
1	1	1	11	3	4.0–35.0
1	2	0	11	2	4.0–35.0
1	2	1	15	3	5.0–38.0
1	3	0	16	3	5.0–38.0
2	0	0	9	1	1.5–35.0
2	0	1	14	2	4.0–35.0
2	0	2	20	0	5.0–38.0
2	1	0	15	1	4.0–38.0
2	1	1	20	2	5.0–38.0
2	1	2	27	0	9.0–94.0
2	2	0	21	1	5.0–40.0
2	2	1	28	3	9.0–94.0
2	2	2	35	0	9.0–94.0
2	3	0	29	3	9.0–94.0
2	3	1	36	0	9.0–94.0
3	0	0	23	1	5.0–94.0
3	0	1	38	1	9.0–104.0
3	0	2	64	3	16.0–181.0
3	1	0	43	1	9.0–181.0
3	1	1	75	1	17.0–199.0
3	1	2	120	3	30.0–360.0
3	1	3	160	0	30.0–380.0
3	2	0	93	1	18.0–360.0
3	2	1	150	1	30.0–380.0
3	2	2	210	2	30.0–400.0
3	2	3	290	3	90.0–990.0
3	3	0	240	1	40.0–990.0
3	3	1	460	1	90.0–1980.0
3	3	2	1100	1	200.0–4000.0
3	3	3	>1100		

Adapted from ISO 7218 [2]. 95%CI, 95% confidence interval.

concentration) yielding three positive tubes together with the next two dilutions. If this is not possible because insufficient dilutions were made beyond the highest dilution yielding three positive tubes, select instead the three highest dilutions. If no dilution contains three positive tubes, select the three highest dilutions in the series amongst which at least one positive result was obtained.

Table 5.7 shows the MPN counts/g or mL obtained when the sample homogenate and two further decimal dilutions are used to inoculate the three sets of tubes. If a liquid sample and its 10^{-1} and 10^{-2} dilutions have been used the MPN value must be multiplied by 10 to obtain the MPN count/mL. This must also be done to obtain the MPN count/g if 10 mL volumes of the sample homogenate are inoculated into double strength medium in the first set of tubes. The MPN/g or mL can be obtained with any set of three dilutions by using the formula:

MPN/g = MPN from Table 5.7 × j/100

where j is the dilution of the middle set of tubes.

The presence of inhibitory substances in the sample may prevent typical reactions taking place in tubes containing the lowest dilution of food or the greatest volume of liquid sample. If this is anticipated the dilution series should be extended. If, however, this is not done, the following examples indicate how to derive the MPN.

EXAMPLES

(a) If the reading is 0,3,1 tubes positive, it is reasonable to assume that the first set of tubes should have been positive.
Adjusted reading = 3,3,1
From Table 5.7, MPN/g = 460
(b) If the reading is 0,3,1 tubes positive, the dilution series might be theoretically extended so that the tubes may be read 0,3,1,0. Use the last three figures to obtain the MPN value, then multiply by 10 to compensate for the further decimal dilution.
Reading = 3,1,0
From Table 5.7, MPN value = 43
MPN/g (MPN value × 10) = 430.

Note: as with other counts, MPN counts should be reported to two significant figures with one figure before and one figure after the decimal point multiplied by the appropriate power of 10.

Interpretation of the probability tables

Wide variations in the results may occur with the MPN technique. Readings at each dilution may vary by one or two tubes, even in tests made separately on the same well-mixed sample. In addition to the MPN value, Table 5.7 shows the category of result and the range defined by 95% confidence limits (95%CI). The category indicates the acceptability of the combination of positive results. Category 1 results are those that have the highest probability of being correct. If combinations belonging to category 1 are obtained they should be used in preference to category 2, and so on. If more than one combination of the same category is obtained the combination with the highest number of positive tubes should be used. When the decision to be taken on the basis of the result is of great importance, only category 1 or at most category 1 and 2 results should be accepted. Category 0 results should be viewed with great suspicion as there is only a 0.1% chance of obtaining a result in this category without anything being wrong. For further information, consult the appropriate ISO standards.

Method 4 Fifteen tube (5,5,5 tube) test [8]

For greater accuracy, a 3×5 tube method can be used, giving a total of 15 tubes incubated. The procedure is the same as described for method 3. The MPN/100 g can be derived from Table 9.2–9.4, pp. 233–7, which gives category 1 and category 2 values for a 15 tube test.

5.8 Surface contact methods

The procedures available in this category are:
- Agar sausage.
- Surface contact plate.
- Dip slide.

The type of medium depends on the organisms sought.

Method 1 Agar sausage

Procedure
(a) Cut one end of an agar sausage and squeeze the agar a little way out of its protective wrapping.
(b) Press the open cut end of the sausage evenly against the test surface.
(c) Cut off a thin slice of the agar sausage and place this, test side face upwards, in a Petri dish.
(d) Replace the lid of the Petri dish and incubate the test slice as appropriate for the organisms sought.
(e) Proceed as for method 3 (p. 124) after incubation.

Method 2 Surface contact plate

Procedure

(a) Remove the lid from a surface contact agar plate and press the surface of the agar evenly against the test surface.

(b) Replace the lid on the plate and incubate as appropriate for the organisms sought.

(c) Proceed as for method 3 (below) after incubation.

Method 3 Dip slide

Procedure

(a) Remove the dip slide from its container and, if necessary, detach the slide from the cap of the container.

(b) Press the agar surface evenly against the test surface.

(c) Reattach the slide to the cap of the container if necessary; return the slide to its container.

(d) Incubate as appropriate for the organisms sought.

After incubation

Count the number of colonies on the agar sausage slice, the central $4\,cm^2$ of the contact plate, or the dip slide.

Calculation

Calculate the number of cfu/cm^2 of surface (N) from the formula:

$$N = C/A$$

where: C is the colony count

A is the area samples (in cm^2).

For the surface contact plate method $A = 4\,cm^2$.

5.9   Surface swabs

This is a procedure for surface swabbing of a known area delineated by a template. The organisms picked up by the swab are recovered in a known volume of fluid and a bacterial count made on the fluid. From this the number of organisms present on the area swabbed can be computed and the count per cm^2 of swabbed area then calculated. If it is likely that sanitizers have been used on the surface, the suspending fluid should contain appropriate neutralizers.

Template

The aluminium template to delineate the test area (e.g. 25 cm^2) is made from thin aluminium sheeting (Fig. 5.1a). Wrap and sterilize the template before use. Alternatively, irradiated wrapped plastic templates are available commercially.

continued

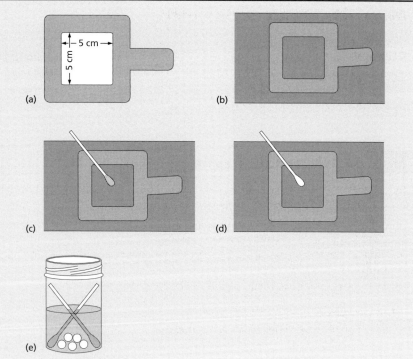

Fig. 5.1 Surface swabs.

Diluent

Neutralizer solution—MRD containing lecithin 3 g/L, polysorbate 80 30 g/L, sodium thiosulphate 5 g/L, L-histidine 1 g/L [10].

Procedure

(a) Hold a sterile template firmly over the surface to delineate the area to be sampled (Fig. 5.1b).

(b) Dip a cotton wool swab into a 10-mL volume of neutralizer solution contained in a small screw-capped bottle with five small glass beads (e.g. 3 mm diameter). Squeeze out the excess fluid against an inner surface of the bottle, and rub the moistened swab thoroughly over the entire test area, turning the swab in order to maximize its ability to pick up organisms (Fig. 5.1c).

(c) Break off the cotton wool end of this swab into the 10 mL neutralizer solution.

(d) Take a second dry cotton wool swab and rub it thoroughly over the entire test area turning as before (Fig. 5.1d).

(e) Break off the end of this swab into the same 10 mL neutralizer solution.

(f) Shake the diluent bottle containing the swabs and beads until the cotton wool has been broken down into fibres (Fig. 5.1e).

(g) Use one of the methods in Sections 5.1–5.7 to count the organisms in suspension.

continued

5.10 Membrane slide cultures

This is a procedure for surface testing using a commercially available kit consisting of a swab in sterile buffer and a sampler consisting of a plastic tab supporting a gridded filter membrane bonded to an absorbent pad containing dehydrated culture medium (Fig. 5.2).*

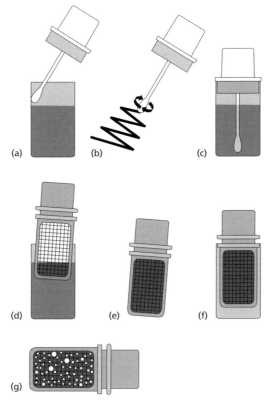

Fig. 5.2 Membrane slide cultures.

*This type of kit can be obtained from Millipore (UK) Ltd, Millipore House, Abbey Road, London NW10 7SP. http://www.millipore.com.

Procedure

(a) Remove the swab from its container and roll the tip against the inner surface of the container to remove excess buffer solution (Fig. 5.2a).

(b) Swab the test surface by rotating the swab while moving it over a defined area (e.g. 10×10 cm) (Fig. 5.2b).

(c) Replace the swab into its container, which contains 18 mL buffer solution (Fig. 5.2c). Seal the container and shake well (at least 30 times). Remove and discard the swab.

(d) Take the sampler from its container and insert it in the test buffer solution from which the swab was removed. Leave for 30 s (Fig. 5.2d,e).

(e) Remove the sampler, allow it to drain and replace it in its original container (Fig. 5.2f).

(f) Incubate the sampler in its container as appropriate for the organisms sought.

After incubation

Count the colonies on the gridded membrane of the sampler (Fig. 5.2g), or compare with the chart supplied with the kit. The sampler absorbs 1 mL of buffer solution; therefore multiply the colony count by 18 to obtain the number of cfu/area sampled.

5.11 Rinse method for watercress, other leaf vegetables and acidic berry fruits [11,12]

The use of a rinse method is suitable for leaf vegetables and may enhance recovery of target organisms from acidic fruits such as berries.

Procedure

(a) Place 100 g of watercress, other leaf vegetables or berry fruit in a large sterile container with a screw cap or other airtight closure and add 200 mL of MRD. Secure the lid.

(b) Shake the container well for 15–30 s so that the diluent wets all the vegetable/fruit surfaces. Leave to stand for 30 min.

(c) Shake well again for 10–15 s.

(d) Examine the rinse fluid for the target organism or group of organisms using an appropriate medium (see Section 6). If counts are expected to be low use membrane filtration or a multiple tube method for enumeration. If counts are likely to be high ($>10^3$/g) a surface plating or pour plating technique can be used.

Calculation

Compute the count per mL of rinse fluid. Multiply this value by two to obtain the count/g of sample.

5.12 Bottle rinse and plate count

This method is most commonly used for determining the effectiveness of milk bottle washing [13]. It may also be used for single use bottles, in which case a neutralizer is not needed in the diluent.

Procedure

(a) Set aside six washed and capped (or stoppered) bottles for testing.

(b) Add 20 mL of MRD (or quarter strength Ringer's solution) containing 0.05% sodium thiosulphate to each bottle and recap.

(c) Thoroughly wet the surfaces of all bottles by rotating gently 12 times in one direction. Allow the bottles to stand for 15–30 min.

(d) Again rotate each bottle gently 12 times in the same direction so that the whole internal bottle surface is thoroughly wetted.

(e) Place 5 mL of the rinse fluid from each bottle into a separate Petri dish.

(f) To each dish add 20 mL of molten milk plate count agar tempered to 44–47°C. Include one plate containing agar only and another plate containing rinsing fluid and agar to act as media sterility controls.

(g) Mix each plate five times in a vertical, clockwise, horizontal and anticlockwise direction (as shown on p. 112), then allow to set.

(h) Incubate the plates at 30°C for 72±3 h.

Calculation

Multiply the colony count in each plate by four to obtain the total colony count per bottle. Add the counts together and divide by six to obtain a mean count per bottle.

If any individual bottle count is more than 25 times greater than the next highest count in the series, it should be omitted from the mean bottle count and a note made to that effect.

> As a general rule, the colony count per bottle should not exceed 1 cfu/mL capacity of the bottle. For 1 pint milk bottles, counts below 200 are considered satisfactory and counts above 600 are considered unsatisfactory.

5.13   References

1 Peterz MEG. Temperature in agar plates and its influence on the results of quantitative microbiological food analyses. *Int J Food Microbiol* 1991; **14**: 59–66.

2 ISO 7218 (BS 5763 Part 0). *Microbiology of Food and Animal Feeding Stuffs—General Rules for Microbiological Examinations*. Geneva: International Organization for Standardization (ISO), 1996; incorporating amendment 1, 2001.

3 ISO 6887-1. *Microbiology of Food and Animal Feeding Stuffs—Preparation of Test Samples, Initial Suspension and Decimal Dilutions for Microbiological Examination. Part 1: General Rules for the Preparation of the Initial Suspension and Decimal Dilutions*. Geneva: International Organization for Standardization (ISO), 1999.

4 LAB 12. *The Expression of Uncertainty in Testing*. Feltham, Middlesex: United Kingdom Accreditation Service, 2000.

5 Standing Committee of Analysts. *Methods for the Examination of Waters and Associated Materials. The Microbiology of Drinking Water (2002)—Part I—Water Quality and Public Health*. Environment Agency, 2002.

6 ISO 4833 (BS 5763 Part 1). *Microbiology—General Guidance for the Enumeration of Microorganisms—Colony Count Technique at 30°C*. Geneva: International Organization for Standardization (ISO), 1991.

7   International Commission on Microbiological Specifications for Foods. *Microorganisms in Foods. 1 Their Significance and Methods of Enumeration*, 2nd edn. London: University of Toronto Press, 1978.

8   ISO 4831 (BS 5763 Part 3). *Microbiology—General Guidance for the Enumeration of Coliforms—Most Probable Number Technique*. Geneva: International Organization for Standardization (ISO), 1991.

9   ISO 7251 (BS 5763 Part 8). *Microbiology—General Guidance for the Enumeration of Presumptive Escherichia coli—Most Probable Number Technique*. Geneva: International Organization for Standardization (ISO), 1993.

10 CCFRA. *Guideline No. 20. Effective Microbiological Sampling of Food Processing Environments*. Chipping Campden, Gloucestershire: Campden and Chorleywood Food Research Association, 1999.

11 Tee GH. Bacteriological examination of watercress. *Mon Bull Min Hlth PHLS* 1962; **21**: 73–8.

12 Public Health Laboratory Service. The hygienic production of watercress: summary of a report by the Watercress Working Party of the Public Health Laboratory Service. *Mon Bull Min Hlth PHLS* 1966; **25**: 146–51.

13 British Standards Institution (BSI). BS 4285. *Microbiological Examination for Dairy Purposes. Part 4. Methods for Assessment of Hygienic Conditions*. London: BSI, 1991.

6 Isolation and enrichment of microorganisms

The procedure used for isolation of a microorganism from a food sample will depend upon a number of factors. If the organism is expected to be found in large numbers, or its presence is only significant when there are large numbers, direct enumeration on a suitable selective solid medium will be sufficient. If, however, only small numbers of that organism are anticipated, or if their presence is significant regardless of the number of cells (e.g. salmonellae) then enrichment culture will be required. This may need to incorporate a pre-enrichment or resuscitation stage if the organism is likely to have suffered injury through freezing, drying, heating, etc. Isolation media and procedures are often a matter of personal choice, but due regard should be given to their suitability for recovery of stressed organisms, which are easily inhibited by many selective agents and also by elevated incubation temperatures. In addition the recovery of spoilage organisms may require adjustments to the isolation medium, such as an increase in the levels of salt or glucose, in order to mimic the nature of the spoiled commodity and thus to allow recovery of the organism.

The quantity of food examined is important; in general for pre-enrichment or direct selective enrichment a 25 g portion should be cultured and the ratio of sample to broth should be 1:9 (or 1/10). For secondary enrichment a 1:10 ratio of inoculum to broth is usually maintained but this may vary depending on the selective broth; for example, the ratio of pre-enrichment broth to Rappaport Vassiliadis broth for isolation of salmonellae should be 1:100.

It is also important to perform internal quality control tests on both the media used for food examination and the whole test procedure. Reference strains derived from a recognized culture collection, such as the National Collection of Type Cultures (NCTC; see Appendix C), are used to compare their ability to grow and the degree of growth on or in the agar or liquid medium under test with results from a non-selective medium. The reference strains can also be used to assess recovery from artificially inoculated foods of different types by the methods used.

Quality control cultures

A wide range of reference cultures is required to test the entire range of liquid and solid culture and test media encountered in the microbiological examination of food. Reference cultures should be obtained on an annual basis in freeze dried form from the appropriate culture collection and developed into reference stock cultures on beads and working cultures according to the suggested procedure shown in Fig. 6.1 [1].

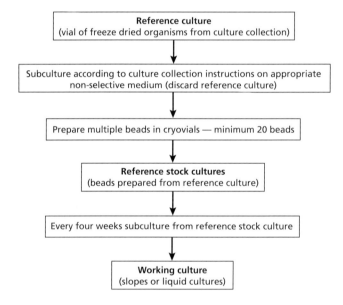

1   Working cultures should not be used to prepare further stocks.
2   Where viability of cultures on slopes or liquid media is poor, a fresh bead from a cryovial may be used as a working culture.
3   Documentation and detailed records on the handling of reference strains from receipt in the laboratory is essential.
4   A new reference culture should be obtained annually.
5   Most working cultures can be maintained at 4°C after incubation to establish sufficient growth for up to four weeks without loss of viability or contamination.
6   The key considerations are the preparation of the reference bead stocks and the life of the working cultures prior to replacement.

Fig. 6.1 Preparation and maintenance of quality control cultures.

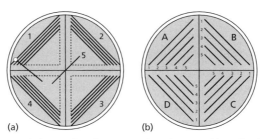

Fig. 6.2 Inoculation of plates using the ecometric technique: (a) method of Mossel *et al.* [2]; (b) modified method.

Quality control testing of solid and liquid media

A standard procedure for testing solid media is the plating out, in a standard, reproducible manner, of the test organism and the recording of the degree of growth. An example of this type of procedure is the 'ecometric' method [2] in which a loopful (1 μL or 5 μL) of an overnight broth culture is spread on to the surface of pre-dried plates in the manner illustrated in Fig. 6.2(a), the loop moving through sections one to five without reloading.

After appropriate incubation the highest rate of dilution that still leads to growth can be assessed and the results expressed as an absolute growth index (AGI). For example growth in all five sectors would give an AGI of 5.0, whereas growth on sections one and two and on only two inoculum lines of section three would give an AGI of 2.4. The relative growth index (RGI), the proportion of the AGI on the test medium compared with that on a control medium, can be used to describe the productive and selective properties of a particular medium.

An alternative method is shown in Fig. 6.2(b). The culture is spread from A1–B1–C1–D1–A2–B2, and so on, finishing at D5 without sterilizing the loop. The AGI can be calculated from the last segment and line at which growth occurs, the figure for each line increasing by five from A1 (5) through to D5 (100). Thus if the last line of growth is B4 then the AGI is 70. The RGI can be calculated by comparing the AGI of the test medium with that of a control medium as described above.

Alternatively a number of consecutive dilutions of the appropriate reference organism can be enumerated on the test medium, for example using the Miles and Misra surface drop method for testing solid media (see Section 5.5), and compared with the results obtained with a control medium.

There are a number of other methods which can be used in the quality assurance of culture media such as dilution to extinction (liquid media), mixed cultures of wanted and unwanted organisms (liquid media) and assessment of growth rate (liquid media). A summary of the available methods has been published [3].

The appropriate positive and negative quality control cultures are listed under each specific method or organism in the different sections of this manual where appropriate.

Quality control of test procedures

The whole test procedure should also be challenged by the use of reference materials or foods known to contain the required target organism. The latter can be achieved by preparing spiked samples or by the re-examination of samples previously found to be positive. Reference materials [4] are available that contain small numbers of the target organism (e.g. *Salmonella* spp., *Listeria monocytogenes*) in an inert substrate (spray-dried milk powder) contained within a gelatin capsule. These reference materials can be used alone to test the efficiency of the medium or in the presence of the relevant food material, with its associated competitive flora, to test the whole procedure.

Quality assurance

This is defined as the total process whereby the quality of laboratory reports can be achieved and is a combination of internal quality control and external quality assessment. Guidelines on the implementation of quality assurance programmes in laboratories involved in food, water and environmental laboratories have been published by an European Union (EU) Working Group [5] with the aim of making available, simply but accurately, procedures that have been developed and applied successfully by the Working Group members.

Internal quality control

This comprises the continual monitoring of working practices, equipment, media and reagents including performance of laboratory personnel. Procedures for the quality control of media are as described earlier in this section. Equipment should be regularly checked to ensure maintenance of optimum performance. The operational techniques and activities used to fulfil the requirements for quality are also referred to as analytical quality control [5], and can be differentiated into three lines of checking as outlined in Table 6.1.

The first line of checking is a means of self-control by the analyst, but it should be supervised by the direct superior responsible for setting criteria and

Table 6.1 Analytical control in microbiology.

Line of checking	Responsibility	Frequency	Purpose
First	Analyst	High	All aspects of the analysis under control and consistent over time
Second	Person independent of the analyst	Less frequent	Different analysts or equipment produce similar results. Individual results not biased
Third	Laboratory management	Regular intervals	To ensure interlaboratory standardization

defining action plans and should be included with every series of examinations. First-line checks should cover equipment and procedures to be undertaken: (a) before the examination (samples, equipment, media, filters and reagents); (b) during the analysis (noting all the information that becomes available such as temperature, anaerobic conditions, confirmation rates, colonial appearance, background flora, etc.); and (c) in addition to the examination. The latter would include internal quality control (IQC) procedures such as examination of additional samples, parallel plating, procedural blanks, positive and negative control samples, colony counts on different volumes/dilutions, use of control charts and use of sufficient colonies for confirmatory tests.

Second-line checks are implemented to assure reproducibility between different analysts or equipment, during training of new workers and evaluation of established staff in order to maintain standards of subjective interpretation. Such checks would include: (a) duplicate counting by the same person to provide the counting error under repeatability conditions, and by different persons, thus including both random and systematic components to the variation; (b) duplicate analytical procedures to test the whole quantitative procedure, by using duplicate samples and plotting control charts; and (c) intensified quality control tests as listed for first-line checks.

Third-line checks should be supervised by the quality assurance officer and include participation in an external quality assurance (EQA) scheme, also known as proficiency testing, and the use of certified reference materials (CRMs). In EQA schemes the samples are examined by different laboratories, the results interpreted retrospectively by the central organization and the performance compared with other participants. It is a flexible approach whereby participants apply their own methods. With CRMs, all laboratories follow a strict protocol and the certified value is valid only for the applied method. Results obtained with other methods can be compared with the certified values.

External quality assessment

Quality assessment acts as a check on the efficiency of the quality control procedures by the introduction of samples of known but undisclosed content for examination by the normal routine methods of the laboratory. This external challenge can be undertaken by participation in a proficiency testing scheme in which such samples, containing a range of food-associated organisms, are distributed on a regular basis. Such a system is offered by the Public Health Laboratory Service (PHLS) Food Microbiology External Quality Assessment Schemes (see Section 4.9 and Appendix C).

Temperature ranges

Incubators and water baths should be capable of maintaining the temperature to within 1°C of the desired temperature. Where more accurate temperature control is required, e.g. to within 0.5°C or 0.2°C, special fan-assisted incubators, or water baths, will be needed. Temperatures should be checked and recorded at least every working day, using thermometers or electronic temperature recording equipment calibrated by techniques traceable to national standards, and records kept for reference. Details of general laboratory practices can be found in ISO 7218 (BS 5763 Part 0) [6].

For tests designated 'recommended' and 'supplementary' in Section 3, the incubation temperatures given in this manual should be maintained to within 1°C and incubation times should not deviate from those stated by more than 2 h. For statutory tests, the temperature and time ranges permitted are quoted in the relevant legislation.

Confirmatory tests

Procedures for the tests most frequently used in confirmation of the identity of the microorganisms included in this section are given in Section 10. Details of other confirmatory tests may be found in standard texts such as *Cowan and Steel's Manual for the Identification of Medical Bacteria* ([1] in Section 10).

In this manual the tests described for the identification of microorganisms are based on traditional methods. However, multi-test micro-methods involving manual biochemical systems using dehydrated substrates (e.g. API®, Minitek®, MicroID®) or agar bases (e.g. Enterotube®) have become established in microbiological practice. These are simple and rapid to use and produce reproducible results. Databases are often provided with computer back-up and a telephone assistance service. Use of such methods is acceptable provided they are fully validated against the traditional tests. Although the standards cited in this manual describe traditional methods, the use of commercially produced biochemical galleries is increasingly permitted.

6.1 *Aeromonas* spp.

Members of the genus *Aeromonas* are Gram negative, facultatively anaerobic, non-sporing rod-shaped bacteria in the family Vibrionaceae. The genus can be divided into two groups of species. One group contains only one species, the psychrophilic fish pathogen *A. salmonicida*. The other group consists of the psychrotrophic, 'motile aeromonads' that includes *A. hydrophila, A. caviae* and *A. sobria*. The oxidase reaction is positive; motility can be variable as can gas production.

The motile aeromonads of the hydrophila group [7,8] have been associated with human disease and are regarded as potential human food-borne pathogens. Illness can range from a mild diarrhoea to a life-threatening cholera-like disease. *A. hydrophila* is the species most frequently implicated but, as there are no simple tests to distinguish between the different strains, they are often referred to as one species. These organisms are ubiquitous and are commonly found in water, sewage, seafood, meat, vegetables and dairy produce, but their significance in the epidemiology of food-borne disease is unclear.

Control cultures

NCTC 8049	*Aeromonas hydrophila*	Positive, growth quantitative
NCTC 9001	*Escherichia coli*	Negative, growth inhibited

Method 1 Direct enumeration

Media

A selective agar: e.g. bile salts irgasan brilliant green agar, Ryan's modification of xylose lysine desoxycholate agar (XLD) agar or ampicillin blood agar (contains ampicillin 10 mg/L).

Procedure

(a) Prepare a 10^{-1} homogenate using 25 g of food sample and 225 mL of maximum recovery diluent (MRD) and further decimal dilutions as described in Section 4.3.

(b) Using a surface counting method selected from Section 5 (eg: 5.4–5.6), enumerate *Aeromonas* spp. on a suitable selective agar.

(c) Incubate at 30°C for 18–24 h.

(d) Examine the plates and count typical colonies; these appear translucent on bile salts irgasan brilliant green agar, dark green, opaque colonies with a darker centre on Ryan's medium and large, colourless, usually haemolytic colonies on ampicillin blood agar.

(e) Subculture five typical colonies (or all if fewer than five) to a non-selective medium such as nutrient agar, then incubate at 30°C for 18–24 h.

(f) Perform an oxidase test (see Section 10.14). Retain oxidase-positive strains and identify by biochemical tests (strains remain viable for up to 20 min after the addition of oxidase reagent).

(g) Calculate the count per g from the proportion of colonies that are identified as *Aeromonas* spp.

Identification

Oxidase-positive strains isolated in this way may be considered to be members of the genus *Aeromonas* if they are fermentative and resistant to vibriostatic agent 0129 (2,4-diamino-6,7-diisopropylpteridine), and capable of growth in 0% but not 6% sodium chloride. Identification of the species can be obtained using the characteristics listed in Table 6.2.

Table 6.2 Identification of *Aeromonas* spp.

Test	A. hydrophila	A. sobria	A. caviae
Voges–Proskauer test	+	+	−
Growth at 42°C	−	+	−
Aesculin hydrolysis	+	−	+
Gas from glucose	V	+	−
Acid from arabinose	+	−	+
Lysine decarboxylase	+	+	−

V, variable.

continued

The 'suicide' test [9] for the speciation of *Aeromonas* based on the fermentation of glucose, with or without gas production, and pelleting of bacteria (suicide phenomenon) has been shown to be both accurate and simple to perform. This test, in combination with a short series of other biochemical tests (Table 6.3), is also recommended for identification of *Aeromonas* spp.

Table 6.3 Short scheme for identification of *Aeromonas* spp.

Test	A. hydrophila	A. sobria	A. caviae
Suicide test*	–	V	+
Gas from glucose	V	+	–
Aesculin hydrolysis	+	–	+
Hydrogen sulphide production	+	+	–

*Aeromonas suicide phenomenon medium [9]: nutrient broth containing 0.5% (w/v) glucose and 0.0015% (w/v) bromocresol purple, dispensed in 5 mL volumes in 125 mm × 16 mm tubes containing inverted Durham tubes.
V, variable.

Method 2 Enrichment culture

Media
Enrichment medium. Alkaline peptone water with electrolyte supplement (contains tryptone peptone 10 g, sodium chloride 10 g, magnesium chloride hexahydrate 4 g, potassium chloride 4 g/L), pH 8.6.

Selective agar: e.g. bile salts irgasan brilliant green agar, Ryan's aeromonas medium or ampicillin blood agar.

Procedure
(a) Prepare a homogenate using 25 g of food sample and 225 mL of enrichment medium.
(b) Incubate at 30°C for 18–24 h.
(c) Subculture to a suitable selective agar and proceed as described from step (c) of method 1.

Specialized reference facilities are available in certain circumstances for identification and serotyping of *Aeromonas* strains (see Appendix C).

6.2 *Bacillus cereus* and other *Bacillus* spp.

The *Bacillus* group includes a large number of Gram positive rod-shaped spore-forming species with a wide variety of properties. The genus is taxonomically non-homogeneous and many characters used for identification are variable including the Gram reaction, motility, ability to grow under anaerobic conditions, the oxidase reaction and method of breakdown of carbohydrates. The best arrangement for subdividing the genus appears to be that of Smith *et al.* [10], which divides the species into three groups based on traditional biochemical tests, spore position and morphology. The main species involved in food-borne illness include *B. cereus* (Group I) and the *B. subtilis/licheniformis* group (Group III), although a number of other species have been incriminated.

Members of the *Bacillus* group are ubiquitous, being found widely in the dust and soil, and are freqently isolated in varying numbers from a wide range of foods especially those containing cereals. The spores may survive many heat processes, and as high numbers are normally required to cause illness low numbers present in foods are not considered significant. Enrichment methods are not normally required. *Bacillus* spp. will grow readily on non-selective media, but for purposes of identification a selective medium should be used [11–14]. The media specified below do not recover all species of *Bacillus*, but do recover the species that are recognized as capable of causing gastrointestinal symptoms. An incubation temperature of 30°C is recommended to ensure the detection of psychrophilic strains of *B. cereus*.

Control cultures

NCTC 7464	*Bacillus cereus*	Positive, growth quantitative
NCTC 10400	*Bacillus subtilis*	Positive, growth qualitative
NCTC 9001	*Escherichia coli*	Negative, growth inhibited

Media

Polymyxin pyruvate egg yolk mannitol bromothymol blue agar (PEMBA)

or

Phenol red egg yolk polymyxin agar (MYP or PREP agar).

Both media contain 1% mannitol, 5% egg yolk emulsion and 100 IU polymyxin/mL. The appropriate ISO method (EN ISO 7932; BS 5763 Part 11) [14] uses MYP agar inoculated by the surface plating method. However international studies have failed to show a significant difference between the performance of the two media [15] and many dairy microbiologists favour the use of PEMBA.

Procedure

(a) Prepare a 10^{-1} homogenate and serial decimal dilutions of the food sample as described in Sections 4.2 and 4.3.

(b) Select a surface counting method from Section 5 (eg: 5.4–5.6), and enumerate using PEMBA or MYP agar.

(c) Incubate aerobically at 30°C for 24 h; if colonies are not clearly visible incubate at 30°C for a further 24 h. If PEMBA is used and a spore stain (see Section 10.4) will be required after incubation the medium should be incubated at 37°C for the first 24 h followed by a further 24 h at room temperature.

(d) Examine plates for characteristic colonies, which will be large (3–7 mm diameter) and dull. Colonies of *B. cereus* appear turquoise/peacock blue on PEMBA agar and

continued

pink on MYP agar due to absence of mannitol fermentation, and are usually surrounded by a zone of opacity due to precipitation of hydrolysed lecithin (see Plate Ia,b, facing p. 150). Most other members of the *Bacillus* group are mannitol positive, appear as green or yellow colonies and do not produce lecithinase (see Plate Ic,d, facing p. 150).

If the food under test is acidic or if the plate contains many colonies that ferment mannitol the characteristic blue (PEMBA) or pink (MYP) colour due to absence of mannitol fermentation may be masked. Further subculture of suspect colonies to PEMBA or MYP will overcome this problem and aid identification.

(e) Select plates containing up to 150 colonies for counting. Count and record the number of colonies with morphology resembling *Bacillus* species to give the presumptive count. If *B. cereus* is also sought count and record blue (PEMBA) or pink (MYP) colonies with and without lecithinase zones.

Note: Some members of the Enterobacteriaceae, such as *Proteus*, and many strains of *Staphylococcus aureus* are able to grow on these selective media. However, they are easily distinguished by colonial morphology and overall appearance, and by egg-yolk clearing, in contrast to egg-yolk precipitation.

Identification

(f) Perform a Gram stain if necessary to confirm cell morphology (large Gram positive bacilli, with or without visible spores). Subculture at least five colonies of each colonial type onto blood agar and incubate for 18–24 h at 30°C. Colonies of *B. cereus* are β-haemolytic, that is they produce complete clearing of the red blood cells around the colony growth.

Confirm the identity of presumptive *B. cereus* and characterize other *Bacillus* strains of different morphology with appropriate biochemical tests The short scheme in Table 6.4 allows distinction of some of the most common strains of *Bacillus* of importance in food poisoning. Details of the biochemical tests can be found in Section 10. To test for anaerobic growth inoculate two blood agar plates; incubate one plate aerobically and the other plate anaerobically at 30°C for 22±2 h, then examine both plates for the presence of growth.

(g) Calculate the total *Bacillus* spp. or *B. cereus* count per g of food.

Table 6.4 Identification of common food poisoning strains of *Bacillus* spp.

	B. cereus	*B. pumilus*	*B. subtilis*	*B. licheniformis*
Glucose (ASS)	+	+	+	+
Arabinose (ASS)	–	+	+	+
Mannitol (ASS)	–	+	+	+
Xylose (ASS)	–	+	+	+
Nitrate reduction	+	–	+	+
Anaerobic growth	+	–	–	+

ASS, ammonium salt sugars. For preparation see [1] in Section 10.

Specialized biochemical, serological and toxin production tests are available (see Appendix C).

6.3   *Brucella* spp.

Brucella spp. are short Gram negative, aerobic or capnophilic, non-motile rods belonging to the *Moraxella-Acinetobacter* Group. The genus comprises a single genospecies *B. melitensis* but the old specific names are still generally used— *B. abortus, B. melitensis* and *B. suis* being the three classical species, all of which cause infections in humans. They are catalase positive, usually oxidase positive and do not show acid production from sugars in peptone-containing media [16–19].

Brucella spp. are Hazard Group 3 pathogens, and samples and cultures must be handled accordingly. Count methods are not normally applicable, the aim being simply to detect the presence of brucellae. The methods described are for the detection of brucellae in milk, but can be adapted for cream, soft cheese and other milk products.

Method 1 Direct culture

Media

A selective agar: e.g. brucella agar base, which contains dextrose; or blood agar or Columbia agar base plus 1% (w/v) sterile dextrose. These media are suitable for use with the addition of 5% inactivated horse serum (i.e. serum held at 56°C for 30 min) and an antibiotic cocktail containing polymyxin 5000 IU, bacitracin 25 000 IU, cycloheximide 100 mg, nalidixic acid 5 mg, nystatin 100 000 IU and vancomycin 20 mg/L.

Procedure

(a) Transfer the milk sample to sterile test tubes (180 mm × 25 mm) and store overnight at 4°C.

(b) Dip a swab into the cream layer and inoculate the surface of a selective agar.

(c) Incubate the plates at 37°C in an atmosphere of air containing 10% carbon dioxide.

(d) Examine the plates every 2 days for up to 10 days. Colonies are usually visible after 4 to 5 days' incubation, and are 1–2 mm in diameter, convex, with round entire edges.

Identification

Brucella spp. can be further identified using antibodies for slide agglutination. Differentiation can also be achieved by the dyes-strip method [18] as follows:

1 Impregnate filter paper strips with 1:200 basic fuchsin or 1:600 thionin and dry.

2 Place a strip of each dye parallel on the surface of a plate of serum dextrose agar and cover with a thin layer of the same medium. Allow the medium to solidify.

continued

3 Make streak inoculations of the *Brucella* strains at right angles to the strips.
4 Incubate in 10% carbon dioxide for 2 to 3 days at 37°C.
5 Examine for growth. Resistant strains grow right across the strip, but sensitive strains show inhibition of growth up to 10 mm from the strip. Typical growth patterns are given in Table 6.5.

Table 6.5 Typical patterns of *Brucella* spp. in the dye-strip tests.

	Basic fuchsin 1:200	Thionin 1:600
B. abortus	Growth	No growth
B. melitensis	Growth	Growth
B. suis	No growth	Growth

Method 2 Enrichment culture

Media
Broth bases: e.g. brucella broth or media suitable for the culture of fastidious organisms such as brain heart infusion broth or tryptone soya broth. Supplement the medium with 5% sterile horse serum and antibiotics as described in method 1. The use of amphotericin B (4 mg/L) and cycloserine (12.5 mg/L) in addition to the antibiotics previously listed has also been recommended.

Procedure
(a) Centrifuge 100 mL of the milk for 30 min at 1500 rev/min.
(b) Transfer the cream layer and deposit from the centrifuged milk to sufficient enrichment broth in a screw-capped container to give an inoculation ratio of 1:10.
(c) Incubate the broth, with screwcap loose, in air containing 10% carbon dioxide at 37°C for 5 days.
(d) Subculture the broth to selective agar and proceed as described from step (c) of method 1.

Facilities are available for the identification and serotyping of *Brucella* spp. (see Appendix C).

6.4 *Campylobacter jejuni, C. coli* and *C. lari*

Thermotolerant, microaerobic campylobacters have only been recognized as important causes of human enteritis since the early 1970s. *Campylobacter jejuni* is responsible for most illness, with *C. coli* causing a small proportion of cases and other species being isolated occasionally. Campylobacters are microaerophilic, Gram negative, small vibrioid or spiral-shaped cells with rapid, darting, reciprocating motility. They reduce nitrate, are unable to oxidize or ferment carbohydrates and mostly reduce nitrite. *C. jejuni*, *C. coli*, *C. upsaliensis* and *C. lari* are thermotolerant, growing at 42°C but not at 25°C. Campylobacters may infect humans after direct contact with animals or indirectly via contaminated water, milk or meat [20].

Many food samples to be examined for the presence of *Campylobacter* spp. [21–26] will have received treatments such as heating, freezing or chilling. These treatments can cause sublethal injury to the organism resulting in increased sensitivity to some antibiotics and lowered resistance to elevated incubation temperatures. The enrichment culture method described below allows resuscitation and recovery of injured organisms. Direct culture of fresh raw foods especially poultry may also be productive. Enumeration of campylobacters is not normally attempted, as the aim of examination is to establish the presence of the organism.

Control cultures

| NCTC 11322 | *Campylobacter jejuni* | Positive, growth quantitative |
| NCTC 9001 | *Escherichia coli* | Negative, growth inhibited |

Method 1 Direct culture

This procedure is likely to be of most value with samples such as chicken skin.

Media
A selective agar: e.g. blood-free modified cefoperazone charcoal deoxycholate agar (CCDA) [22], Exeter [23], Preston [21] or Skirrow [24].

Procedure
(a) Take a swab of the food sample and inoculate on to the surface of a suitable selective agar.
(b) Incubate the plates at 37°C for 4 h and then at 41.5°C for a further 44–68 h in an atmosphere of nitrogen containing 5–15% carbon dioxide and 5–10% oxygen.
(c) Examine the plates for typical colonies, which have the following characteristics [20]:

C. jejuni (and *C. lari*)—flat, glossy, effuse colonies, with a tendency to spread along the inoculation track. Well-spaced colonies resemble droplets of fluid. On moist agar a thin, spreading film may be seen. With continued incubation colonies become low and convex with a dull surface. A metallic sheen will eventually develop (see Plate II, facing p. 150).

C. coli—less effuse, often umbonate colonies with the surface usually remaining shiny.

continued

Identification

(d) Identification to genus level can be made by the following tests:

    1 Oxidase test: positive (see Section 10.14).

    2 Growth on blood agar incubated at 41.5°C for 24–48 h under microaerobic conditions described in step (b) but no growth following incubation under aerobic conditions.

    3 Microscopy showing Gram negative, highly motile rods with S-shaped or spiral morphology. This rapidly degenerates to a coccal form with exposure to oxygen.

(e) *C. jejuni, C. coli* and *C. lari* can be differentiated by the biochemical tests shown in Table 6.6.

Table 6.6 Differentiation of *Campylobacter* spp.

	Hippurate hydrolysis	Nalidixic acid sensitivity
C. jejuni	+	S
C. coli	–	S
C. lari	–	R

R, resistant; S, sensitive.

Method 2 Enrichment culture

Suitable enrichment broths contain FBP supplement (ferrous sulphate, sodium metabisulphite and sodium pyruvate, each at 0.025% concentration) to improve aerotolerance and allow aerobic incubation. A mixture of antibiotics is also required to prevent overgrowth by competing organisms and are included in the formulation of Preston [21], Exeter [23] and Bolton [26] broths. Preston broth is based on the formulation of Preston agar. Exeter broth is similar but also includes cefoperazone for greater selectivity. Exeter broth has been shown to produce superior isolation rates to that of Preston broth. Sensitivity to some of the ingredients demonstrated by sublethally injured campylobacters can be overcome by incubating the broths at 37°C [25]. Bolton broth has been elaborated to optimize recovery of injured cells (see method 3).

The method described below is similar to that described in one part of ISO 10272 (BS 5763 Part 17) [27].

Media

Exeter campylobacter-selective medium [23] *of the following composition:*

Nutrient broth (Oxoid No. 2)	1000 mL
Lysed blood	50 mL
Trimethoprim	10 mg
Rifampicin	10 mg
Cefoperazone	15 mg

continued

Polymyxin		4 mg
Amphotericin		2 mg
Sodium pyruvate		250 mg
Sodium metabisulphite	FBP	250 mg
Ferrous sulphate		250 mg

For plates add 15 g of agar.

FBP can be made as a combined 2.5% solution of each additive in water. Ten millilitres of this can then be added to 1 L of medium. Discard stock solution after 7 days. Antibiotics have to be made as separate solutions.

Selective agars: e.g. blood-free modified CCDA [22], Preston [21], Exeter [23] or Skirrow [24].

Procedure

(a) Homogenize 25 g of the food sample in 225 mL of Exeter enrichment broth. The broth should be at room temperature on inoculation. Transfer the homogenate to a screw-topped jar leaving very little headspace, and close the top tightly.

(b) Incubate at 37°C for 18–48 h preferably in a fan-assisted incubator to obtain rapid heat transfer. Adjust the incubation period according to the expected degree of contamination of the sample: for samples such as chicken skin, incubate at 37°C for 18 h; for water samples, where cells will be severely damaged, incubate for 48 h.

(c) Subculture onto a suitable selective agar.

(d) Incubate the plates at 41.5°C for 24–48 h in a microaerobic atmosphere (see step (b) of method 1).

(e) Proceed as described in steps (c)–(e) of method 1.

Specialized tests for biotyping and serotyping of campylobacters are available (see Appendix C).

Method 3 Enrichment culture for isolation of injured cells

A number of changes have been proposed to the current version of ISO 10272. The new version (in preparation) contains a more convenient method for the recovery of stressed *Campylobacter* cells, such as those that might be found in frozen foods. The new method is oulined below.

Media

Enrichment broth: Bolton broth [26]
Selective agars: blood-free modified CCDA and a second selective agar of choice.

Procedure

(a) Homogenize 25 g of sample in 225 mL of Bolton broth. Transfer the homogenate to a screw-topped jar leaving very little headspace, and close the top tightly.

(b) Incubate at 37°C for 4 h; transfer to 41.5°C for a further 42–44 h.

(c) Subculture onto modified CCDA agar and one other agar of choice.

(d) Incubate the plates at 41.5°C for 40–48 h.

(e) Proceeed as described in steps (c)–(e) of method 1.

6.5 *Clostridium perfringens* and other sulphite-reducing clostridia [28–32]

Clostridium perfringens is commonly found in human and animal faeces and is widespread in the environment in soil, dust, flies and vegetation. Because of current slaughtering practices it is difficult to obtain animal carcasses free of gut contamination; the organism is therefore a common contaminant of meat and poultry. It was associated with diarrhoea as early as 1895 and first reports of its role in food poisoning date from 1943. It is a Gram positive, square ended, anaerobic (but relatively oxygen tolerant) non-motile member of the genus *Clostridium*. It forms oval, central spores rarely seen in culture unless specially formulated media are used. The spores are readily formed in the intestine; an enterotoxin is produced on sporulation in the gut. *C. perfringens* produces a capsule, it reduces sulphite and nitrate and produces a lecithinase (β-toxin activity). Sugar reactions may be irregular but lactose fermentation can help differentiate the organisms from *C. sordelli* and *C. novyi*, while the lack of motility and inability to sporulate freely can be used to separate *C. perfringens* from *C. bifermentans* and also *C. sordelli*, to which it is antigenically related [31].

Foods contaminated with large numbers of vegetative cells of *C. perfringens* can give rise to illness characterized by diarrhoea and abdominal pain. The vegetative cells are very sensitive to chilling and freezing, and only the spore form may survive in chilled and frozen foods. Other sulphite-reducing clostridia are implicated in food spoilage, especially of poorly processed canned food. The first method described for direct enumeration will detect almost all sulphite-reducing clostridia and is capable of good recovery of both vegetative cells and spores. The second method is useful for investigating food poisoning outbreaks, but may not recover some strains.

Control cultures

NCTC 8237	*Clostridium perfringens*	Positive, growth quantitative
NCTC 9001	*Escherichia coli*	Negative, growth inhibited (tryptose sulphite cycloserine: TSC)
NCTC 10975	*Proteus mirabilis*	Negative, growth inhibited (neomycin blood agar)
NCTC 532	*Clostridium sporogenes*	Positive, growth quantitative

Method 1 Direct enumeration

This method is based on BS EN 13401 and ISO 7937 [31]. The difference between these two international methods lies in the confirmation technique. The revision of ISO 7937 will allow either method to be used instead of only lactose sulphite medium.

Media

Tryptose sulphite cycloserine agar [28,29,32] (TSC): perfringens agar base plus D-cycloserine (400 mg/L); for spoilage clostridia sensitive to cycloserine, use perfringens agar base containing kanamycin sulphate (12 mg/L) and polymyxin B (30 000 IU/L).

Reagents

Nitrite reagents: equal volumes of 5-amino-2-naphthalene sulphonic acid (0.1% solution in 15% by volume acetic acid solution) and sulfanilic acid solution (0.4% in 15% by volume acetic acid solution) mixed just before use.

Procedure

(a) Prepare a 10^{-1} homogenate and serial decimal dilutions of the food as described in Sections 4.2 and 4.3.

(b) Place 1 mL of the 10^{-1} homogenate and each dilution into separate sterile Petri dishes. Add 10–15 mL of molten, cooled agar. Rotate gently to mix the agar and the inoculum and allow to solidify. (Modification of method is described in Section 5.3.)

(c) Overlay the solidified agar with a further 10 mL of molten, cooled agar and allow to set.

(d) Incubate the plates anaerobically at 37°C for 20±2 h.

(e) Count the black colonies on plates containing up to 150 such colonies. These are presumptive sulphite-reducing clostridia (see Plate IIIa, facing p. 150).

(f) Subculture at least five black colonies to two blood agar plates; incubate one plate aerobically and the other anaerobically at 37°C for 18–24 h to ensure absence of aerobic growth. Colonies which fail to grow aerobically are confirmed as sulphite-reducing clostridia.

(g) Confirm the identity of black colonies that have grown anaerobically either by the nitrate motility/lactose gelatin method (g)–(i) or by use of lactose sulphite (LS) medium at 46°C (j)–(m).

Nitrate motility/lactose gelatin method

(h) Stab-inoculate the colonies into nitrate-motility and lactose-gelatin media in screw-capped bottles that have been steamed and cooled just prior to use. Incubate anaerobically with the bottle tops loose at 37°C for 24 h. If *C. perfringens* is specifically sought and the headspace in the bottles is small, aerobic incubation with the bottle tops tightly closed will help select for this relatively aerotolerant species.

(i) Examine the nitrate-motility bottle for motility. *C. perfringens* is non-motile and produces a distinct line of growth along the stab (as opposed to diffuse growth

continued

through the medium). Add the nitrite reagents to the nitrate-motility bottle; *C. perfringens* usually reduces nitrate to nitrite with formation of a red colour on the agar surface after addition of the reagents. If no red colour is produced after addition of the nitrite reagent add a small amount of powdered zinc. Continued absence of a red colour indicates that the nitrate in the original medium has been reduced completely by the organism, and denotes a positive result. If a red colour is detected, the nitrate in the medium has been reduced by the zinc rather than by the organism.

(j) Examine the lactose-gelatin medium for the presence of acid and gas, then refrigerate the bottle for 30 min. If no liquefaction is noted after 24 h, reincubate the lactose-gelatin medium for a further 24 h and re-examine. *C. perfringens* is lactose-positive and liquefies gelatin.

Bacteria that produce black colonies in the TSC medium, are non-motile, reduce nitrate to nitrite, produce acid and gas from lactose and liquefy gelatin in 48 h are considered to be *C. perfringens*. However, the confirmatory tests described above will not distinguish between *C. perfringens* and other closely related but less commonly encountered *Clostridium* spp. such as *C. paraperfringens* and *C. absonum*.

Lactose sulphite method

(h) Inoculate each selected colony into fluid thioglycollate medium and incubate anaerobically at 37°C for 18–24 h.

(i) Immediately after incubation use a sterile pipette to transfer five drops of the thioglycollate culture to lactose sulphite medium containing an inverted Durham tube, that has been steamed and cooled just prior to use.

(j) Incubate at 46°C for 18–24 h in a water bath.

(k) Tubes of LS medium containing a black precipitate and with Durham tubes more than a quarter full of gas are considered positive. If the Durham tube, in a blackened medium, is less than one-quarter full of gas, transfer five drops of the growth from this tube to a further tube of LS medium and incubate at 46°C. Read as described above. Colonies giving the typical appearance in the TSC medium and positive confirmation with the LS medium are considered to be *C. perfringens*.

Colonies may be confirmed as *C. perfringens* type A by the Nagler reaction, i.e. by demonstrating the ability of *C. perfringens* type A antitoxin to inhibit lecithinase production using an egg yolk agar. A few strains do not produce lecithinase. However, care must be taken not to confuse the reaction with that produced by other closely related species of clostridia such as *C. bifermentans* and *C. sordelli*.

Method 2 Enrichment culture

This method can be used to determine the presence or absence of clostridia when the number of cells is likely to be small or when only spores are present.

Procedure

(a) Weigh two 1 g samples of the food into separate screw-capped bottles containing 25 mL volumes of cooked meat medium or reinforced clostridial medium that has been boiled to expel oxygen and cooled immediately before use.

(b) Heat one bottle to 60–65°C for 15 min to heat shock the spores. Do not heat the other bottle.

(c) Incubate both bottles at 37°C for 20–24 h.

(d) Subculture both bottles to a suitable selective agar to confirm the presence of clostridia as described in steps (a)–(i) of method 1. (Bottles of reinforced clostridial medium that have grown clostridia will have blackened.)

Cooked meat medium and reinforced clostridial medium may be used to enumerate clostridia by a multiple tube (most probable number) method (see Section 5.7).

Specialist tests for identification of clostridia and *C. perfringens* serotyping and toxin testing are available (see Appendix C).

6.6 Coliforms, thermotolerant (faecal) coliforms and *Escherichia coli*

Coliforms, thermotolerant (faecal) coliforms and *Escherichia coli* have long been used as marker (index and indicator) organisms in the examination of a variety of foods. These organisms are very sensitive to heat and so their presence in heat processed foods indicates post-processing contamination. The coliform (coliaerogenes) group, defined as lactose-positive members of the Enterobacteriaceae, is frequently used by the dairy industry as an indicator of hygiene. However, it is an ill-defined group and tests to demonstrate Gram negative bacteria growing on media containing bile salts and which produce acid from lactose would also include all sorts of entirely different bacteria depending on the medium and incubation conditions and the criteria used for reading results. They would also sometimes erroneously exclude organisms on the basis of aberrant biochemical behaviour or unusual colonial type [33]. The term faecal coliform is used to denote a coliform of faecal origin and those that can grow at 44°C have been referred to as thermotolerant faecal coliforms. However, not all thermotolerant coliforms are of faecal origin and not all faecal coliforms are thermotolerant. Thus tests which determine the presence of well defined groups or species are much more useful. For foods processed for safety a test for the whole of the Enterobacteriaceae group is the test of choice, but there is limited scope in the examination of fresh foods such as salad ingredients.

Escherichia coli originates from the intestinal tract of humans and animals. It is a clear-cut taxonomic entity and can be used as a marker to demonstrate that faecal pollution may have occurred at some stage during the production of a food. Tests have traditionally been based on the detection of organisms that produce indole and gas from lactose at 44°C. However, most strains of *E. coli* are also glucuronidase positive, and methods have latterly been introduced which detect the presence of β-glucuronidase producing organisms by the cleavage of fluorogenic or chromogenic substrates such as methylumbelliferyl β-D-glucuronide (MUG) and 5-bromo-4-chloro-3-indolyl β-D-glucuronide (BCIG) media (see method 7). The pathogenic strains of *E. coli* such as verocytotoxin producing O157 are not usually sought routinely but only in instances of food poisoning and in high-risk foods. Tests for this organism are dealt with in method 10 of this section.

Control cultures

NCTC 9001	*Escherichia coli*	Positive, growth quantitative β-glucuronidase positive
NCTC 12900 (non-toxigenic)	*Escherichia coli* O157	Sorbitol negative
NCTC 13216	*Escherichia coli*	β-glucuronidase weak positive

Negative controls will vary with test media and conditions:

NCTC 6571	*Staphylococcus aureus*	Brilliant green bile broth, MacConkey agar, MacConkey broth, lauryl sulphate tryptose broth, violet red bile agar
NCTC 9528	*Klebsiella aerogenes*	Brilliant green bile broth at 44°C, peptone/tryptone water (indole), MUG media, BCIG media
NCTC 11047	*Staphylococcus epidermidis*	Membrane enriched broths
NCTC 9001	*Escherichia coli*	Sorbitol positive

Method 1 Coliforms—pour plate

This method is based on ISO 4832 (BS 5763 Part 2) [34]. Coliforms detected by this method are defined as lactose fermenting Gram negative bacilli capable of growth in the presence of bile. It can be used for liquid samples and food homogenates, and a modification of the method is widely used by the dairy industry (see Section 7, method 2). For dairy products and hygiene investigations incubation at 30°C is recommended; for other foods and public health investigations an incubation temperature of 37°C is preferable.

continued

The following illustrations (Plates I–XIII) show the typical colonial morphology of a range of food-borne organisms on the media most commonly used for their isolation and identification. Plates XIV–XVIII relate to the confirmatory tests in Section 10.

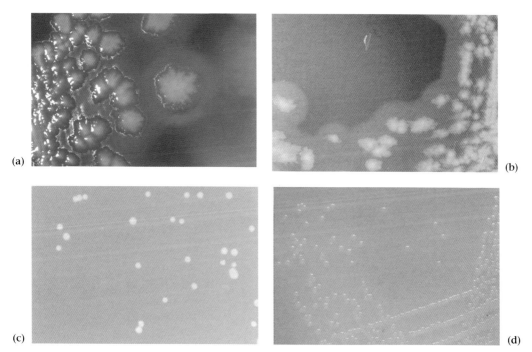

(a) (b) (c) (d)

Plate I *Bacillus* spp. on selective agars: (a) *B.cereus* on polymyxin pyruvate egg yolk mannitol bromothymol blue agar (PEMBA); (b) *B.cereus* on phenol red egg yolk polymyxin agar (MYP); (c) *B.subtilis* on PEMBA; (d) *B.subtilis* on MYP.

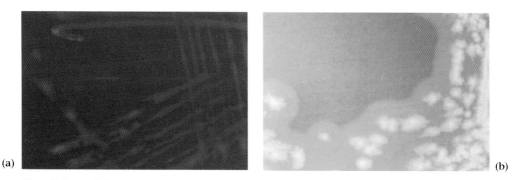

(a) (b)

Plate II Campylobacters on selective agars: (a) blood containing agar (Preston); (b) blood-free agar containing charcoal (CCDA).

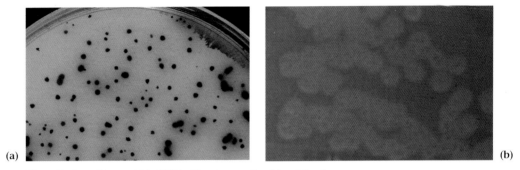

(a)
(b)

Plate III *C. perfringens*: (a) in TSC (without egg yolk); (b) on blood agar.

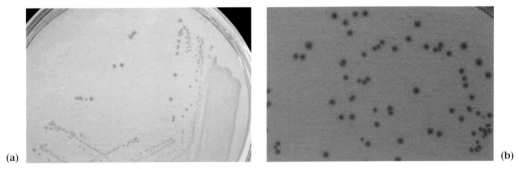

(a)
(b)

Plate IV (a) *Escherichia coli* O157 on sorbitol MacConkey agar; (b) beta-glucuronidase producing *E.coli* on methylumbelliferyl α-D-glucuronide (MUG) agar.

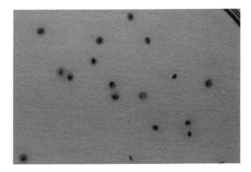

Plate V Enterobacteriaceae in violet red bile glucose agar.

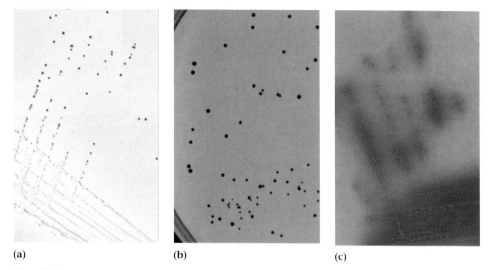

(a)   (b)   (c)

Plate VI Enterococci on selective agars: (a) *KF.streptococcus* agar; (b) Slanetz and Bartley agar; (c) bile aesculin agar.

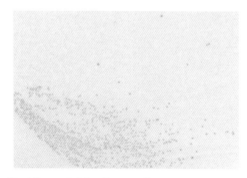

Plate VII *Lactobacillus acidophilus* on de Man, Rogosa, Sharpe agar.

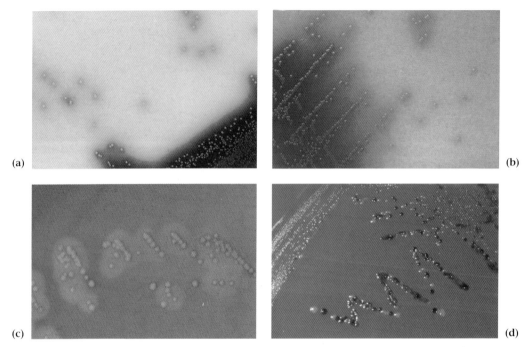

Plate VIII *Listeria monocytogenes* on: (a) Oxford agar; (b) PALCAM agar; (c) ALOA agar—blue colonies with haloes are *L. monocytogenes*, blue colonies without haloes are *L. innocua*; (d) Rapid L Mono agar—blue colonies are *L. monocytogenes*, white colonies are *L. innocua*.

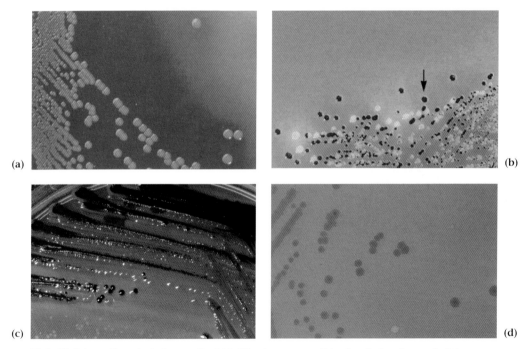

Plate IX *Salmonella* on isolation media: (a) brilliant green agar; (b) xylose lysine desoxycholate agar; (c) mannitol lysine crystal violet brilliant green agar. Arrows indicate typical *Salmonella* colonies on plates of mixed cultures; (d) Rambach agar. Arrows indicate typical *Salmonella* colonies on plates of mixed cultures.

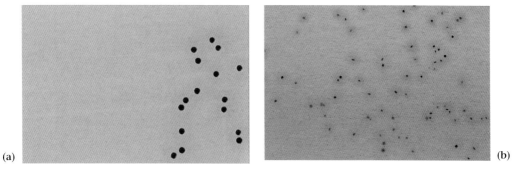

Plate X *Staphylococcus aureus* on: (a) Baird–Parker agar; (b) rabbit plasma fibrinogen agar.

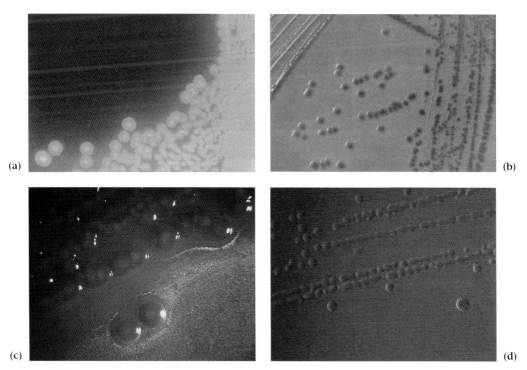

Plate XI *Vibrio* on selective agars: (a) *V. alginolyticus* on TCBS agar; (b) *V. parahaemolyticus* on TCBS agar; (c) *V. vulnificus* on SDS agar; (d) *V. furnissi* on SDS agar.

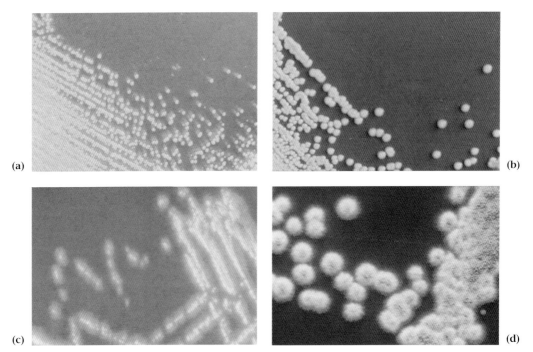

(a)

(b)

(c)

(d)

Plate XII Yeasts and moulds: (a) yeast on dichloran-glycerol agar; (b) yeast on rose-bengal chloramphenicol agar; (c) mould on dichloran-glycerol agar; (d) mould on rose-bengal chloramphenicol agar.

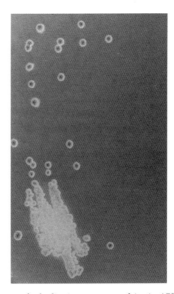

Plate XIII *Yersinia enterocolitica* on cefsulodin-irgasan-novobiocin (CIN) agar.

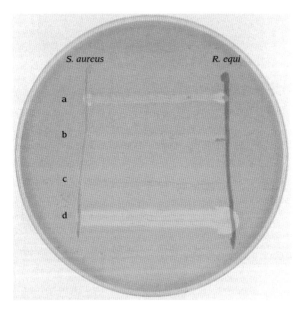

Plate XIV CAMP test for *Listeriae*: (a) *L. monocytogenes*; (b) *L. seeligeri*; (c) *L. innocua*; (d) *L. ivanovii*.

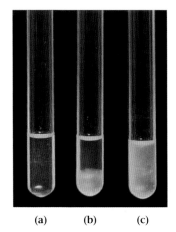

(a)   (b)   (c)

Plate XV Coagulase test: (a) uninoculated; (b) weak positive;(c) strong positive.

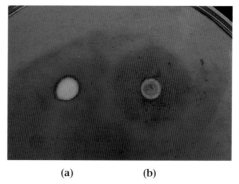

(a)   (b)

Plate XVI Desoxyribonuclease (Dnase) test using toluidine blue solution: (a) negative; (b) positive.

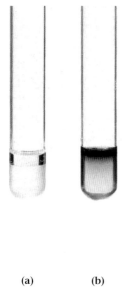

(a)   (b)

Plate XVII Hippurate test for *Campylobacter*: (a) negative; (b) positive.

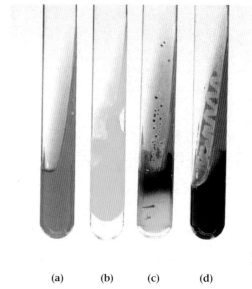

(a)   (b)   (c)   (d)

Plate XVIII Hydrogen sulphide test, TSI slope: (a) uninoculated; (b) acid and gas, no hydrogen sulphide; (c) young culture of *Salmonella* showing acid butt and hydrogen sulphide production; (d) old culture of *Salmonella*.

Media

Violet red bile agar (VRBA).

Procedure

(a) Place 1 mL of liquid sample or 10^{-1} homogenate into each of two Petri dishes; repeat with each dilution prepared.

(b) To each plate add 15 mL of molten VRBA cooled to 44–47°C. Mix carefully and allow to set. Overlay each plate with a further 4–5 mL of molten, cooled VRBA and allow to set. Incubate the plates at 30°C or 37°C for 24 ± 2 h.

(c) Select dishes that contain not more than 150 colonies and count purplish red colonies that have a diameter of 0.5 mm or greater, usually surrounded by a reddish zone.

(d) Calculate the count per g or mL as described in Section 5.3.

Method 2 Coliforms, thermotolerant (faecal) coliforms and *Escherichia coli* — surface plate

This method is convenient in that it uses pre-poured plates. It will only detect aerogenic coliforms, thermotolerant coliforms and *E. coli*. If the ratio of *E. coli* to other organisms in the sample is low, the method may not detect *E. coli*.

Media

Violet red bile agar (VRBA)
Brilliant green bile (lactose) broth (BGBB)
1% tryptone water.

Procedure

(a) Prepare a 10^{-1} homogenate and serial decimal dilutions of the food as described in Sections 4.2 and 4.3.

(b) Select a surface counting method from Section 5 (eg: 5.4–5.6) and enumerate using pre-poured VRBA plates. Incubate the plates at 37°C for 24 ± 2 h.

(c) Count the purplish-red colonies. This will give the presumptive coliform count.

(d) Confirm the identity of at least five of the purplish-red colonies by subculturing into two tubes of BGBB containing an inverted Durham fermentation tube, and into 1% tryptone water. Incubate one tube of BGBB at 37°C for 48 h, and the second tube of BGBB and the tryptone water at 44 ± 0.5°C for 24 h.

(e) After incubation, add 0.2–0.3 mL of Kovac's reagent to the tryptone water to detect indole production, shown by a red surface layer, and examine the tubes of BGBB for gas production (Table 6.7).

continued

Table 6.7 Differentiation of coliforms, thermotolerant coliforms and *Escherichia coli* type 1.

	Gas in BGBB 37°C (48 h)	Gas in BGBB 44°C (24 h)	Indole production
Coliforms	+	–	+ or –
Thermotolerant (faecal) coliforms	+	+	+ or –*
E. coli (type 1)	+	+	+

*Escherichia coli are thermotolerant (faecal) coliforms. If thermotolerant (faecal) coliforms are sought, colonies identified as *E.coli* should be included.

Full identification of the organisms can be made if required after subculture of the BGBB broths to an agar medium. Coliforms, thermotolerant coliforms and *E. coli* are oxidase negative.

Method 3 Coliforms, thermotolerant (faecal) coliforms and *Escherichia coli*—most probable number [35–37]

Although this method will only detect aerogenic strains, it will allow the enumeration of low levels of *E. coli* in the presence of high levels of other coliforms. Some liquid media also allow the growth of other organisms such as *Bacillus* species that may give rise to false positive results. ISO 4831 [36] allows incubation of the primary liquid medium at either 30°C or 37°C, depending on the reason for seeking coliforms.

Media

Suitable liquid enrichment media containing Durham tubes for gas detection: e.g. lauryl sulphate tryptose broth; minerals modified glutamate broth (MMGB) [37].

Selective confirmatory medium: e.g. brilliant green bile broth or *Eserichia coli* (EC) broth. 1% tryptone water.

Both ISO 48317 and ISO 7251 [36] specify the use of lauryl sulphate tryptose broth as the enrichment medium and ISO 7251 specifies confirmation in EC broth.

Procedure

(a) Prepare a 10^{-1} food homogenate and further serial decimal dilutions as described in Sections 4.2 and 4.3.
(b) Using Section 5.7, method 3 or 4, inoculate the tubes of media with suitable dilutions of the food sample. Incubate the tubes at 30°C or 37°C for 48 h.
(c) Examine the tubes after 24 h and 48 h for gas production (acid and gas production in MMGB). Tubes showing gas production may be considered presumptively positive for coliforms.

continued

(d) Confirm the presence of coliforms, faecal coliforms and *E. coli* type 1 by subculturing tubes showing the presence of gas (or acid and gas) to EC broth or BGBB as described in steps (d) and (e) of method 2.

(e) Use the number of positive tubes at each dilution to compute the number of coliforms, thermotolerant coliforms and *E. coli* type 1 using Table 5.7 (pp. 121–2) for three tubes per dilution and Table 9.2 (pp. 233–4) for five tubes per dilution.

Method 4 Coliforms, thermotolerant (faecal) coliforms and *Escherichia coli*—presence/absence

If only information on presence or absence of the organisms is required, the following method can be used.

Procedure

(a) Inoculate 10 mL of the sample if liquid or 10^{-1} food homogenate if solid to 10 mL of double strength liquid medium containing an inverted Durham fermentation tube, as described in method 3.

(b) Proceed as described in steps (b)–(e) of method 3.

Method 5 *Escherichia coli*—direct enumeration using membranes

The use of membranes and solid media allows rapid enumeration of *E. coli* and incorporates a resuscitation stage to permit recovery of injured *E. coli* cells [38]. The method described is based on ISO 6391 (BS 5763 Part 13) [39] and BS ISO 11866-3 [36,40].

Media

Non-selective agar: e.g. minerals modified glutamate agar (MMGB solidified with agar) or tryptone soya agar.

Selective agar: tryptone bile agar.

Procedure

(a) Prepare a 10^{-1} food homogenate and serial decimal dilutions as described in Sections 4.2 and 4.3.

(b) Using sterile forceps place cellulose ester membranes, 85 mm diameter and 0.45–1.2 µm pore size with working surface (dull side) uppermost, onto the surface of plates of a non-selective agar taking care to avoid trapping air bubbles beneath the membrane. Smooth over the membrane surfaces with a sterile spreader. Use sufficient plates for the range of decimal dilutions selected for testing.

(c) Inoculate 1 mL of the 10^{-1} food homogenate or dilution on to the centre of the membrane. Spread this inoculum over the whole membrane surface, using a sterile spreader, taking care not to spill over the membrane edge. Allow the inoculum to soak in by leaving at room temperature for 15 min

(d) Incubate plates with the membrane/agar surface uppermost at 37°C for 4 h.

continued

(e) Transfer the membranes aseptically to plates of tryptone bile agar (do NOT smooth over the membrane surface).

(f) Incubate at 44±1°C for 18–24 h. Do not invert the plates.

(g) Remove the Petri dish lid, and place 2 mL of Vracko and Sherris [41] indole reagent (5% *p*-dimethylaminobenzaldehyde in 1 M hydrochloric acid) in the lid.

(h) Remove the membrane from the agar surface and lower it on to the indole reagent so that the whole of the lower surface of the membrane is wetted. After 5 min, pipette off the excess indole reagent.

(i) Develop the indole reaction by exposing the treated membrane to strong sunlight or ultraviolet light (366 nm) for 30 min.

(j) Count the number of pink-red (indole positive) colonies, selecting plates containing up to 150 pink colonies, and calculate the level of *E. coli* per g of food sample.

Method 6 β-glucuronidase positive *Escherichia coli*

Most strains of *E. coli* express the enzyme β-glucuronidase, the activity of which can be demonstrated by the cleavage of fluorogenic or chromogenic substrates. Fluorogenic methods use the substrate 4-methylumbelliferyl β-D-glucuronide (MUG), which is cleaved to form 4-methylumbelliferone with the production of blue/white fluorescence under ultraviolet light at 366 nm (see Plate IV, facing p. 150). The addition of MUG to conventional media for the detection of *E. coli* at a concentration of 50 mg/L for liquid media and 100 mg/L for agar media can be used to provide presumptive evidence of the presence of *E. coli* which should be confirmed by further biochemical tests. An example of the use of MUG is described in Section 7.4, method 1. Chromogenic methods use the substrate 5-bromo-4-chloro-3-indolyl β-D-glucuronide (BCIG or X-β-D-glucuronide) which when cleaved forms insoluble coloured hydrolysis products and glucuronic acid. *E. coli* absorbs the substrate and strains producing β-glucuronidase form coloured colonies on agar media containing the substrate (see Plate IVb). Incubation at 44°C in the presence of bile salts provides highly specific conditions.

Method 7 Detection of β-glucuronidase positive *Escherichia coli* — membrane method

The procedure in Part 1 of BS ISO 16649 [42] is identical to that in ISO 6391 [39] and BS ISO 11866-3 [40] except that the trypone bile agar is supplemented with BCIG. If glucuronidase positive *E. coli* is present, blue colonies are formed. No confirmation is required.

Media
As for method 5, and in addition:
Tryptone bile agar containing 144 μmol BCIG (e.g. 0.075 g/L of cyclohexammonium salt) (TBX/TBG agar).

Procedure
Follow method 5 from step (a) to step (f). Count the number of blue or blue-green colonies in plates containing up to 300 colonies in total (blue and colourless). Calculate the count per g of β-glucuronidase positive *E. coli*.

Method 8 Detection of β-glucuronidase positive *Escherichia coli* — pour plate method

Part 2 of BS ISO 16649 [43] describes a pour plate method using TBX agar for detection of β-glucuronidase positive *E. coli*. Incubation is performed throughout at 44°C, although the option is given of initial incubation at 37°C for 4 h if stressed organisms are likely to be present. Because of this the method may not recover stressed organisms; for example, those present in frozen foods and dried foods.

Media
TBX agar.

Procedure
(a) Prepare a 10^{-1} food homogenate and serial decimal dilutions as described in Sections 4.2 and 4.3.
(b) Transfer 1 mL volumes of each dilution to Petri dishes. To each plate, add 15–20 mL of molten TBX agar cooled to 44–47°C. Mix carefully and allow to set.
(c) Incubate at 44°C for 20–24 h (or at 37°C for 4 h followed by incubation at 44°C for 16–20 h).
(d) Count the number of blue or blue-green colonies in plates containing up to 300 colonies in total.
(e) Calculate the count per g as described in Section 5.3.

Method 9 Enumeration of β-glucuronidase positive *Escherichia coli* — surface plate method

For routine purposes, pre-poured plates of TBX agar may be used in conjunction with a surface method of enumeration [44].

Media
TBX agar.

Procedure
(a) Prepare a 10^{-1} food homogenate and serial decimal dilutions if required as described in Sections 4.2 and 4.3.
(b) Select a surface counting method from Section 5 (eg: 5.4–5.6) and enumerate using pre-poured TBX plates.
(c) Incubate the plates at 30°C for 4 h, followed by incubation at 44°C for 16–20 h.
(d) Count the number of blue or blue-green colonies in plates containing up to 300 colonies in total.
(e) Calculate the count per g as described in Section 5.

> If it is not possible to transfer plates between the two incubation temperatures the plates may be incubated at 37°C throughout. However any blue colonies that are formed should be subjected to confirmation by indole testing (see Section 10.10).

Method 10 *Escherichia coli* — specific detection of O157

The verocytotoxin producing strain *E. coli* O157 (VTEC) is a food-borne pathogen causing symptoms ranging from mild diarrhoea to haemorrhagic colitis (HC) and haemolytic uraemic syndrome (HUS). Most outbreaks have been linked with consumption of undercooked beef or dairy products [45], including raw milk. This serotype of *E. coli* is unusual in that it grows poorly at 44°C and does not possess the enzyme β-glucuronidase. The methods described are relevant when suspect foods are being investigated following the diagnosis of HC or HUS or if surveillance of foods is being undertaken specifically for this organism. Enrichment methods are recommended as illness may be caused by very low levels of the organism in food. Recovery is enhanced by the use of immunomagnetic separation (IMS), which separates and concentrates the target O157 cells by the use of immunomagnetic beads coated with *E. coli* O157 antiserum [46].

Safety note

Escherichia coli O157 is a Hazard Group 3 organism. Appropriate containment conditions should be used when handling food samples that are likely to contain this organism. Containment conditions are also recommended if a manual IMS technique is used.

Enrichment culture [47]

Media

Selective broth: tryptone soya broth containing bile salts no. 3 1.5 g, dipotassium hydrogen orthophosphate 1.5 g, novobiocin 20 mg/L.

Selective agars: tellurite cefixime sorbitol MacConkey agar (TC-SMAC) [48]; sorbitol MacConkey agar containing potassium tellurite 2.5 mg/L and cefixime 0.05 mg/L; sorbitol MacConkey agar; chromogenic O157 agars.

Non-selective agar: Nutrient agar; MacConkey agar; cystine-lactose-electrolyte-deficient (CLED) agar.

Procedure

(a) Prepare a 10^{-1} food homogenate in selective broth as described in Sections 4.2 and 4.3.

(b) Incubate at 41.5°C for 18–24 h.

(c) After 6 h and 18–24 h, subculture directly to TC-SMAC and a second selective agar of choice. In addition perform immunomagnetic separation (see below) and subculture the beads to TC-SMAC and a second medium of choice.

(d) Incubate the plates at 37°C for 18–24 h.

(e) Examine the plates for the presence of typical colonies, which on TC-SMAC and SMAC appear as transparent and almost colourless with a pale yellowish-brown tinge (see Plate IVa, facing p. 150). If present subculture five such colonies to a non-selective agar and incubate at 37°C for 18–24 h.

continued

(f) Confirm the growth obtained biochemically by performing an indole test (see Section 10.10).

(g) Perform serological tests on indole positive strains using O157 antiserum or a suitable latex kit.

(h) Send strains that give a positive agglutination to a reference laboratory for confirmation and determination of verocytotoxin production (see Appendix C).

Immunomagnetic separation (immunocapture)

(i) Transfer 20 μL of resuspended paramagnetic beads coated with *E. coli* O157 antiserum to a 1.5 mL screw top Eppendorf tube.

(ii) Add 1 mL of enrichment culture obtained in step (c) to the tube and close with a screw cap.

(iii) Vortex each tube briefly and place on the sample mixer. Rotate the tubes gently at 12–20 rev/min for 10 min at room temperature.

(iv) Place the tube in a magnetic rack with the magnet in place and allow the magnetic particles to congregate against the magnet (about 3 min).

(v) Gently rotate and invert the rack through 180° to concentrate the beads into a small pellet.

(vi) Remove the screw cap carefully and remove the liquid from the bottom of the tube using a fine-tipped pipette, taking care not to disturb the magnetic particles.

(vii) Add 1 mL of wash buffer (phosphate buffered saline pH 7.4 containing 0.05% Tween 20) and replace cap. Remove the magnet from the rack and gently rotate and invert the rack through 180°.

(viii) Return the magnet to the rack, then repeat steps (iii) to (vii) at least twice more.

(ix) Aspirate the liquid and remove the magnet. Add 100 μL of wash buffer and resuspend by using a vortex mixer.

(x) Transfer 50 μL of the contents to TC-SMAC and 50 μL to the second selective agar of choice and proceed as described in steps (d)–(h).

Enumeration

Enumeration is not normally performed unless there is a desire to establish the infective dose following reported illness. In most instances the organisms in the food are likely to be stressed and so a liquid enrichment procedure is more suitable.

Procedure

(a) Prepare a 10^{-1} homogenate of the food and decimal dilutions (if required) in selective broth (see enrichment culture method) as described in Sections 4.2 and 4.3.

(b) Select a multiple tube counting method from Section 5.7 and proceed as described for enrichment culture.

(c) Calculate the number of *E. coli* O157/g of food from the number of tubes yielding positive growth.

6.7 Enterobacteriaceae

Coliform tests will only detect organisms capable of fermenting lactose. If large numbers of lactose-negative bacilli are also present, the performance of coliform tests may lead to falsely assuring results. In addition, many food pathogens do not ferment lactose. Thus, examining a sample for the presence of members of the family Enterobacteriaceae, a well-defined group of organisms, instead of for coliforms, an ill-defined group, may give a better indication of the likelihood of pathogen presence, as well as providing more accurate information about the handling and storage of the food commodity.

Control cultures

NCTC 9001	*Escherichia coli*	Positive, growth quantitative
NCTC 10975	*Proteus mirabilis*	Positive, growth quantitative
NCTC 6571	*Staphylococcus aureus*	Negative, growth inhibited

Method 1 Colony count method

The following pour plate method helps to suppress the growth of non-fermentative organisms. It is based on BS 5763 Part 10 [49] and ISO 21528-3 [50]. Surface methods are also suitable using pre-poured plates of VRBGA, but may allow greater growth of competing non-fermentative bacilli.

Media
Violet red bile glucose agar (VRBGA)
Tubes of glucose agar
Non-selective medium: e.g. nutrient agar.

Procedure
(a) Prepare a 10^{-1} homogenate and decimal dilutions of the food as described in Sections 4.2 and 4.3.
(b) Transfer 1 mL aliquots of each dilution to separate Petri dishes, add 10–15 mL of molten, cooled VRBGA, mix and allow to set. Overlay the solidified medium with a further 10 mL of molten, cooled VRBGA and allow to set.
(c) Invert the plates and incubate at 37°C for 24 ± 2 h.
(d) Count pink to red-purple colonies of diameter 0.5 mm or more with or without haloes of precipitation (see Plate V, facing p. 150).
(e) Confirm the identity of five such colonies by subculture onto a non-selective medium and incubation at 37°C for 24 ± 4 h.
(f) Test each strain for oxidase reaction (see Section 10.14). Perform a fermentation test on oxidase-negative strains by stab inoculating tubes of glucose agar and incubating at 37°C for 24 ± 4 h. If the medium changes colour throughout the tube the strain is fermentative and may be considered to be a member of the family Enterobacteriaceae.
(g) Use the proportion of five colonies confirmed as Enterobacteriaceae to calculate the number of Enterobacteriaceae present as described in Section 5.3, using plates containing up to 150 colonies.

Method 2 Detection method with pre-enrichment

ISO 8523 [51] describes the detection of Enterobacteriaceae using a pre-enrichment step to aid resuscitation. It is suitable for presence/absence testing in a defined weight of sample. The method can be adapted for enumeration by using the same media in a nine-tube test as described in Section 5.7.

Media

Pre-enrichment medium: buffered peptone water.
Enrichment medium: buffered brilliant green bile glucose broth (EE broth).
Plating medium: violet red bile glucose agar (VRBGA).

Procedure

(a) Weigh a known amount of sample and add to 10 times its weight of buffered peptone water.
(b) Incubate this suspension at 37°C for 18±2h.
(c) Transfer 1 mL of the pre-enrichment culture to 10 mL of EE broth. Incubate at 37°C for 18–24 h.
(d) Subculture the incubated EE broth to a pre-poured plate of VRBGA. Incubate at 37°C for 24 h.
(e) Examine the VRBGA plate for the presence of characteristic pink to red-purple colonies.
(f) If present, confirm the identity of the colonies following steps (e) and (f) of method 1.

Method 3 Multiple tube method for enumeration

ISO 21528 Part 2 [52] describes an enumeration method for Enterobacteriaceae using a multiple tube procedure without pre-enrichment.

Media

Buffered brilliant green bile glucose broth (EE broth)
Violet red bile glucose agar (VRBGA).

Procedure

(a) Prepare a 10^{-1} homogenate and decimal dilutions of the food as described in Sections 4.2 and 4.3.
(b) Inoculate 1 mL aliquots of the 10^{-1} homogenate and dilutions into EE broth as described in Section 5.7, method 3. Incubate the tubes at 37°C for 24±2h.
(c) Subculture each tube to a pre-poured plate of VRBGA. Incubate at 37°C for 24±2h.
(d) Examine the VRBGA plates for the presence of characteristic pink to red-purple colonies. If present confirm their identity following steps (e) and (f) of method 1.
(g) Compute the count per g from the number of tubes yielding growth of Enterobacteriaceae.

6.8 Enterococci

The enterococci mainly originate in the intestinal tracts of many animals, and so are sometimes used as marker organisms of faecal contamination, although their use is not as straightforward as *E. coli* [53,54]. This group of organisms includes some of the strains formerly known as Lancefield Group D streptococci. Enterococci are more resistant to adverse conditions than Enterobacteriaceae and so may survive longer in the food processing environment. In particular they are relatively heat resistant and can grow over a wide temperature range, sometimes leading to food spoilage. They are used as an index of sanitation and proper holding conditions.

Enterococci are Gram positive cocci that occur in pairs or short chains. They are aerobic, facultatively anaerobic, non-sporing, generally non-motile, catalase and oxidase negative and attack carbohydrates fermentatively. The most common strains in food are *E. faecalis* and *E. faecium*. The enumeration method described below is based on the method described in BS 4285 Section 3.11 [55].

Control cultures

NCTC 775	*Enterococcus faecalis*	Positive, growth quantitative
NCTC 9001	*Escherichia coli*	Negative, growth inhibited

Media

Detection: KF streptococcus agar or Slanetz and Bartley glucose azide agar.
Confirmation: Aesculin-containing agar, e.g. kanamycin aesculin azide agar.

Procedure

(a) Prepare a 10^{-1} food homogenate and serial decimal dilutions as described in Sections 4.2 and 4.3.

(b) Using the 10^{-1} homogenate and suitable dilutions enumerate by either the pour plate (see Section 5.3) or a suitable surface method chosen from Section 5 (eg: 5.4–5.6) with the selected detection medium.

(c) Incubate the plates at 37°C for 48±2 h.

(d) Count all red, maroon or pink colonies (see Plate VIa,b, facing p. 150.). This will give the presumptive enterococci count per g.

continued

(e) Confirm the identity of the colonies by subculture to an aesculin-containing agar followed by incubation at 44°C for 18–24 h (see Plate VIc, facing p. 150). Test aesculin positive colonies for their catalase reaction (see Section 10.3). Enterococci are catalase negative, Gram positive cocci that can grow at 44°C in the presence of bile and hydrolyse aesculin.

(g) Count the confirmed colonies of enterococci and calculate the number of colony forming units per g.

Warning note

The media contain sodium azide. Precautions must be taken to prevent inhalation or ingestion of dust. Always wear a mask, gloves and eye protection when handling these powders.

Sodium azide reacts with many metals to form explosive metal azides. Copious water should be used when disposing of azide-containing compounds down sinks, drains or waste disposal units.

6.9 Lactobacilli and the lactic acid bacteria

The lactic acid bacteria are a group of Gram positive, catalase negative, fermentative organisms that produce large amounts of lactic acid. They include members of the genera *Lactobacillus*, *Streptococcus*, *Leuconostoc* and *Pediococcus*. Owing to their widespread distribution, their microaerophilic nature, and their ability to grow at low temperatures and at low pH, they play a major role in the spoilage of meat and a wide range of other food, especially vacuum-packaged commodities [56]. Certain strains of lactobacilli and streptococci are also used in the manufacture of fermented foods including yoghurt, cheese, continental sausages and fermented vegetables. The relative proportions of lactobacilli and streptococci usually need to be similar to produce the required flavour and acidity.

Control cultures

NCTC 6681	*Lactococcus lactis*	Positive, growth quantitative *Lactobacillus streptococcus* (L-S, differential medium)
NCTC 12712	*Lactobacillus delbrueckii Ssp. bulgaricus*	Positive, growth quantitative
NCTC 6571	*Staphylococcus aureus*	Negative, growth inhibited
NCTC 9001	*Escherichia coli*	Negative, growth inhibited (de Man, Rogosa, Sharpe: MRS agar)

Enumeration of lactobacilli or lactic acid bacteria

Recovery of lactic acid bacteria will depend on the temperature of incubation and the pH of the medium. BS ISO 15214 [57], on which this method is based, specifies a medium of pH 5.7 and an incubation temperature of 30°C. These conditions may not recover all lactic acid bacteria; incubation at 22–25°C may be used for psychrotrophic organisms whilst the use of a medium at pH 6.2–6.5 may increase recovery. Growth may also be enhanced by incubation under microaerobic conditions or addition of an overlay to the poured plates.

Media

de Man, Rogosa, Sharpe (MRS) agar.

Procedure

(a) Prepare a 10^{-1} homogenate and serial decimal dilutions of the food as described in Sections 4.2 and 4.3.

(b) Place 1 mL of the 10^{-1} homogenate and each dilution into separate Petri dishes. Add 15 mL of molten MRS agar cooled to 45°C to each plate. Mix thoroughly and allow to set.

(c) Incubate at 30°C for 72 ± 3 h.

(d) Count the colonies of each colonial type on plates containing up to 150 colonies. Perform Gram staining if necessary to confirm morphology. Compute the number of lactobacilli/lactic acid bacteria per g of food.

MRS agar will recover lactic acid bacteria (see Plate VIIc, facing p. 150) and will also allow the growth of yeasts. Differentiation of the lactic acid group and lactobacilli in particular can be achieved by examining films of different colonial forms by optical microscopy.

6.10 *Listeria monocytogenes* and other *Listeria* spp. [58–65]

Listeriae are Gram positive, short, non-sporing rods, catalase positive, oxidase negative and facultatively anaerobic. They are motile at 22°C, showing a characteristic tumbling motility, but non-motile at 37°C. Of the six species currently recognized, *L. monocytogenes* is the most important causing a range of infections in humans and animals. The organism can be found in a wide variety of habitats including the soil, food processing environments and raw foods. The ability of the organism to grow at refrigeration temperatures is of importance in food production.

Microbiological specifications for food items often stipulate absence of *L. monocytogenes* in 25 g of food sample. Enrichment culture is therefore necessary to determine this low level. Members of the genus *Listeria* are ubiquitous in the environment and so this specification is stringent. For foods with a remaining short shelf-life of a few days and when a food item has been incriminated as a source of *L. monocytogenes* infection it may also be useful to assess the extent of contamination. This may be done by direct enumeration of the organism on solid media, which may not recover injured cells, or by a most probable number method in liquid media. While other members of the *Listeria* genus are not implicated in disease, their presence indicates an increased risk of contamination by *L. monocytogenes*.

Numerous enrichment and isolation media have been described for the isolation of *Listeria* spp.

Chromogenic plating media have now been developed that allow good differentiation between *L. monocytogenes* and other *Listeria* species. The methods described below are those most commonly used.

Control cultures

NCTC 11994	*L. monocytogenes*	Positive, growth quantitative
NCTC 775	*Enterococcus faecalis*	Negative, growth inhibited
NCTC 9528	*Klebsiella aerogenes*	Negative, growth inhibited

Method 1 Enrichment culture

BS EN ISO 11290-1 [58] describes a two-stage enrichment method for detection of *L. monocytogenes* with isolation on PALCAM [59] agar and Oxford [60] agar. It will also recover other strains of *Listeria*. It is currently being rewritten to include the use of a chromogenic medium to allow better detection of *L. monocytogenes* in the presence of other *Listeria* species (see below).

Media
Selective primary enrichment medium: half Fraser broth (contains nalidixic acid sodium salt 10 mg/L and acriflavine hydrochloride 12.5 mg/L).

Selective secondary enrichment medium: Fraser broth (contains nalidixic acid sodium salt 20 mg/L and acriflavine hydrochloride 25 mg/L).

Selective agars: polymyxin, acriflavin, lithium chloride, ceftazidime, aesculin, mannitol (PALCAM) agar and Oxford agar.

Non-selective agar: e.g. blood agar, nutrient agar, tryptone soya yeast extract agar.

Procedure
(a) Homogenize 25 g of food sample with 225 mL of half Fraser broth as described in Section 4.2.
(b) Incubate the half Fraser broth at 30°C for 24±2 h.
(c) Subculture to Oxford agar and PALCAM agar; incubate the plates at 30°C or 37°C for a total of 42–48 h. Note: incubation at 37°C may inhibit the growth of some strains of *Listeria* species other than *L. monocytogenes* [61].
(d) Subculture 1 mL of half Fraser broth to 10 mL of Fraser broth; incubate at 37°C for 48±2 h.
(e) Subculture Fraser broth to Oxford and PALCAM agar; incubate the plates at 30°C or 37°C.
(f) Examine all agar plates after 24 h and 42–48 h of incubation for the presence of typical colonies.

continued

Strains of *Listeria* species hydrolyse aesculin, producing black zones around the colonies (see Plate VIIIa,b, facing p. 150). After 48 h incubation, typical colonies are 2–3 mm diameter with a sunken centre.

(g) Subculture five typical colonies (or all if fewer than five) onto a non-selective agar; incubate at 30°C or 37°C for 18–24 h. Ensure that representatives of each colonial form are selected.

(h) Confirm the identity of these strains using appropriate biochemical tests (see Section 10). Typical reactions are shown in Table 6.8.

(i) Strains identified as *Listeria* spp. can be further characterized using the reactions shown in Table 6.9.

Table 6.8 Reactions of the genus *Listeria*.

Test	Result
Gram stain	Gram positive rods
Voges Proskaüer test	+
Urease	−
Catalase	+
Oxidase	−
Aesculin hydrolysis	+
D-glucose fermentation	Acid no gas
D-salicin fermentation	Acid no gas
Motility at 22°C	+ tumbling

Table 6.9 Differentiation of *Listeria* spp.

	β-haemolysis on blood agar	Nitrate reduction	Acid produced from: D-mannitol	L-rhamnose	D-xylose	MM	CAMP test with: S. aureus	R. equi
L. monocytogenes*	+	−	−	+	−	+	+	−
L. ivanovii	++	−	−	−	+	−	−	+
L. innocua	−	−	−	V	−	+	−	−
L. welshimeri	−	−	−	V	+	+	−	−
L. seeligeri	(+)	−	−	−	+	V	(+)	−
L. grayi	−	−	+	−	−	NS	−	−
L. murrayi (now a subspecies of L. grayi)	−	+	+	V	−	NS	−	−

*A few strains of *L. monocytogenes* are rhamnose negative while 60% of *L. innocua* are rhamnose positive.

MM, α methyl-D-mannoside (methyl α-D-mannopyranoside); V, variable reaction; NS, not stated; (+), weak reaction.

Note that *L. denitrificans* has been reclassified, it is now in a separate genus and known as *Jonesia denitrificans*.

Method 2 Enrichment culture

This method is based on an International Dairy Federation (IDF) method [62] for milk and dairy products and is similar to BS 4285 Section 3.15 [63] except that the content of acriflavine hydrochloride has been reduced to 10 mg/L.

Media

Selective primary enrichment medium: Modified tryptone soya broth containing yeast extract 6 g/L made selective by the addition of acriflavine hydrochloride (10 mg/L), nalidixic acid sodium salt (40 mg/L) and cycloheximide (50 mg/L).

Selective agar: Oxford agar (PALCAM agar may also be used if desired).

Non-selective agar: e.g. blood agar, nutrient agar, tryptone soya yeast extract agar.

Procedure
(a) Homogenize 25 g of food sample with 225 mL of modified tryptone soya broth as described in Section 4.2.
(b) Incubate at 30°C for 48±2 h.
(c) Subculture from the enrichment broth after 24 h and 48 h incubation on to Oxford agar (and PALCAM agar if desired).
(d) Incubate plates at 37°C for 48 h. If species other than *L. monocytogenes* are sought, incubate plates at 30°C. Examine for the presence of typical colonies after 24 h and 48 h.
(e) Subculture five typical colonies (or all colonies if fewer than five) onto a non-selective agar, and incubate at 37°C or 30°C for 24±2 h.
(f) Confirm the identity of these strains as described in method 1.

Method 3 Enumeration by plate method

Part 2 of ISO 11290 [64] describes enumeration of *L. monocytogenes* on PALCAM agar; however, international studies [65] were unable to demonstrate a significant difference in performance between Oxford and PALCAM media, and studies in the editors' own laboratory (Greenwood, pers. comm.) have demonstrated greater recovery using Oxford agar for enumeration.

Procedure
(a) Prepare a 10^{-1} homogenate of food sample and serial decimal dilutions as described in Sections 4.2 and 4.3, or use the homogenate prepared in step (a) of method 1 or method 2. Stand for 1 h±5 min at 20±2°C to allow resuscitation of stressed organisms.
(b) Select a surface counting method from Section 5 (eg: 5.4–5.6), and enumerate on Oxford or PALCAM agar. Incubate at 37°C or 30°C for 42–48 h.
(c) Count the number of typical colonies on plates containing up to 150 colonies.
(d) Subculture five typical colonies and confirm as described in steps (g)–(i) of method 1.
(e) Use the number of *L. monocytogenes* or total *Listeria* species (including *L. monocytogenes*) to calculate the count per g of food.

Method 4 Enumeration by multiple tube method

If it is likely that the food product contains highly stressed cells of *Listeria*, it may be preferable to use a liquid culture method for enumeration to allow resuscitation. Use a most probable number method selected from Section 5.7 and the procedure described in method 1 to obtain a most probable number/g.

Specialist tests for serotyping and phage typing of *L. monocytogenes* are available (see Appendix C).

> **Precautionary note**
> The pregnant woman should be prohibited from working with known cultures of *Listeria* spp. Cycloheximide is a Schedule 1 poison, and both cycloheximide and acriflavine may cause skin and eye irritation. Powders should be weighed in a fume cupboard, and gloves worn when handling. Antibiotic supplements are available commercially, which will obviate the need to weigh the powders. Although these substances are less hazardous when in solution, contact should be avoided.

Use of chromogenic media

Chromogenic media are available for isolation of *Listeria* species and distinction of *L. monocytogenes* from other strains. These media enhance the detection of *L. monocytogenes*, particularly in food products that contain more than one species of *Listeria*. One type of medium produces blue colonies due to β-glucosidase activity if *Listeria* species are present with differentiation between the species on the basis of phospholipase activity. Strains possessing phospholipase activity require further testing for the presence of an aminopeptidase that acts on alanine substituted substrates; this enzyme is absent in strains of *L. monocytogenes* but present in other species of *Listeria*. The other type of medium produces blue colonies due to phospholipase activity and distinguishes between phospholipase producing strains on the basis of xylose fermentation.

6.11 *Pseudomonas aeruginosa* and other pseudomonads

Pseudomonas species are aerobic, oxidase positive, catalase positive, non-fermentative Gram negative rods that are motile with polar flagella. Some species attack sugars by oxidation and produce a diffusible fluorescent pigment; others produce alkali. The psychrotrophic strains are low-temperature spoilage organisms of fresh egg, fish, meat and milk and are found widely in the soil, water and vegetation. *Ps. aeruginosa* is a thermotrophic organism that commonly causes eye and ear infections as well as wound infections in other sites. It can sometimes be found in food, soil and water and should be regarded as a hygiene parameter; it is not thought to cause gastrointestinal illness.

Council Directive 80/777/EEC [66] requires that *Ps. aeruginosa* is absent in any 250 mL of mineral water sample examined. It is also desirable that water used in the production of food and drink should be free of *Ps. aeruginosa*. The detection of pseudomonads other than *Ps. aeruginosa*, such as the psychrophilic strains found in chilled foods and processing plants, is also described.

Control culture

NCTC 10662	*Pseudomonas aeruginosa*	Positive, growth quantitative
NCTC 10661	*Pseudomonas cepacia*	Positive, growth quantitative
NCTC 9001	*Escherichia coli*	Negative, growth inhibited
NCTC 10038	*Pseudomonas fluorescens*	Negative, growth inhibited (cetrimide milk agar at 42°C)

Method 1 Enumeration of *Ps. aeruginosa* in water [51]

Media
Pseudomonas cetrimide, malidixic acid (CN) agar: pseudomonas agar base containing glycerol 10 mL/L and made selective by inclusion of cetyltrimethyl ammonium bromide (cetrimide; 200 mg/L) and nalidixic acid sodium salt (15 mg/L).

Milk cetrimide agar: milk agar containing cetrimide (200 mg/L) [53].

Procedure
(a) Filter the test volume of water through a membrane having a pore size of 0.45 μm using membrane filtration apparatus as described in Section 5.2.
(b) Transfer the membrane to the surface of a pseudomonas CN plate.
(c) Incubate in a closed container at 37°C for 44–48 h

> If problems are encountered due to the high level of other pseudomonads in the sample, incubation may be performed at 30°C for 4 h followed by incubation at 42°C for the remainder of the incubation period to improve selectivity for *Ps. aeruginosa*.

(d) Count all colonies that produce pyocyanin or pyorubin (blue–green or reddish-brown pigment), and those which fluoresce under ultraviolet light.
(e) Colonies that exhibit these characteristics may be regarded as *Ps. aeruginosa*. Non-pigmented, non-fluorescing strains may be confirmed by subculture to milk cetrimide agar followed by incubation at 42°C for 24 h. Parallel incubation at 37°C may be desirable to demonstrate casein hydrolysis which appears as clearing around the growth.
(f) Organisms that grow at 42°C within 24 h and hydrolyse casein are confirmed as *Ps. aeruginosa*.

Method 2 Enumeration of other pseudomonads (food and environmental samples) [67]

Media

Pseudomonas cetrimide fucidin cephaloridine (CFC) agar: pseudomonas agar base containing glycerol (10 mL/L) and the selective agents cetrimide (10 mg/L), cephaloridine (50 mg/L) and fucidin (10 mg/L).

Procedure

(a) Prepare a 10^{-1} homogenate and serial decimal dilutions of the food as described in Sections 4.2 and 4.3.

(b) Use the 10^{-1} homogenate and suitable dilutions with a surface method of enumeration (eg: Section 5, method 5.4–5.6) on pseudomonas CFC agar.

(c) Incubate at 25°C for 48±2 h.

(d) Count all the colonies that develop on this medium and confirm their identity as pseudomonads by oxidase testing (see Section 10.14).

(e) Test oxidase positive colonies by stab inoculating tubes of glucose agar and incubating at 25°C for 24 h. Tubes that show no colour change or only show a colour change at the top surface of the agar are regarded as *Pseudomonas* spp.

6.12   *Salmonella* spp.

The salmonellae belong to a genus of the family Enterobacteriaceae. They are Gram negative, facultatively anaerobic, non-spore forming rods. Motile forms have peritrichous flagella. They are usually catalase positive, oxidase negative and reduce nitrates to nitrites. Currently a single species, *S. enterica*, is recognized and has been subdivided into seven subspecies. Each subspecies is divided into serovars based on O and H antigens. Subspecies 1, enterica, which corresponds to the old subgenus 1, contains the typical pathogenic salmonellae isolated from the intestinal contents of warm blooded animals. Salmonellae are recognized as a major cause of enteric fever and gastroenteritis. Many foods, particularly those of animal origin, have been recognized as vehicles for transmitting the organisms to humans and to the food processing and preparation environment.

The presence of salmonellae in food that is ready to eat is considered significant regardless of the level of contamination. Isolation is therefore achieved by enrichment culture of a defined mass or volume of food. The level of contamination in dried foods may be very low; therefore the mass of food examined should be increased accordingly. Incorporation of a pre-enrichment resuscitation stage is recommended in the examination of frozen, dried or otherwise processed foods, to allow recovery of injured cells. Numerous media are available for isolation of salmonellae; the following methods include those media most commonly used.

Control cultures

NCTC 4840	*Salmonella poona*	Positive, growth quantitative
NCTC 9001	*Escherichia coli*	Negative, growth inhibited
NCTC 9750	*Citrobacter freundii*	Negative, growth inhibited (bismuth sulphite agar)
NCTC 10975	*Proteus mirabilis*	Negative, growth inhibited (brilliant green agar)

Method 1 Pre-enrichment and enrichment culture

RV @ 42°C/SC @ 37°C

This method is based on BS EN 12824 [68]. The method will recover all strains of *Salmonella* likely to cause illness.

Media

Pre-enrichment broth: buffered (1%) peptone water.

Enrichment broths: Rappaport Vassiliadis (RV) broth.
Selenite cystine (SC) broth.

Selective agar media: modified brilliant green agar (BGA) and a second agar selected from xylose lysine desoxycholate agar (XLD), desoxycholate citrate agar (DCA, Hynes modification), salmonella-shigella agar (SS), brilliant green MacConkey agar (BGM), bismuth sulphite agar (BS), mannitol lysine crystal violet brilliant green agar (MLCB) and chromogenic media specific for salmonellae. Bismuth sulphite and MLCB agars also detect lactose-fermenting salmonellae.

Procedure

(a) Homogenize 25 g of food sample with 225 mL of buffered peptone water. If a larger food sample is required, maintain a sample-to-broth ratio of 1 : 9. Incubate at 37°C for 18±2 h.

> For certain products the addition of various substances to the pre-enrichment broth or adjustment of the ratio of sample to broth can improve isolation. Examples of these are listed in Table 6.10.

(b) Subculture to RV and SC broths; add 0.1 mL to 10 mL of RV medium, and 1 mL to 10 mL of SC broth. Incubate the RV at 42°C and the SC at 37°C for 20–24 h.

(c) Subculture a loopful of each broth to two selective agar media.

> Extension of incubation time of the inoculated enrichment media to 48 h with subculture to selective agar plates after 24 h and 48 h may improve recovery of salmonellae.

(d) Incubate plates at 37°C for 20–24 h. Bismuth sulphite agar plates should be incubated for up to 48 h.

continued

Table 6.10 Additions/adjustments to *Salmonella* enrichment broths.

Product	Addition/adjustment	Purpose
High-fat foods, e.g. cheese	Surfactant (e.g. tergitol 7, 1.0% with lactose broth 0.22% with BPW)	Aids dispersion of food
Onion and garlic	Potassium sulphite (0.5% final concentration)	Reduces natural bactericidal properties
Cocoa powder and chocolate confectionery	Casein (5% final concentration); 10% (w/v) non-fat dried milk	Reduces natural bactericidal properties
High-salt/sugar	Reduce sample : broth ratio (amount will depend on initial salt/sugar concentration)	Maintains salts or sugar foods concentration at <2%
Oregano, cinnamon, cloves, allspice	Reduce sample : broth ratio to 1:100 or 1:1000	Reduces inhibitory properties
High-acid/alkaline products	Adjust pH to 6.6–7.0 prior to incubation	Neutralizes effect of acid/alkali

BPW, buffered peptone water.

(e) Examine the plates for typical colonies. (See Plate IX, facing p. 150.) Select at least five suspect colonies a   propertiesnd subculture to a non-selective agar. Incubate at 37°C for 18–24 h.

(f) Screen biochemically using triple sugar iron (TSI) agar or lysine iron (LI) agar slopes in conjunction with urease and sucrose/lactose media. Incubate at 37°C for 24±2 h. Typical strains of salmonellae produce an acid (yellow) butt and an alkaline (red) slope in TSI agar and an alkaline (purple) reaction throughout the LI medium, both with blackening due to hydrogen due to hydrogen sulphide production, are urease negative and do not ferment sucrose or lactose.

(g) Presumptive isolates of *Salmonella* spp. should be further characterized biochemically, and serological tests performed using salmonella agglutinating sera.

Method 2 Pre-enrichment and enrichment culture

RVS @ 41.5°C/SC @ 37°C

This method is also based on BS EN 12824 [68] and is identical to method 1 except that it replaces Rappaport Vassiliadis broth by Rappaport Vassiliadis soya peptone broth (RVS), and the incubation temperature of the RVS medium has been reduced to 41.5°C by international agreement.

This protocol is widely used in the UK [69].

Method 3 Pre-enrichment and enrichment culture

RVS @ 41.5°C/MRTTn @ 37°C

The following method is based on ISO 6579 [70], which replaces the teratogenic selenite enrichment medium in BS EN 12824 by a tetrathionate medium. Muller–Kauffmann tetrathionate medium has been chosen to aid recovery of *Salmonella enterica* subspecies Typhi and Paratyphi.

Media

Pre-enrichment broth: buffered (1%) peptone water.

Enrichment broths: Muller–Kauffmann tetrathionate broth containing novobiocin (20 mg/L) (MKTTn); Rappaport Vassiliadis soya peptone (RVS) broth.

Selective agar media: XLD agar and a second medium of choice (see method 1).

Procedure

(a) Follow step (a) of method 1.
(b) Subculture 0.1 mL of the pre-enrichment broth to RVS broth and 1 mL to the MKTTn broth. Incubate RVS broth at 41.5°C and MKTTn broth at 37°C for 24±3 h.
(c) Subculture to XLD agar and a second medium of choice. Incubate the plates at 37°C for 24±3 h (48 h if bismuth sulphite agar is used).
(d) Follow steps (d)–(g) in method 1.

Method 4 Pre-enrichment and enrichment

If recovery of *S. enterica* subspecies Typhi and Paratyphi is not required, the Muller–Kauffmann tetrathionate medium used in method 4 can be replaced by the tetrathionate formulation specified in the US *Pharmacopoeia* [71].

Method 5 Direct enrichment

If the food to be examined is likely to be heavily contaminated a pre-enrichment stage may not be necessary.

Media

Enrichment broth: select from any of the enrichment broths given in methods 1, 2 and 3.

Selective agars: select two agars from those given in method 1.

Procedure

(a) Homogenize 50 g of food sample in 450 mL of a suitable enrichment medium. Divide the homogenate into two portions. Incubate one portion at 37°C and the other portion at 41.5°C for 48 h.

continued

(b) Subculture from the two portions after 24 h and 48 h to two selective agar media and proceed as described in steps (c)–(g) of method 1.

or

(a) Homogenize 25 g of food sample in 225 mL each of two different enrichment media. Incubate at the temperatures appropriate to the media for up to 48 h.

(b) Subculture from the two media after 24 h and 48 h to two selective agar media and proceed as described in steps (c)–(g) of method 1.

Method 6 Enumeration

Occasionally it may be desirable to quantify the level of *Salmonella* contamination in a food. The following method may be used.

Media

Pre-enrichment broth: buffered (1%) peptone water.

Enrichment broth: Rappaport Vassiliadis soya peptone broth (RVS).

Selective agar media: XLD and a second medium of choice (see method 1).

Procedure

(a) Prepare a 10^{-1} homogenate of the food in buffered peptone water, ensuring that sufficient quantity is prepared for the test.

(b) Choose a multiple tube method from Section 5.7, then aliquot the homogenate appropriately. If method 1 or 2 is chosen, aliquot into six or 10 separate volumes of 10 mL each (equivalent to 1 g per aliquot) or 100 mL each (equivalent to 10 g per aliquot). If method 3 (or method 5) is chosen the homogenate should be aliquoted into three (five) 100 mL aliquots, three (five) 10 mL aliquots and three (five) 1 mL aliquots.

(c) Incubate the aliquots at 37°C for at least 18 h and up to 24 h, depending on the nature of the product (food types of low water activity should be incubated for up to 24 h).

(d) Subculture 0.1 mL from each tube to a separate tube of RVS broth. Incubate all RVS broths at 41.5°C.

(e) Follow steps (e) to (g) described in method 1.

(h) Compute the most probable number of salmonellae per g from the appropriate table (Tables 5.5–5.7 (pp. 119–22) and 9.2–9.4 (pp. 233–8)), remembering to adjust the most probable number (MPN) value according to the weight of sample examined.

Specialized reference facilities are available for serotyping and phage typing of *Salmonella* (see Appendix C).

6.13 *Shigella* spp.

Shigella is a genus of the family Enterobacteriaceae. The organisms are Gram negative, facultatively anaerobic, non-motile and non-sporing rods. They are oxidase negative, urease negative, lactose and sucrose negative, and do not produce hydrogen sulphide. Four species are recognized—*S. sonnei*, *S. dysenteriae*, *S. flexneri* and *S. boydii*.They all cause enteritis with varying degrees of severity, including dysentery that may be fatal. The serotypes are characterized by somatic O antigens; some strains also possess heat stable K envelope antigens.

The most important reservoir of infection is the intestinal tract of humans and primates and transmission is mainly person to person by the faecal–oral route. However contaminated water and food are also significant causes of illness and a number of food-borne outbreaks have been described [72]. Very few organisms are required to cause illness, therefore they are sought by enrichment. The method described below is based on EN ISO 21567 [72].

Media

Selective enrichment medium: Shigella enrichment broth containing peptone 20 g, potassium hydrogen phosphate 2 g, potassium dihydrogen phosphate 2 g, sodium chloride 5 g, glucose 1 g, polyoxyethylenesorbitan monooleate 1.5 mL, novobiocin 0.55 mg/L.

Selective agar media: XLD, MacConkey agar and Hektoen enteric agar.

Non-selective agar: e.g. nutrient agar.

Procedure
(a) Prepare a 10^{-1} homogenate of food in shigella enrichment broth as described in Section 4.2.
(b) Incubate the enrichment broth at 41.5°C under anaerobic conditions (with the container closure loose) for 18±2 h.
(c) Subculture the enrichment broth to XLD, MacConkey and Hektoen enteric agar. Incubate the plates at 37°C for 20–24 h.
(d) Examine the plates for characteristic colonies, which appear red/cerise on XLD, colourless and lactose negative on MacConkey agar and green and moist on Hektoen agar. Subculture five suspect colonies (or all colonies if less than five) from each plate to a non-selective agar, then incubate at 37°C for 18–24 h.
(e) Screen biochemically using TSI slopes, oxidase test and motility (see Section 10). Oxidase negative, non-motile strains that form a yellow butt and red or unchanged slope without production of hydrogen sulphide should be considered as presumptive *Shigella* species. Further biochemical characterization is required to confirm their identity.
(f) Perform serological tests on presumptive isolates using shigella agglutinating sera.

Specialized reference facilities are available for serotyping and phage typing (see Appendix C).

6.14 *Staphylococcus aureus* and other coagulase positive staphylococci

Staphylococcus aureus is the type species of the genus *Staphylococcus*, which are Gram positive, facultatively anaerobic, catalase positive, coagulase positive cocci that divide in more than one plane to produce irregular clusters of cells. *Staphylococcus aureus* is a common cause of skin and wound infection in humans, and a significant proportion of the population also carries the organism as a commensal of the skin and nose. It is therefore frequently introduced into food by food handlers and indirectly by equipment. Some strains of *S. aureus* can produce a heat stable enterotoxin that may cause vomiting if high levels of an enterotoxin-producing strain are allowed to develop in food. Staphylococcal enterotoxins A–J are currently recognized. A number of other toxins are also produced. *S. aureus* may be further subdivided into biotypes and by phage and serotyping.

Other coagulase positive strains have also been identified, including *S. intermedius* from dogs and some birds and *S. hyicus* from pigs, poultry and some beef animals [73]. Differentiation requires extensive biochemical testing. The methods described below apply to coagulase positive staphylococci and not specifically *S. aureus*.

Control cultures

NCTC 6571	*Staphylococcus aureus*	Positive, growth quantitative
NCTC 11047	*Staphylococcus epidermidis*	Negative, growth inhibited
NCTC 7464	*Bacillus cereus*	Negative, growth inhibited

Method 1 Enumeration — colony count on Baird–Parker agar

This method is based on BS EN ISO 6888-1 [74], which describes the enumeration of coagulase positive staphylococci using Baird–Parker medium with confirmation of colonies by a positive coagulase test result. The medium allows resuscitation of stressed cells with the formation of characteristic colonies.

Procedure
(a) Prepare a 10^{-1} food homogenate and serial decimal dilutions as described in Sections 4.2 and 4.3.
(b) Select a suitable surface counting method from Section 5 and enumerate on Baird–Parker agar.
(c) Incubate plates at 37°C for 48±4 h. Examine for the presence of typical colonies, which appear grey black, shiny and convex, of diameter 1–1.5 mm (24 h incubation) or up to 3 mm (48 h incubation), surrounded by a zone of clearing. After at least 24 h an opalescent ring immediately in contact with the colony may appear within the zone of clearing (see Plate X, facing p. 150). Bovine strains do not always produce these zones. Count the number of colonies of each type.
(d) Confirm the identity of the colony types by using the coagulase test and desoxyribonuclease (DNase) test (Section 10.5), subculturing to a non-selective agar medium first if necessary. Include positive and negative controls.
(e) Use the proportion of colonies confirmed as *S. aureus* to calculate the count per g.

Method 2 Enumeration—colony count using RPFA

This method is based on BS EN ISO 6888-2 [71] and is similar to method 1 except that it uses a medium, rabbit plasma fibrinogen agar (RPFA), from which the coagulase reaction can be read directly, eliminating the need for confirmation tests.

Procedure

(a) Prepare a 10^{-1} food homogenate and serial decimal dilutions as described in Sections 4.2 and 4.3.

(b) Use the pour plate method as described in Section 5.3 to enumerate using RPFA medium.

(c) Incubate the plates at 37°C for up to 48 h. Examine after 18–24 h for black, grey or even white small colonies surrounded by a halo of precipitation, indicating coagulase activity. *Proteus* colonies may show a similar appearance at the beginning of incubation but after 24 h or 48 h of incubation they may appear spreading and brownish allowing them to be distinguished from staphylococci.

(d) Count the typical colonies in each plate containing a maximum of 300 colonies and up to 100 typical colonies, and compute the count per g.

Method 3 Enumeration—most probable number technique

Part 3 of ISO 6888 [76] describes a most probable number method for enumeration of coagulase positive staphylococci (*S. aureus* and other species). It is particularly suitable if the numbers of coagulase-positive cocci are expected to be low or the organisms are stressed, for example in dried products.

Media

Enrichment broth: Giolitti–Cantoni broth containing 0.1% tween 80, single and double strength, dispensed in 10 mL volumes. Steam and cool just before use, then add 0.1 mL (single strength) or 0.2 mL (double strength) of 1% potassium tellurite solution.

Selective agar: Baird–Parker agar or rabbit plasma fibrinogen agar (RPFA).

Procedure

(a) Prepare a 10^{-1} homogenate and further decimal dilutions of the food sample as described in Sections 4.2 and 4.3.

(b) Transfer 10 mL of 10^{-1} homogenate to each of three tubes of double strength enrichment broth, 1 mL of 10^{-1} homogenate to each of three tubes of single strength enrichment broth, and 1 mL of each subsequent dilution to each of three tubes of single strength enrichment broth. Overlay the tubes with liquid paraffin.

(c) Incubate the tubes at 37°C for 24 ± 2 h. If any tubes show blackening, remove the liquid paraffin and subculture to Baird–Parker agar or RPFA. Reincubate all other tubes for a further 24 ± 2 h, then subculture all tubes (whether blackened or not) as before.

continued

(d) Incubate the plates at 37°C for up to 48 h, then proceed as described in steps (c) and (d) of method 1 or step (c) of method 2 as appropriate.

(e) Use Table 5.7 (pp. 121–2) to compute the most probable number per g from the number of tubes that have yielded growth of coagulase positive staphylococci, multiplying the MPN value shown by 10.

Method 4 Enrichment culture

If demonstration of presence or absence of coagulase positive staphylococci is required in a specific weight of food, the medium described in method 3 can be used (Giolitti Canloni broth). For 1 g of sample, add 10 mL of 10^{-1} food homogenate to 10 mL of double strength enrichment medium. For 10 g of sample, use 100 mL volumes of both food homogenate and double strength enrichment broth (containing 2 mL of 1% potassium tellurite solution). Then proceed as described in method 3.

Specialized reference facilities are available for phage typing and toxin production testing (see Appendix C).

6.15 *Vibrio* spp.

Members of the genus *Vibrio* [7,8,77] are commonly found in aquatic environments. The group are oxidase positive, Gram negative, often curved, facultatively anaerobic rods usually motile by a sheathed polar flagellum. They can be distinguished from the Enterobacteriaceae by their positive oxidase reaction and from the *Aeromonas* group by their failure to produce gas and by sensitivity to O129 compound. The type species is *V. cholerae*, which can be subdivided into a number of serogroups based on the O somatic antigen. Serogroup O1 produces a cytotoxin and is the main cause of true cholera, but serogroup O139 is also pathogenic due to cytotoxin production. *Vibrio cholerae* is normally water-borne but may be food-borne, often as a result of poor hygiene. *Vibrio parahaemolyticus*, a halophilic member of the genus, is a well-recognized food poisoning pathogen usually associated with fish and shellfish originating from warm and temperate coastal waters. *Vibrio vulnificus* is also halophilic and can cause gastroenteritis, septicaemia and wound infections. Other *Vibrio* species have also been implicated in human disease but infections are less common and less severe.

The main source of pathogenic vibrios is seafood. The presence of any *Vibrio* spp. in cooked food is of significance, as they are easily destroyed by heat.

Control cultures

NCTC 11218	*Vibrio furnissii*	Positive, growth quantitative
NCTC 10885	*Vibrio parahaemolyticus*	Positive, growth quantitative
NCTC 9001	*Escherichia coli*	Negative, growth inhibited

Method 1 Enrichment culture for pathogenic *Vibrio* spp.

This method is based on a proposed ISO method for the detection of all pathogenic strains of *Vibrio* [78]. Although the method allows a second selective agar medium of choice, SDS agar [79] (see below) has been shown to recover cold-stressed cells well and is specified here.

Media

Enrichment broth: Alkaline peptone water containing yeast extract 3 g, neutralized peptone 10 g, sodium chloride 20 g/L, pH 8.6±0.2.

Selective agar media: thiosulphate citrate bile salt sucrose (TCBS) agar and one other selective agar of choice, e.g. sodium dodecyl sulphate polymixin sucrose (SDS) agar, containing proteose peptone 10 g, beef extract 5 g, sucrose 15 g, sodium dodecyl (lauryl) sulphate 1 g, bromothymol blue 0.04 g, cresol red 0.04 g, polymyxin B sulphate 100 000 IU, agar 15 g/L, pH 7.6±0.2.

Non-selective agar media (containing sodium chloride): e.g. blood agar.

> If *V. cholerae* is specifically sought, the use of polymyxin mannose tellurite agar [80] may help to differentiate strains of serogroup O1 from other serogroups. However strains which are sensitive to polymyxin such as the classical biotype of *V. cholerae* O1 and some non-O1 strains may be missed.

Procedure

(a) Prepare a 10^{-1} homogenate of food in alkaline peptone water as described in Section 4.2.

(b) For frozen, chilled, salted or otherwise processed food incubate the homogenate at 37°C for 6 h. For fresh fish incubate the homogenate at 41.5°C for 6 h.

(c) After 6 h, subculture the homogenate to TCBS and SDS agar. Incubate the plates at 37°C for 18–24 h. Also subculture the food homogenate to a new 100 mL volume of alkaline peptone water (secondary enrichment) and incubate at 41.5°C for 18 h. Reincubate the food homogenate at 41.5°C for 18 h.

(d) At the end of incubation, subculture both the food homogenate and the secondary enrichment broth to TCBS and SDS agar. Incubate the plates at 37°C for 18–24 h.

(e) Examine the TCBS and SDS plates for characteristic colonies (Table 6.11 and plate XI).

(f) Subculture five suspect colonies from each agar to a non-selective agar containing sodium chloride. Incubate at 37°C for 18–24 h.

(g) Characterize the suspect colonies according to the properties shown in Table 6.12, performing further biochemical tests as necessary.

Table 6.11 Appearance of *Vibrio* spp. on TCBS, SDS and PMT agars.

	TCBS		SDS	PMT	
V. cholerae O1	Yellow[1]	2–3 mm	Yellow, often with opaque halo	Yellow[3]	2–3 mm
V. cholerae non-O1*	Yellow/green	2–3 mm	Yellow/cream, sometimes with opaque halo	Dark violet[4]	2–3 mm
V. parahaemolyticus	Green[2]	2–5 mm	Purple/green	Yellow	3–4 mm
V. vulnificus	Green	2–3 mm	Purple/green centre, often with opaque halo	Yellow	1–3 mm
V. alginolyticus	Yellow	2–5 mm	Yellow	Dark violet§	1–2 mm
V. metschnikovii	Yellow	2–4 mm	Yellow	No growth	2–3 mm
V. mimicus	Green	2–3 mm	Purple/green	Yellow	2–3 mm
V. furnissii	Yellow	2–5 mm	Yellow	Yellow§	3–4 mm
V. fluvialis	Yellow	2–5 mm	Yellow	Yellow	3–4 mm
Aeromonas spp.	Yellow	Variable colony size	Variable	Variable§	2–5 mm

1, sucrose positive; 2, sucrose negative; 3, mannose positive; 4, mannose negative; PMT, polymyxin mannose tellurite; SDS, sodium dodecyl sulphate polymyxin sucrose; TCBS, thiosulphate citrate bile salt sucrose.

*An insignificant number of non-O1 *V. cholerae* strains are mannose positive and will therefore give a colonial appearance identical to *V. cholerae* O1 on PMT.

§ Partial inhibition.

Organisms other than vibrios that can grow on TCBS form colonies of 1 mm diameter or less.

Table 6.12 *Characteristics of Vibrio* spp.

	Sucrose (TCBS or SDS)	Oxidase	O129* disc 10 µg	O129* disc 150 µg	0% NaCl (CLED)
V. cholerae† (all serotypes)	+	+	S	S	+
V. parahaemolyticus	−	+	R	S	−
V. vulnificus	−	+	S	S	−
V. alginolyticus	+	+	R	S	−
V. metschnikovii	+	−	S	S	V
V. mimicus	−	+	S	S	+
V. fluvialis	+	+	R	S	V
V. furnissii‡	+	+	R	S	V
Aeromonas spp.	+	+	R	R	V
Pseudomonas spp.	+	+	R	R	V

S, sensitive; R, resistant; SDS, sodium dodecyl sulphate polymyxin sucrose; TCBS, thiosulphate citrate bile salt sucrose; V, variable.

*O129 denotes 2,4-diamino 6,7-di-isopropyl pteridine phosphate.

†All isolates of *V. cholerae* should be tested for agglutination with O1 antiserum to identify the cholera vibrio, *V. cholerae* O1. A few strains of *V. cholerae*, e.g. serotype O139, show resistance to O129. These can be differentiated from *Aeromonas* on the basis of decarboxylase tests.

‡*V. furnissii* produces gas from glucose, *V. fluvialis* does not.

Method 2 Enrichment culture for *V. parahaemolyticus*

This method is based on ISO 8914 (BS 5763 Part 14) [81].

Media

Enrichment media: salt polymyxin broth (SPB) and either alkaline salt peptone water (ASPW) containing peptone 20 g, sodium chloride 30 g/L, pH 8.6, or saline glucose medium with sodium dodecyl sulphate (GST), containing peptone 10 g, meat extract 3 g, sodium chloride 30 g, gluose 5 g, methyl violet 0.002 g, sodium dodecyl sulphate 1.36 g/L, pH 8.6.

Selective agar media: thiosulphate citrate bile salt sucrose (TCBS) agar and triphenyl tetrazolium chloride soya tryptone (TSAT) agar.

Procedure

(a) Prepare separate 10^{-1} homogenates of the food sample with 25 g of food and 225 mL of SPB and ASPW or GST.

(b) Incubate the homogenates at 37°C for 18±2 h.

continued

(c) Subculture to TCBS agar and TSAT agar after 7–8 h and after 18 h. Incubate the plates for 20–24 h

(d) Examine TCBS plates for presence of green colonies (see Plate XIb, facing p. 150) and TSAT plates for dark red colonies with a diameter of more than 2 mm.

(e) Confirm the identity of suspect colonies as described in steps (f) and (g) of method 1.

Method 3 Direct enumeration of *Vibrio* spp.

Procedure

(a) Prepare a 10^{-1} homogenate as described in step (a) of method 1 or 2 and further decimal dilutions in peptone saline diluent. Use a surface counting method chosen from Section 5 (eg: 5.4–5.6) to enumerate on TCBS agar. If organisms are likely to be stressed enumeration should also be performed on SDS agar.

(b) Incubate the plates at 37°C for 20–24 h.

(c) Count the number of colonies of each type suspected to be vibrios.

(d) Confirm suspect colonies as described in steps (f) and (g) of method 1.

(e) Calculate the count per g from the proportion of colonies that were confirmed as *Vibrio* spp.

Method 4 Enumeration of *Vibrio* spp. by multiple tube method

Procedure

(a) Prepare a 10^{-1} homogenate and serial decimal dilutions of the food sample as described in Sections 4.2 and 4.3.

(b) Select a multiple tube method described in Section 5.7 and a liquid medium from method 1 or 2.

(c) Proceed as described in method 1 or 2, as appropriate.

(d) Calculate the most probable number per g from the number of tubes that yield growth of *Vibrio* spp.

Specialized reference facilities are available for the identification and serotyping of *Vibrio* spp. (see Appendix C).

6.16 Viruses

In theory any enteric virus could be transmitted by food, but in practice nearly all food-borne viral illness is either hepatitis A or viral gastroenteritis. The Norwalk-like viruses (NLV), previously known as small round structured viruses (SRSV), are most frequently implicated in viral gastroenteritis [82]. Food-borne transmission of other viruses causing gastroenteritis, such as rotavirus, appears rare. Although the clinical features differ, the food-borne mode of transmission of both hepatitis A and viral gastroenteritis is essentially the same. Viruses do not replicate in foods.

Viral contamination of food

Primary contamination

Food may be contaminated at source by polluted water. Bivalve molluscs are a particular problem, as they take up and concentrate microorganisms from the surrounding water during feeding. Cleansing of molluscs in depuration tanks can effectively eliminate bacterial contamination, but does not necessarily remove viruses.

Vegetable, salad and fruit crops may be contaminated during fertilization and irrigation. Soft fruits, such as raspberries, have been implicated in outbreaks of hepatitis A. Salad items are often implicated in outbreaks of viral gastroenteritis, although in these cases contamination is usually thought to occur at the time of preparation.

Secondary contamination

Food may become contaminated during preparation by infected food handlers. Usually cold foods, such as salads and sandwiches that require much handling during preparation, are implicated. Transfer of virus is passive only and levels of viral contamination will be low. However, both hepatitis A virus (HAV) and the gastroenteritis viruses are believed to be infectious in very low doses.

Virus detection

Identification of a food-borne viral infection usually depends on diagnosis in the patient and good epidemiology to link infection to a food source. It is rarely feasible to attempt detection of virus in food samples, even when a food item is implicated in causing illness. Routine testing of foods for viruses, even shellfish, is impractical.

Bivalve molluscs can concentrate virus and hence the levels of virus contamination may be expected to be higher than in other foods. However, virus sticks avidly to shellfish meat and complex extraction methods are required. Many methods have been published, but recovery rates in all are poor and none can be regarded as satisfactory.

Hepatitis A virus

Suspect food samples are infrequently available, because of the long incubation period (3–6 weeks) of hepatitis A. Identification depends on epidemiological investigation and diagnosis in the patient, usually by detection of anti-HAV specific IgM antibody. HAV can be cultured, usually in FRhk cells (a continuous line of fetal rhesus monkey kidney cells), but primary isolation is unreliable and a lengthy procedure. In a water-borne outbreak in the USA, virus was successfully isolated, but only after culture for 26 weeks. Radioimmunoassays for HAV are available and have been applied to heavily contaminated shellfish. On most occasions, however, the level of virus is too low for detection.

Gastroenteritis viruses

NLV, which include SRSV, cannot be cultured and their identification is mainly by electron microscopy of faecal specimens from patients. Specimens, which need to be collected within 48 h of onset of symptoms, may contain only small numbers of virus particles, detection of which requires considerable skill on the part of the microscopist. It is not practical to test food samples for NLVs. Molecular methods based on the cloning of the Norwalk virus genomes are now available and are used for diagnostic tests in outbreaks but these methods are usually only available in reference laboratories.

Other viruses causing gastroenteritis are rarely transmitted by food. Their identification similarly depends on detection of virus in the patient and good epidemiology to link infection to a specific food item.

Specialist reference facilities are available for advice on viruses in relation to food-borne illness (see Appendix C).

6.17   Yeasts and moulds

Yeasts and moulds may play an important part in spoilage of food; in addition some moulds can produce harmful mycotoxins. These organisms will grow readily on many types of agar media, but may require prolonged incubation at a lower temperature than necessary for most bacteria. Use of a surface method of enumeration in conjunction with the media described below will allow recovery and enumeration of yeasts and moulds from all types of food [83–85].

Control cultures

NCYC 568	*Zygosaccharomyces rouxii*	Positive, growth quantitative
NCPF 2275	*Aspergillus niger*	Positive, growth quantitative
NCPF 3178	*Saccharomyces cerevisiae*	Positive, growth quantitative
NCTC 7464	*Bacillus cereus*	Negative, growth inhibited

Method 1 Direct enumeration

Inclusion of dichloran helps to restrict the size of mould colonies, facilitating counting. Addition of glycerol reduces the water activity (a_w) of the medium and allows recovery of xerophilic yeasts and moulds as well as osmophilic strains.

Media

Dichloran glycerol chloramphenicol (DG) agar
Dichloran rose bengal chloramphenicol (DRBC) agar or oxytetracycline glucose yeast extract (OGYE) agar.

continued

Procedure

(a) Prepare a 10^{-1} food homogenate and serial decimal dilutions as described in Sections 4.2 and 4.3.

(b) Use this homogenate and its decimal dilutions with a surface counting method selected from Section 5 (eg: 5.4–5.6) to enumerate on DG agar, DRBC agar or OGYE agar.

(c) Incubate the plates at 25°C for 5 days (some fungi may need up to 14 days' incubation).

(d) Count the colonies of yeasts and moulds (see Plate XII, facing p. 150) after 3 and 5 days (in order to avoid problems from overgrowth) in plates containing up to 150 colonies.

(e) Calculate the count per g of yeasts and moulds separately.

Method 2 Enumeration of xerophilic yeasts and moulds

Osmophilic yeasts and moulds are capable of growth in high sugar concentrations. In order to obtain recovery of these strains it may be necessary to adjust the water activity (a_w) of both the diluent and the isolation medium. The use of a diluent containing 50% (w/w) glucose has been recommended. An agar medium containing 35–50% glucose will allow recovery of xerotolerant strains whilst inhibiting osmophilic strains; failure to grow under these conditions precludes the strain as a potential cause of spoilage of high sugar commodities such as confectionery. The reduced a_w of the medium may necessitate prolonged incubation for several weeks [86,87].

Procedure

(a) Prepare a 10^{-1} homogenate and serial decimal dilutions of the food in 50% (w/w) glucose solution.

(b) Use suitable aliquots of this homogenate and dilutions and spread them over the surface of malt extract yeast extract 40% (w/w) glucose agar.

(c) Incubate the plates at 20–25°C for moulds and 25–30°C for yeasts for up to 3 weeks.

(d) Count the colonies of yeasts and moulds and calculate the count per g.

6.18 *Yersinia* spp.

The genus *Yersinia*, a member of the family Enterobacteriaceae, contains at least 11 species including *Y. pestis*, *Y. pseudotuberculosis* and *Y. enterocolitica*, which are pathogenic for humans and animals [88,89]. The organisms are Gram negative, facultatively anaerobic, catalase positive, oxidase negative rod-shaped bacteria that produce oval or coccoid cells in young culture at 25°C. *Y. enterocolitica*, the species most often associated with food-borne yersinisosis, is psychrotrophic and can grow in food at refrigeration temperatures. *Y. enterocolitica* can be subdivided into a number of biotypes, and can be further subdivided by serotyping.

   Yersinia enterocolitica and related species are widespread in the environment, and are also found in a wide range of foods. Pathogenic strains are particularly associated with pigs, but other strains found in processed, heat-treated foods are significant as indicators of poor hygiene or cross-contamination. Enumeration of the organisms in food is not usually attempted: isolation is performed by enrichment culture.

Control cultures

| NCTC 10460 | *Yersinia enterocolitica* | Positive, growth quantitative |
| NCTC 9001 | *Escherichia coli* | Negative, growth inhibited |

Method 1 Enrichment culture

This method is capable of detecting all biotypes and serovars from a wide range of dairy, food and environmental sources [90–93].

Media
Enrichment medium: tris buffered peptone water: peptone 10 g, sodium chloride 5 g, tris (hydroxymethyl) methylamine 12.1 g, distilled water 1 L, adjusted to pH 8.0.

Selective agar: cefsulodin-irgasan-novobiocin (CIN) agar.

Procedure
(a) Homogenize 25 g of food sample in 225 mL of tris buffered peptone water.
(b) Incubate the homogenate at 9°C for 2 weeks (or at 21–25°C).

> Incubation at 21 ± 3°C is a satisfactory alternative to 9°C for all food items except pasteurized milk. If this is done, subculture should be performed after 1 and 2 weeks' incubation to obtain optimal recovery. Pasteurized milk may also be incubated at 4°C for 3 weeks with subculture at the end of the incubation period.

(c) Subculture after 2 weeks at 9°C (or after 1 and 2 weeks at 21–25°C) as follows: add 1 mL of the incubated homogenate to 9 mL of 0.5% potassium hydroxide/0.5% sodium chloride solution and mix. After 15–30 s subculture a loopful of the mixture to CIN agar.
(d) Incubate CIN plates at 30°C for 24 h.
(e) Examine CIN plates for the presence of colonies. Typical colonies have a bullseye appearance with a red centre surrounded by a transparent border (see Plate XIII, facing p. 150), and are usually smaller than colonies of other coliforms capable of growth on CIN agar. Colonies may also appear very small and dry, or much larger with irregular edges and a large amount of colourless periphery relative to the red centre.
(f) Confirm the identity of suspect colonies. *Yersinia* spp. are urease-positive (occasionally negative), produce an acid butt without production of gas or hydrogen sulphide in TSI agar slopes, and are non-motile at 37°C but motile below 28°C. Some strains can produce acid from lactose. *Y. enterocolitica* and related strains can

continued

decarboxylate ornithine but not lysine; strains of *Y. pseudotuberculosis* do not possess decarboxylase activity.

(g) Colonies may be further characterized using the biochemical reactions shown in Table 6.13.

Table 6.13 Characteristics of *Yersinia* spp.

	Sucrose	Rhamnose	Melibiose	Xylose	Indole	Lipase
Y. enterocolitica						
Biotype 1	+	−	−	+	+	+
Biotype 2	+	−	−	+	(+)	−
Biotype 3	+	−	−	+	−	−
Biotype 4	+	−	−	−	−	−
Y. frederiksenii	+	+	−	+	+	V
Y. intermedia	+	+	+	+	+	V
Y. kristensenii	−	−	−	+	+	V
Y. pseudotuberculosis	−	+	+	+	−	−

V, variable; (+) weak reaction.

Method 2 Enrichment procedure

Dual isolation procedure

The method described in ISO 10273 (BS 5763 Part 16) [94] uses two enrichment media and different isolation protocols. Enrichment in a buffered peptone sorbitol bile salts broth will recover all strains of *Y. enterocolitica* and related species; the other enrichment procedure is targeted at the pathogenic serotypes common in Europe (O3, O9 and O5,27).

Media

Enrichment media: peptone sorbitol bile salts broth (PSB), containing 1% sorbitol and 0.15% bile salts pH 7.6 and irgasan ticarcillin potassium chlorate broth (ITC).

Selective agar media: cefsulodin irgasan novobiocin (CIN) agar and salmonella shigella agar supplemented with 1% sodium desoxycholate and 0.1% calcium chloride (SSDC).

Procedure (i)

(a) Prepare a 1/10 homogenate of food in PSB broth.

(b) Incubate the homogenate at 22–25°C for 3 days with agitation or 5 days without agitation.

(c) Subculture directly to CIN agar. Also subculture 1 mL to 9 mL of 0.25% potassium hydroxide/0.85% sodium chloride solution. After 20 s, subculture a loopful to CIN agar.

(d) Incubate the plates at 30°C for 24 h.

(e) Examine the plates for suspect colonies and proceed as described in steps (e)–(g) of method 1.

continued

Specialized reference facilities are available for identification and serotyping (see Appendix C).

6.19 References

1 DD ENV ISO 11133. *Microbiology of Food and Animal Feeding Stuffs—Guidelines on Quality Assurance and Performance Testing of Culture Media. Part 1. General Guidelines on Quality Assurance of Culture Media in the Laboratory*. Geneva: International Organization for Standardization (ISO), 2000.

2 Mossel DAA, van Rossem F, Koopmans M, Hendriks M, Verdouden M, Eelderink L. Quality control of solid culture media: a comparison of the classic and the so-called ecometric technique. *J Appl Bacteriol* 1980; **49**: 439–54.

3 Working Party on Culture Media (WPCM). Pharmacopoeia of culture media for food microbiology. *Int J Food Microbiol* 1987; **5**: 291–6.

4 Mooijman KA, in't Veld PH, Hoekstra JA, *et al*. Development of microbiological reference materials. BCR information chemical analysis. *Report EUR; 14375EN*. Luxembourg: Commission of the European Communities, 1992.

5 Lightfoot NF, Maier EA, eds. *Microbiological Analysis of Food and Water. Guidelines for Quality Assurance*. Chapter 8. Analytical quality control in microbiology. Amsterdam: Elsevier Science, 1998: 149–89.

6 ISO 7218 (BS 5763 Part 0). *Microbiology of Food and Animal Feeding Stuffs—General Rules for Microbiological Examinations*. Geneva: International Organization for Standardization (ISO), 1996.

7 Furniss AL, Lee JV, Donovan TJ. *The Vibrios. Public Health Laboratory Service Monograph Series. No. 11*. London: HMSO, 1978.

8 Lee JV. *Vibrio, Aeromonas* and *Plesiomonas*. In: Parker MT, Duerden BI, eds. *Principles of Bacteriology, Virology and Immunity*, 8th edn. Vol. 2: *Systematic Bacteriology*. London: Edward Arnold, 1990: 513–30.

9 Wilcox MH, Cook AM, Thickett KJ, Eley A, Spencer RC. Phenotypic methods for speciating clinical *Aeromonas* isolates. *J Clin Path* 1992; **45**: 1079–83.

10 Gordon RE, Haynes WC, Pang CH. The genus *Bacillus. Agriculture Handbook No. 427*. Washington DC: US Department of Agriculture. 1973.

11 Holbrook R, Anderson JM. An improved selective and diagnostic medium for the isolation and enumeration of *Bacillus cereus* in foods. *Can J Microbiol* 1980; **26**: 753–9.

12 Mossel DAA, Koopman MJ, Jongerius E. Enumeration of *Bacillus cereus* in foods. *Appl Microbiol* 1967; **15**: 650–3.

13 Kramer JM, Turnbull PCB, Munshi G, Gilbert RJ. Identification and characterisation of *Bacillus cereus* and other *Bacillus* species associated with foods and food poisoning. In: Corry JEL, Roberts D, Skinner FA, eds. *Isolation and Identification Methods for Food Poisoning Organisms*. London: Academic Press, 1982: 261–86.

14 EN ISO 7932 (BS 5763 Part 11). *Microbiology—General Guidance for the Enumeration of Bacillus cereus—Colony Count Technique at 30°C*. Geneva: International Organization for Standardization (ISO), 1993.

15 Schulten SM, in't Veld PH, Nagelkerke NJD, *et al*. Evaluation of the ISO 7932 standard for the enumeration of *Bacillus cereus* in foods. *Int J Food Microbiol* 2000; **57**: 53–61.

16 Brodie J, Sinton GP. Fluid and solid media for the isolation of *Brucella abortus*. *J Hyg* 1975; **74**: 359–67.

17 Farrell ID, Robinson L. A comparison of various selective media, including a new selective medium, for the isolation of brucellae from milk. *J Appl Bacteriol* 1972; **35**: 625–30.

18 Robertson L, Farrell ID, Hinchliffe PM, Quaife RA. *Benchbook on Brucella. Public Health Laboratory Service Monograph Series. No. 14*. London: HMSO, 1980.

19 Cruickshank R, Duguid JP, Marmion BP, Swan RHA. *Medical Microbiology*, 12th edn, Vol. 2. Edinburgh: Churchill Livingstone, 1975: 455.

20 Skirrow MB. *Campylobacter*, *Helicobacter* and other motile, curved Gram negative rods. In: Parker MT, Collier LH, eds. *Principles of Bacteriology, Virology and Immunity*, 8th edn. Vol. 2: *Systematic Bacteriology*. London: Edward Arnold, 1990: 531–49.

21 Bolton FJ, Robertson L. A selective medium for isolating *Campylobacter jejuni/coli*. *J Clin Pathol* 1982; **35**: 462–7.

22 Hutchinson DN, Bolton FJ. Improved blood-free selective medium for the isolation of *Campylobacter jejuni* from faecal specimens. *J Clin Pathol* 1983; **37**: 956–7.

23 Humphrey TJ. Techniques for the optimum recovery of cold injured *Campylobacter jejuni* from milk and water. *J Appl Bacteriol* 1986; **61**: 125–32.

24 Skirrow MB. *Campylobacter* enteritis: a 'new' disease. *Br Med J* 1977; **2**: 9–11.

25 Humphrey TJ, Muscat I. Incubation temperature and the isolation of *Campylobacter jejuni* from food, milk and water. *Lett Appl Microbiol* 1989; **9**: 137–9.

26 Bolton FJ, Gibson DM. Automated electrical techniques in microbiological analysis. In: Patel P, ed. *Rapid Analysis in Food Microbiology*. Glasgow: Blackie Academic and Professional, 1994: 131–69.

27 ISO 10272: 1995 as amended 1998 (BS 5763 Part 17). *Microbiology of Food and Animal Feeding Stuffs—Horizontal Method for Detection of Thermotolerant Campylobacter*. Geneva: International Organization for Standardization (ISO), 1998.

28 Harmon SM, Kautter DA, Peeler JT. Improved medium for enumeration of *Clostridium perfringens*. *Appl Microbiol* 1971; **22**: 688–92.

29 Hauschild AHW, Hilsheimer R. Enumeration of food-borne *Clostridium perfringens* in egg-yolk free tryptose sulphite cycloserine agar. *Appl Microbiol* 1974; **27**: 521–6.

30 Mead GC, Adams BW, Roberts TA, Smart JL. Isolation and enumeration of *Clostridium perfringens*. In: Corry JEL, Roberts D, Skinner FA, eds. *Isolation and Identification Methods for Food Poisoning Organisms*. London: Academic Press, 1982: 99–110.

31 International Commission on Microbiological Specifications in Foods. *Micro-organisms in Foods 5. Microbiological Specifications of Food Pathogens.* London: Blackie Academic and Professional, 1996, p. 112.

32 BS EN 13401. *Microbiology of Food and Animal Feeding Stuffs—Horizontal Method for the Enumeration of Clostridium perfringens—Colony Count Technique (ISO 7937: 1997 modified).* Brussels: European Committee for Standardization (CEN), 1999.

33 Mossell DAA, Corry JEL, Struijk CB, Baird RM. *Essentials of the Microbiology of Foods. A Textbook for Advanced Studies.*

34 ISO 4832 (BS 5763 Part 2). *Microbiology—General Guidance for the Enumeration of Coliforms—Colony Count Technique.* Geneva: International Organization for Standardization (ISO), 1991.

35 International Commission on Microbiological Specifications for Foods. *Microorganisms in Foods I. Their Significance and Methods of Enumeration,* 2nd edn. Toronto: University of Toronto Press, 1978: 125–39.

36 ISO 4831 (BS 5763 Part 3). *Microbiology—General Guidance for the Enumeration of Coliforms—Most Probable Number Technique.* Geneva: International Organization for Standardization (ISO), 1991.

37 ISO 7251 (BS 5763 Part 8). *Microbiology—General Guidance for the Enumeration of Presumptive Escherichia coli—Most Probable Number Technique.* Geneva: International Organization for Standardization (ISO), 1993.

38 Holbrook R, Anderson JM. The rapid enumeration of *Escherichia coli* in foods by using a direct plating method. In: Corry JEL, Roberts D, Skinner FA, eds. *Isolation and Identification Methods for Food Poisoning Organisms.* London: Academic Press, 1982: 238–54.

39 ISO 6391 (BS 5763 Part 13). *Meat and Meat Products—Enumeration of Escherichia coli—Colony Count Technique at 44°C Using Membranes.* Geneva: International Organization for Standardization (ISO), 1997.

40 BS ISO 11866-3. *Milk and Milk products—Enumeration of Presumptive Escherichia coli—Colony Count Technique at 44°C Using Membranes.* Geneva: International Organization for Standardization (ISO), 1997.

41 Vracko R, Sherris JC. Indole spot test in bacteriology. *Am J Clin Pathol* 1963; **39**: 429–32.

42 BS ISO 16649. *Microbiology of Food and Animal Feeding Stuffs—Horizontal Method for the Enumeration of β-glucuronidase Positive Escherichia coli. Part 1: Colony Count Technique at 44°C Using Membranes and 5-bromo-4-chloro-3-indolyl β-ᴅ-glucuronide.* Geneva: International Organization for Standardization (ISO), 2001.

43 BS ISO 16649. *Microbiology of Food and Animal Feeding Stuffs—Horizontal Method for the Enumeration of β-glucuronidase Positive Escherichia coli. Part 2: Colony Count Technique at 44°C Using 5-bromo-4-chloro-3-indolyl β-ᴅ-glucuronide.* Geneva: International Organization for Standardization (ISO), 2001.

44 Public Health Laboratory Service (PHLS). *Methods for Food Products. Standard Method F20. Direct Enumeration of Escherichia coli.* London: PHLS, 1998.

45 Chapman PA, Siddons CA, Wright DJ, Norman P, Fox J, Crick E. Cattle as a possible source of verocytotoxin-producing *Escherichia coli* O157 infections in man. *Epidemiol Infect* 1993; **111**: 439–47.

46 Padhye NV, Doyle MP. Rapid procedure for detecting enterohaemorrhagic *Escherichia coli* O157: H7 in food. *Appl Environ Microbiol* 1991; **57**: 2693–8.

47 BS EN ISO 16654. *Microbiology of Food and Animal Feeding Stuffs—Horizontal Method for*

the *Detection of Escherichia coli O157*. Geneva: International Organization for Standardization (ISO), 2001.

48 Zadik PM, Chapman PA, Siddons CA. Use of tellurite for the selection of verocyto-toxigenic *Escherichia coli* O157. *J Med Microbiol* 1993; **39**: 155–8.

49 British Standards Institution (BSI). BS 5763. *Microbiological Examination of Food and Animal Feeding Stuffs. Part 10 Enumeration of Enterobacteriaceae*. London: BSI, 1986.

50 ISO 21528-3. *Microbiology of Food and Animal Feeding Stuffs—Horizontal Method for the Detection and Enumeration of Enterobacteriaceae—Colony Count Technique*. Geneva: International Organization for Standardization (ISO), in preparation.

51 ISO 8523 (BS 5763 Part 15). *Microbiology—General Guidance for the Detection of Enterobacteriaceae with Pre-Enrichment*. Geneva: International Organization for Standardization (ISO), 1991.

52 ISO 21528-2. *Microbiology of Food and Animal Feeding Stuffs—Horizontal Method for the Detection and Enumeration of Enterobacteriaceae—MPN Technique Without Pre-enrichment*. Geneva: International Organization for Standardization (ISO), in preparation.

53 Standing Committee of Analysts. *Methods for the Examination of Waters and Associated Materials. The Microbiology of Drinking Water (2002)—Part I—Water Quality and Public Health*. Environment Agency, 2002.

54 Hartman PA, Deibel RH, Sieverding LM. Enterococci. In: Vanderzant C, Splittstoesser DF, eds. *Compendium of Methods for the Microbiological Examination of Foods*, 3rd edn. Washington, D.C.: American Public Health Association, 1992: 523–31.

55 British Standards Institution (BSI). BS 4285. *Microbiological Examination for Dairy Purposes. Section 3.1. Detection and Enumeration of Faecal Streptococci*. London: BSI, 1985.

56 Vedamuthu ER, Raccah M, Glatz BA, Seitz EW, Reddy MS. Acid producing organisms. In: Vanderzant C, Splittstoesser DF, eds. *Compendium of Methods for the Microbiological Examination of Foods*, 3rd edn. Washington, D.C.: American Public Health Association, 1992: 225–38.

57 BS ISO 15214. *Microbiology of Food and Animal Feeding Stuffs—Horizontal Method for the Enumeration of Mesophilic Lactic Acid Bacteria—Colony Count Technique at 30°C*. Geneva: International Organization for Standardization (ISO), 1998.

58 BS EN ISO 11290-1. *Microbiology of Food and Animal Feeding Stuffs—Horizontal Method for the Detection and Enumeration of Listeria monocytogenes. Part 1. Detection Method*. Geneva: International Organization for Standardization (ISO), 1997.

59 Van Netten P, Perales I, van de Moosdijk A, Curtis GDW, Mossel DAA. Liquid and solid selective differential media for the detection and enumeration of *L.monocytogenes* and other *Listeria* spp. *Int J Food Microbiol* 1989; **8**: 299–316.

60 Curtis GDW, Mitchell RG, King AF, Griffin EJ. A selective differential medium for the isolation of *Listeria monocytogenes*. *Lett Appl Microbiol* 1989; **8**: 95–8.

61 Curtis GDW, Nicholls WW, Falla TJ. Selective agents for listeria can inhibit their growth. *Lett Appl Microbiol* 1989; **8**: 169–72.

62 IDF Standard 143a. *Milk and Milk Products. Detection of Listeria monocytogenes*. Brussels: International Dairy Federation, 1995.

63 British Standards Institution (BSI). BS 4285. *Microbiological Examination for Dairy Purposes. Section 3.15. Detection of Listeria monocytogenes*. London: BSI, 1993.

64 BS EN ISO 11290-2. *Microbiology of Food and Animal Feeding Stuffs—Horizontal Method for the Detection and Enumeration of Listeria monocytogenes. Part 2. Enumeration Method*. Geneva: International Organization for Standardization (ISO), 1998.

65 Scotter SL, Langton S, Lombard B, *et al.* Validation of ISO method 11290 part 1 — detection of *Listeria monocytogenes* in foods. *Int J Food Microbiol* 2001; **64**: 295–306.

66 Council of the European Communities. Directive No. 80/777/EEC on the approximation of the laws of the Member States relating to the exploitation and marketing of natural mineral waters. *Off J Eur Comm* 1980; **L229**: 1–10.

67 ISO 13720 (BS 7857 Part 1). *Meat and Meat Products — Enumeration of Pseudomonas spp.* Geneva: International Organization for Standardization (ISO), 1995.

68 BS EN 12824. *Microbiology of Food and Animal Feeding Stuffs — Horizontal Method for the Detection of Salmonella.* Brussels: European Committee for Standardization (CEN), 1998.

69 Public Health Laboratory Service (PHLS). *PHLS Methods for Food and Dairy Products. Standard Method F13.* London: PHLS, 1998.

70 ISO 6579. *Microbiology of Food and Animal Feeding Stuffs — Horizontal Method for the Detection of Salmonella spp.* Geneva: International Organization for Standardization (ISO), in preparation.

71 US Pharmacopoeia XXI. *Microbial Limit Tests.* Rockville, MD: United States Pharmacopial Convention, Inc, 1985.

72 EN ISO 21567. *Microbiology of Food and Animal Feeding Stuffs — Horizontal Method for the Detection of Shigella spp.* Geneva: International Organization for Standardization (ISO), in preparation.

73 International Commission on Microbiological Specifications in Foods. *Microorganisms in Foods 5. Microbiological Specifications of Food Pathogens.* London: Blackie Academic and Professional, 1996, pp. 301–11.

74 EN ISO 6888. *Microbiology of Food and Animal Feeding Stuffs — Horizontal Method for the Enumeration of Coagulase-positive Staphylococci (Staphylococcus aureus and Other Species). Part 1. Technique Using Baird–Parker Agar Medium.* Geneva: International Organization for Standardization (ISO), 1999.

75 EN ISO 6888. *Microbiology of Food and Animal Feeding Stuffs — Horizontal Method for the Enumeration of Coagulase-positive Staphylococci (Staphylococcus aureus and Other Species). Part 2. Technique Using Rabbit Plasma Fibrinogen Agar Medium.* Geneva: International Organization for Standardization (ISO), 1999.

76 EN ISO 6888. *Microbiology of Food and Animal Feeding Stuffs — Horizontal Method for the Enumeration of Coagulase-positive Staphylococci (Staphylococcus aureus and Other Species). Part 3. Most Probable Number Technique.* Geneva: International Organization for Standardization (ISO), in preparation.

77 International Commission on Microbiological Specifications for Foods. *Microorganisms in Foods 1. Their Significance and Methods of Enumeration,* 2nd edn. Toronto: University of Toronto Press, 1988: 201–7.

78 ISO. *Microbiology of Food and Animal Feeding Products. Detection of Pathogenic Vibrio.* Geneva: International Organization for Standardization (ISO), in preparation.

79 Acuff GR. Media, reagents and stains. In: Vanderzant C, Splittstoesser DF, eds. *Compendium of Methods for the Microbiological Examination of Foods,* 3rd edn. Washington, D.C.: American Public Health Association, 1992: 1167–208.

80 Shimala T, Sakazaki R, Fujimura S, Niwano K, Mishima M, Takizawa K. A new selective, differential agar medium for isolation of *Vibrio cholerae* 01: PMT (polymyxin mannose tellurite) agar. *Jpn J Med Sci Biol* 1990; **43**: 37–41.

81 ISO 8914 (BS 5763 Part 14). *Microbiology — General Guidance for the Detection of Vibrio parahaemolyticus.* Geneva: International Organization for Standardization (ISO), 1990.

82 Public Health Laboratory Service (PHLS) Working Party on Viral Gastroenteritis. Food-borne viral gastroenteritis (with a brief comment on hepatitis A). *PHLS Microbiol Dig* 1988; **5**: 69–75.

83 Hocking AD, Pitt JI. Dichloran-glycerol medium for enumeration of xerophilic fungi from low moisture foods. *Appl Environ Microbiol* 1980; **39**: 488–92.

84 King AD, Hocking AD, Pitt JI. Dichloran-rose bengal medium for enumeration and isolation of moulds from foods. *Appl Environ Microbiol* 1979; **37**: 959–64.

85 Mossel DAA, Kleynen-Semmeling AM, Vincentie HM, Beerens H, Catsaras M. Oxytetracycline glucose yeast extract agar for selective enumeration of moulds and yeasts in foods and clinical material. *J Appl Bacteriol* 1970; **33**: 454–7.

86 Lenovich LM, Konkel PJ. Confectionery products. In: Vanderzant C, Splittstoesser DF, eds. *Compendium of Methods for the Microbiological Examination of Foods*, 3rd edn. Washington, D.C.: American Public Health Association, 1992: 1007–18.

87 Pitt JI, Hocking AD. *Fungi and Food Spoilage*. London: Academic Press, 1985.

88 Corbel MJ. *Yersinia*. In: Parker MT, Duerden BI, eds. *Principles of Bacteriology, Virology and Immunity*, 8th edn. Vol. 2: *Systematic Bacteriology*. London: Edward Arnold, 1990: 496–512.

89 Wauters G, Janssens M, Steigerwalt AG, Brenner DJ. *Yersinia mollaretii* sp.nov. and *Yersinia bercovieri* sp.nov., formerly called *Yersinia enterocolitica* biogroups 3A and 3B. *Int J Syst Bacteriol* 1988; **38**: 424–9.

90 Greenwood MH, Hooper WL. Improved methods for the isolation of *Yersinia* species from milk and foods. *Food Microbiol* 1989; **6**: 99–104.

91 Greenwood MH. Comparison of enrichment at 9°C and 21°C for recovery of *Yersinia* species from food and milk. *Food Microbiol* 1993; **10**: 23–30.

92 Aulisio CCG, Mehlman IJ, Sanders AC. Alkali method for rapid recovery of *Yersinia enterocolitica* and *Yersinia pseudotuberculosis* from foods. *Appl Environ Microbiol* 1980; **39**: 135–40.

93 Schiemann DA. Synthesis of a selective agar medium for *Yersinia enterocolitica*. *Can J Microbiol* 1979; **25**: 1298–304.

94 ISO 10273 (BS 5763 Part 16). *Microbiology—General Guidance for the Detection of Presumptive Pathogenic Yersinia enterocolitica*. Geneva: International Organization for Standardization (ISO), 1994.

7 Milk and dairy products

7.1 Pasteurized milk
7.2 Untreated milk
7.3 Ultra heat treated milk and sterilized milk
7.4 Dairy products

The tests and methods given in this section are based mainly on those for milk and dairy products stipulated in European and UK legislation. EC Directive 92/46/EEC [1] lays down health rules for the production and placing on the market of raw milk, heat treated milk and milk-based products. This Directive was incorporated into UK law as the Dairy Products (Hygiene) Regulations 1995 [2], Code of Practice number 18 of the Food Safety Act 1990 [3] and associated Guidance Notes [4]. The Regulations and Guidance Notes contain microbiological standards and guidelines for products sampled at any point in a production, holding or heat treatment establishment. The methods to be used for examination of liquid milk are described in Commission Decision 91/180/EEC [5]. Methods for other dairy products are specified in the UK Regulations. All methods specified are recognized internationally; the legislation also states that any other internationally recognized method that gives equivalent results may be used. The regulations apply to milk and milk products of any animal origin (cow, goat, sheep, buffalo).

7.1 Pasteurized milk

The Dairy Products (Hygiene) Regulations 1995 [2] specify tests for coliforms, pre-incubated plate count, phosphatase and peroxidase for pasteurized milk. In addition, the regulations require the absence of pathogens in 25 mL of product but do not specify which organisms should be investigated. However, Commission Decision 91/180/EEC [5] states that if the other tests are satisfactory, a specific test for pathogens is only necessary if the milk is thought to be associated with an outbreak of food poisoning.

Sampling

Conditions for sampling, transport and storage of samples can be found in Commission Decision 91/180/EEC [5]. Sample units of pasteurized milk in complete sealed packages should be taken from the packaging machine or cold room as soon as possible after processing and on the same day as processing. For routine testing, three separate samples should be taken:

• Sample 1—to measure temperature on receipt at the laboratory.

- Sample 2—to be used for the coliform, phosphatase and peroxidase tests.
- Sample 3—to be kept intact at 6°C for the pre-incubated plate count test.

For statutory purposes each test is performed on five separate samples; therefore at least 12 separate samples are required for the coliform and pre-incubated plate count tests, to allow for one bottle per insulated sample transport container for temperature monitoring.

Samples should be transported to the testing laboratory in an insulated container with the least possible delay and should be transported and stored between 0°C and 4°C. The time between sampling and examination should be as short as possible and should not exceed 24 h.

Colony count

A colony count (referred to in the legislation as a plate count) is no longer specified in UK legislation for the testing of pasteurized milk as this was not a requirement of Directive 92/46/EEC [1]. However, this test can be a useful tool for quality assurance purposes. The standard specified in the 1989 UK Dairy Regulations [6] was 2.0×10^4/mL. In practice freshly pasteurized milk usually has a colony count below 10^4/mL. The methods described in Sections 5.3–5.6 are suitable for performing colony counts but milk plate count agar should be used with incubation at 30°C for 72 h. Dilutions to 10^{-3} may be required.

Method 1 Pre-incubated colony count

This method is described in Commission Decision 91/180/EEC [5].

> **Special note**
> For routine purposes, other methods of colony counting such as spiral plating (Section 5.4) are acceptable. If results are required for referee purposes the pour plate method described below should be used.

Equipment
Incubator at 6±0.5°C
Incubator at 21±1°C
Water bath at 44–47°C
Pipettes or pipettors and sterile tips, to deliver 1 mL.

Media
Milk plate count agar
Peptone saline solution (maximum recovery diluent).

Procedure
(a) On arrival in the laboratory, incubate the sample (consisting of an intact container) at a temperature of 6±0.5°C for 120±2 h (i.e. 5 days) together with an

continued

---

identical container used to monitor temperature during incubation. Check the temperature of the milk during the incubation period using the control container.

(b) After incubation mix the contents of the container thoroughly by inverting the container 25 times.

(c) Prepare serial decimal dilutions of the milk sample to 10^{-4} using peptone saline solution as diluent.

(d) Prepare molten milk plate count agar and temper to 44–47°C before use.

(e) Place 1 mL aliquots of each dilution in sterile Petri dishes. Inoculate two dishes for each dilution. Use a separate pipette for each dilution.

(f) Within 15 min of preparation of the dilutions, add 15–18 mL of molten, tempered agar to each dish. Mix carefully and allow to set.

(g) Add 15–18 mL of agar to an empty Petri dish to act as an agar control and to a dish containing 1 mL of peptone saline solution as a diluent control.

(h) Invert the set plates and incubate at 21±1°C for 25 h. Record the start and finish times.

Calculation

(i) Count the colonies in plates that contain 10–300 colonies. If a plate is overgrown, count the colonies in the half of the plate that is clear and multiply the count by two. Reject any plate that is more than half overgrown. If no plate produces fewer than 300 colonies, calculate the result from the plate with the lowest number of colonies and report the estimated number of organisms per mL. If the primary dilution fails to produce any colonies, report the result as less than 10 organisms/mL.

(j) Calculate the number of organisms, N, per mL as follows:

$$N = \frac{\text{total number of colonies counted}}{\text{total volume plated} \times \text{dilution.}}$$

If there are plates containing 10–300 colonies at more than one dilution, apply the following formula:

$$N = \frac{C}{V(n_1 + 0.1n_2)d}$$

where: C is the sum of colonies on all plates counted

V is the volume applied to each plate

n_1 is the number of plates counted for the first dilution

n_2 is the number of plates counted for the second dilution

d is the dilution from which the first counts were obtained.

Note: all counts from plates of the selected dilutions should be included unless the count exceeds 300 or is overgrown.

(k) Report the result in floating point form to two significant figures raised to the power of 10. When the digit to be rounded off is five with no further significant figures, round off so that the figure immediately to the left is even, e.g. 28 500 becomes 2.8×10^4.

continued

EXAMPLE

Volume applied   1 mL

Dilution 10^{-2} 173 and 145 colonies

Dilution 10^{-3} 15 and 8 colonies

$$\text{Number} = \frac{173+145+15+8}{[2+(0.1+2)]10^2}$$

$$= \frac{341}{0.022}$$

$$= 15500 \text{ expressed as } 1.6 \times 10^4$$

Interpretation

Refer to Section 3 for criteria. Counts below 5×10^4 colony forming units (cfu)/mL are satisfactory; counts above 5×10^5 cfu/mL are unsatisfactory.

For enforcement purposes five samples taken at the same time are required. Guidance Notes [4] on the Dairy Products (Hygiene) Regulations indicate that action should not be taken on unsatisfactory results in the pre-incubated test unless another parameter is also unsatisfactory.

Method 2 Coliform test

Coliform tests on milk and dairy products are performed at 30°C.

The method described below is that described in Commission Decision 91/180/EEC [5]. It is similar to BS 4285 Section 3.7 [7] but uses three 1 mL aliquots of undiluted milk instead of two.

Equipment
Water bath at 44–47°C

Incubator at 30 ± 1°C

Pipettes or pipettors and sterile tips, to deliver 1 mL.

Media
Violet red bile (lactose) agar (VRBA)

Brilliant green bile(2%) broth, containing Durham tube.

Procedure
(a) Prepare molten VRBA, cool to 44–47°C and use within 3 h of preparation. Do not sterilize the medium in an autoclave and avoid reheating or overheating.

(b) Place 1 mL of undiluted milk into each of three Petri dishes.

(c) Add about 12 mL of molten tempered VRBA to each dish, mix carefully and allow to set.

(d) Pour at least 4 mL of molten tempered VRBA over the surface of the plate and allow to set.

(e) Prepare control plates containing only VRBA to check the sterility of the medium.

continued

(f) Invert the set plates and incubate at $30 \pm 1°C$ for 24 ± 2 h.

(g) Count red colonies having a diameter of at least 0.5 mm, characteristic of coliforms. Also count atypical red colonies.

Confirmation

(h) Typical colonies do not require confirmation. Confirm atypical colonies by inoculating five colonies of each type (if available) into separate tubes of brilliant green bile broth.

(i) Incubate the tubes at $30 \pm 1°C$ for 24 ± 2 h. Consider colonies which show gas formation in the Durham tube as coliforms.

Calculation

(j) Calculate the coliform count, taking into account the confirmatory test if carried out, by totalling the coliform colonies in the three plates and dividing by three to give a coliform count/mL of milk.

Interpretation

Refer to Section 3 for criteria. Results are satisfactory if no coliform colonies are found. If the count exceeds 5 cfu/mL results are unsatisfactory. The specification for m is 0 so if any colonies are present at all this specification has been exceeded. If the average number of coliforms/mL is between 0 and 1, report the coliform count as present; <1 cfu/mL.

If pasteurization has been properly performed, coliform presence will be due to post-pasteurization contamination.

Method 3 Phosphatase test

The enzyme alkaline phosphatase is normally found in mammalian milk. Levels of phosphatase vary with the time of year and between mammalian species. Ewes' milk contains similar or higher levels to bovine milk but goats' milk contains levels around one third of those found in cows' milk. The enzyme is destroyed by conditions close to the time/temperature combinations used in pasteurization and so its absence is used to indicate adequate pasteurization.

Commission Decision 91/180/EEC [5] states that samples for phosphatase tests should be kept in the refrigerator (0–4°C) before analysis for not more than 2 days after sampling.

Method 3a Spectrophotometric method

This method of phosphatase detection is specified in Commission Decision 91/180/EEC [5] and is therefore regarded as the reference method. It is also known as the Scharer method. The method uses disodium phenylphosphate as substrate, from which the enzyme liberates phenol which is then coupled with a colour reagent to

continued

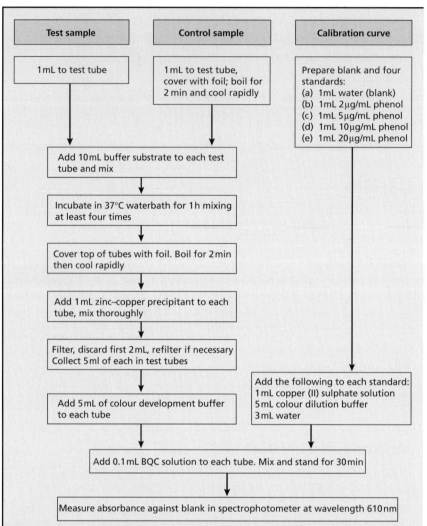

Fig. 7.1 Flow chart for spectrophotometric detection of alkaline phosphatase activity in milk.

form an indophenol. Interfering turbidity is removed by precipitating the proteins and lipids with zinc and barium salts. A spectrophotometer is used to determine the intensity of the blue colour produced. The method is time consuming to perform and at best can only detect levels of around 0.1% raw milk. The method is summarized in Fig. 7.1.

Equipment
Analytical balance
Water bath at $37 \pm 1°C$
Spectrophotometer, 610 nm wavelength
Test tubes 16 mm or 18 mm × 150 mm, preferably graduated at 5 mL and 10 mL
Cuvettes

continued

Pipettes or pipettors and tips, to deliver 10 mL and 1 mL

Glass funnels, e.g. 5 cm in diameter

Folded filters at least 9 cm in diameter for medium filtration speed (Whatman no. 42, no. 2 or equivalent)

Volumetric flasks, 100 mL and 1000 mL.

> All glassware, stoppers and sampling tools must be carefully cleaned. Soak in hot running water and rinse with freshly distilled or deionized water after cleaning.

Reagents

Barium borate-hydroxide buffer: dissolve 50.0 g barium hydroxide in water, make up to 1000 mL. Dissolve 22.0 g of boric acid in water, make up to 1000 mL. Warm 500 mL of each solution to 50°C, mix the solutions, stir and cool rapidly to about 20°C. Adjust pH if necessary to 10.6±0.1. Filter, then store solution in a tightly stoppered bottle. Dilute the solution before use with an equal volume of water.

Colour development buffer: dissolve 12.6 g of sodium metaborate tetrahydrate or 6.0 g of anhydrous sodium metaborate and 20.0 g of sodium chloride in water and make up to 1000 mL.

Colour dilution buffer: dilute 10 mL of the colour development buffer to 100 mL with water.

2,6-Dibromoquinonechlorimide (BQC) solution: dissolve 40±1 mg of BQC in 10 mL of 96% ethanol. Store in a dark-coloured bottle in a refrigerator. Discard if it is discoloured or more than 1 month old.

Buffer substrate: dissolve 0.1 g of phenyl phosphate disodium salt dihydrate (phenol free) in 100 mL of barium borate-hydroxide buffer. Note: if the hydration of phenyl phosphate disodium salt is not specified, the water content will be stated on the label. It is usually 11–12%, which is equivalent to the dihydrate.

If the salt is not phenol free, dissolve 0.5 g of phenyl phosphate disodium salt in 4.5 mL of colour development buffer, add two drops of BQC and stand at room temperature for 30 min. Extract the colour so formed with 2.5 mL of butan-1-ol and stand until the alcohol separates; remove the alcohol and discard. The solution may be stored in the refrigerator for a few days; develop the colour and re-extract before use. Prepare the buffer substrate immediately before use by diluting 1 mL of this solution to 100 mL with the barium borate-hydroxide buffer.

Zinc-copper precipitant: dissolve 3.0 g of zinc sulphate septahydrate and 0.6 g of copper (II) sulphate pentahydrate in water and make up to 100 mL.

Copper (II) sulphate solution: dissolve 0.05 g of copper (II) sulphate pentahydrate in water and make up to 100 mL.

Phenol standards — stock solution: weigh 200±2 mg of pure anhydrous phenol, transfer to a 100-mL volumetric flask, add water, mix and make up to the mark. This stock solution remains stable for several months if kept in a refrigerator. For use, dilute 10 mL

continued

of stock solution to 100 mL with water and mix. One millilitre of this solution contains 200 µg of phenol.

Procedure

> Note: avoid the influence of direct sunlight during the determination.

Preparation of calibration curve

Prepare a calibration curve each time the test is performed.

(a) Using the standard phenol solution (200 µg/mL), prepare a range of diluted standards containing 2 µg, 5 µg, 10 µg and 20 µg/mL. Keep these standards in the refrigerator for no more than 1 week.

(b) Into each of five test tubes, pipette, respectively, 1 mL of water (control or blank) and 1 mL each of the four diluted phenol standard solutions.

(c) Add to each tube 1 mL of copper (II) sulphate solution, 5 mL of colour dilution buffer, 3 mL of water and 0.1 mL of BQC solution, then mix.

(d) Allow the colour to develop at room temperature for 30 min.

(e) Measure the absorbance of each tube against the control or blank in the spectrophotometer at a wavelength of 610 nm.

(f) Using the procedure of least squares, calculate the regression line from the values of absorbance obtained from each quantity of phenol added.

Preparation of the test sample

Bring the sample to room temperature before testing commences.

(g) Pipette 1 mL of the test sample into each of two test tubes; use one tube as control or blank.

(h) Heat the blank for 2 min in boiling water; cover the test tube and beaker of boiling water with aluminium foil to ensure that the entire tube will be heated. Cool rapidly to room temperature. Treat the heated blank and the test sample in a similar manner for the rest of the procedure.

(i) Add 10 mL of the buffer substrate to each tube and mix.

(j) Immediately incubate the samples in the 37°C water bath for 60 min, mixing the contents at least four times during incubation.

(k) Heat the samples in boiling water for at least 2 min as described before, then cool rapidly to room temperature.

(l) Add 1 mL of zinc-copper precipitant to each tube and mix thoroughly.

(m) Filter through dry filter paper, discard the first 2 mL. Refilter if necessary until the filtrate is completely clear, then collect 5 mL in a test tube.

(n) Add 5 mL of colour development buffer to each tube.

(o) Add 0.1 mL of BQC solution to each tube, mix and allow the colour to develop for 30 min at room temperature.

(p) Measure the absorbance against the control or blank in the spectrophotometer at a wavelength of 610 nm.

(q) If the absorbance of the test sample exceeds the absorbance of the 20 µg phenol standard, repeat the determination using an appropriate dilution of the sample.

continued

Bring a portion of the same test sample carefully to the boil to inactivate the phosphatase, then use this as the diluent for the diluted sample.

(r) Using the regression line obtained in (f), calculate the quantity of phenol from the absorbance reading of the test sample.

Interpretation

Levels below 4 µg of phenol/mL are regarded as satisfactory. However this may represent more than 0.1% raw milk. If levels above 1 µg are detected further investigations at the dairy are recommended.

Method 3b Fluorimetric method

The fluorimetric method is an automated method requiring the use of a dedicated fluorimeter. It can detect very low levels of phosphatase activity (below 0.005%) and so is of more use in public health terms than methods 3a and 3c of this Section. The method is internationally recognized and has been published as BS EN ISO 11816 Part 1 [8]. The phosphatase activity is measured by a continuous fluorimetric kinetic assay. In the presence of any active alkaline phosphatase enzyme in the sample a non-fluorescent aromatic monophosphoric ester substrate is hydrolysed to produce a highly fluorescent product. The amount of fluorescence produced is measured at 38°C in a fluorimeter. The result is expressed as milliunits per litre, where one unit is defined as the amount of enzyme that catalyses the transformation of 1 µmol of substrate/min/L of sample. The lower limit of detection is 10 mU/L.

Equipment

Filter fluorimeter with thermostatted cuvette holder maintained at $38 \pm 1°C$, with right-angle optics, allowing excitation at a wavelength of 440 nm and emission at 560 nm, e.g. Fluorophos®* fluorimeter model FLM 200 containing programmable calculator and associated printer

Incubator block (20 well dry block) set at $38 \pm 0.5°C$

Vortex mixer

Positive displacement pipettor to deliver 75 µL

Pipette/pipettor to deliver 1 mL

Fixed volume dispenser, to deliver 2 mL

Disposable cuvettes, non-fluorescent glass, diameter 12 mm, length 75 mm.

Reagents

Substrate: e.g. Fluorophos® substrate (a water-soluble, non-fluorescent aromatic monophosphoric ester). This is stable for 1 year when crystallized and stored in glass vials at 4°C.

Substrate diluent: diethanolamine (DEA) buffer, pH 10.0, 2.4 mol/L solution. This is stable for 1 year at 4°C.

---

*The Fluorophos® system is available from Advanced Instruments Inc. Two Technology Way, Norwood, MA 02062, US. Tel: 00 1617 320 90 00; Fax: 00 1617 320 36 39; E-mail: www.aitests.com.

continued

Working substrate: Add a volume of the substrate diluent to the substrate to give a concentration of 1044 mmol/L and mix well by inversion. Use amber glass to protect against light. This solution is stable for 8 weeks when stored in the dark at 4°C. Do not store at 38°C for more than 2 h.

Working calibrators: fluoroyellow in DEA buffer.
   Calibrator solution A, containing 0 µmol/L of fluoroyellow.
   Calibrator solution B, containing 17.24×10^{-3} µmol/L of fluoroyellow.
   Calibrator solution C, containing 34.48×10^{-3} µmol/L of fluoroyellow.

These calibrator solutions are stable for 1 year when stored at 4°C.

Procedure

Preparation of calibration curve

Establish a calibration curve using the appropriate assigned channel. Use separate channels for full-cream, semi-skimmed and skimmed milk. Also use separate channels for milks from different animals. If the Fluorophos® system is used the following procedure will automatically calculate the calibration ratio for the product type under test.

(a) Gently invert each bottle of calibrator solution before use.
(b) Label two cuvettes for each calibrator.
(c) Dispense 2 mL of each calibrator in duplicate into the appropriately labelled cuvettes.
(d) Place the cuvettes in the heating block and pre-warm to 38°C for 10 min.
(e) Dispense 75 µL of well mixed test sample to each of the cuvettes, then mix the cuvette contents.
(f) Replace the cuvettes in the heating block. Complete the calibration within 10 min of adding the sample to the calibrators.
(g) Set the fluorimeter to zero fluorescence using the two cuvettes of calibrator A, then read and record the amount of fluorescence obtained with calibrator B and calibrator C. Once calibration is completed proceed with the analysis of the sample.

Determination of alkaline phosphatase activity

(h) Dispense 2 mL of Fluorophos® substrate into a new cuvette, then pre-warm to 38°C in the heating block for 10 min.
(i) Mix the milk sample thoroughly, then transfer 75 µL to the pre-warmed substrate. Mix thoroughly again.
(j) Place the cuvette in the fluorimeter and close the lid.
(k) Choose the appropriate calibrated channel and start the reading. Allow 1 min for temperature equilibration, then record the fluorescence at the beginning of the 2nd min and the end of the 3rd min.
(l) Divide the difference of the two values by two to obtain the average amount of fluorescence produced per min.
(m) Use this value to calculate the alkaline phosphatase activity produced per min. Results obtained in steps (j), (k) and (l) may be calculated automatically by the fluorimeter. Manual calculation can be performed using the formula:

continued

$$\frac{\text{Average fluorescence/min}}{\text{Calibration ratio for product}} \times 459.7$$

(n) Repeat the test using positive and negative controls. Commercial preparations may be used or produced in house. Prepare a negative control by heating 5 mL of product to 95°C for 1 min. A result of less than 10 mU/L should be obtained. Prepare a positive control by adding 0.2 mL of fresh, mixed-herd raw milk to 100 mL of a sample that has previously been heated to 95°C for 1 min and rapidly cooled. This should give a value of around 500 mU/L, but may vary with the herd and the time of year.

Interpretation

Levels below 500 mU/L are considered to satisfy the statutory requirement. However this level may represent more than 0.1% of raw milk. Because the method is so sensitive it will also detect reactivated phosphatase and microbial phosphatase. An action level of 100 mU/L has been suggested; if phosphatase levels exceed this value microbial phosphatase and reactivation should be ruled out as the cause. If the level is due to mammalian phosphatase investigations should be undertaken at the dairy to identify the reasons for its presence.

Microbial phosphatase

Microbial phosphatase is more resistant than mammalian phosphatase to the temperatures used for pasteurization. If residual phosphatase is still present after laboratory pasteurization has been performed, the reading is due to the presence of microbial phosphatase and the original sample was properly pasteurized. Presence of microbial phosphatase is usually due to poor plant hygiene with build up of milk residues on the equipment. It may also be due to high numbers of certain psychrotrophic organisms in the raw milk.

(o) Pipette 1–5 mL of sample into a labelled bijou or test tube, then replace cap. Place the container in a water bath set at 63 ± 1°C so that the water level is at least 4 cm above the sample level.

(p) Heat for 30 min, then cool rapidly.

(q) Re-test the sample for phosphatase activity as described in (h) to (l).

Reactivation

Reactivation of alkaline phosphatase activity may occur if milk is pasteurized at a higher than normal temperature or if the storage temperature after pasteurization is elevated. The test for detecting reactivation is based on the ability of magnesium ions to catalyse reactivation of phosphatase and significantly increase phosphatase activity. If reactivation has occurred, incubation of the sample with magnesium ions before repeating the test will result in at least a six-fold increase in phosphatase activity [9]. This procedure is summarized in Fig. 7.2.

(r) Place 10 mL of the sample in a suitable glass container and heat in a boiling water bath for 1 min. Cool rapidly.

(s) Place 5.0 mL of unheated sample in each of two test tubes. Label one tube 'blank' and add 0.1 mL of deionized water. Label the second tube 'test' and add 0.1 mL of

continued

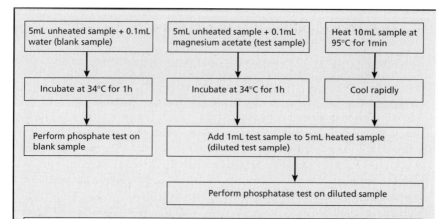

5mL unheated sample + 0.1mL water (blank sample)	5mL unheated sample + 0.1mL magnesium acetate (test sample)	Heat 10mL sample at 95°C for 1min
Incubate at 34°C for 1h	Incubate at 34°C for 1h	Cool rapidly
Perform phosphate test on blank sample	Add 1mL test sample to 5mL heated sample (diluted test sample)	

Perform phosphatase test on diluted sample

If phosphatase level of diluted test sample = blank sample, reactivation has been demonstrated
If phosphatase level of diluted test sample < blank sample, original result is due to mammalian phosphatase

Fig. 7.2 Flow chart for demonstrating reactivation of alkaline phosphatase activity in milk.

magnesium acetate solution. Cap both test tubes and mix well. Incubate at $34 \pm 1°C$ for 1 h. Remove the test tubes and cool rapidly.

Magnesium acetate solution (40.1 mg of Mg^{++}/mL)
Dissolve 35.4 g of $Mg(C_2H_3O_2)_2.4H_2O$ in about 50 mL of deionized water, with warming, then bring to 100 mL with additional deionized water. This solution is stable for 1 year at 3–5°C.

(t) Perform a phosphatase test on the 'blank' sample as described in steps (h)–(m).
(u) Add 1 mL of the 'test' sample to 5 mL of heated, cooled test product (1+5 dilution). Perform a phosphatase test on this 'diluted test' sample.

If the phosphatase activity of the 'diluted test' sample (1+5 dilution) containing magnesium ions has equal or greater activity than the undiluted sample containing no magnesium ions (the 'blank' sample), the phosphatase level originally measured is of reactivated origin. If the 'diluted test' sample contains less phosphatase activity than the undiluted sample, the original phosphatase level is considered to be of mammalian origin.

Note: the phosphatase level may be due to both reactivation and microbial phosphatase. In addition, reactivation may mask the presence of mammalian phosphatase. If reactivation is demonstrated it is not possible to rule out the presence of mammalian phosphatase.

Method 3c Aschaffenberg and Müllen (A–M) test

This method for the phosphatase test was described in full in Statutory Instrument No. 2383 [6], which has now been revoked. The method is not internationally recognized and so has no legal standing but it is a useful method for screening purposes. It is a simple colourimetric method that uses disodium *p*-nitrophenol phosphate as the substrate. This is broken down by phosphatase activity to *p*-nitrophenol. The presence of this compound is indicated by a yellow coloration, the level of which is determined using a colour comparator and appropriate disc. The integrity of this comparator disc is of paramount importance; the disc should be stored away from light and replaced at regular intervals. This method is not capable of detecting low levels of phosphatase activity; any presence of yellow coloration indicates the possible presence of underpasteurized milk. The sample should be raised to room temperature just before testing.

Equipment
Lovibond 'all purposes' comparator with comparator disc APTW or APTW 7
Water bath at $37 \pm 0.5°C$
Glassware kept aside from other laboratory glassware and used only for the phosphatase test. Clean it carefully and thoroughly before use to remove substances that may interfere with the test.

Reagents
Buffer solution: dissolve 3.5 g of anhydrous sodium carbonate and 1.5 g of sodium bicarbonate in distilled or deionized water and dilute to 1 L.

Substrate: disodium *p*-nitrophenyl phosphate. The solid substrate should be kept in the refrigerator.

Buffer-substrate solution: place 0.15 g of the substrate in a measuring cylinder and make up to 100 mL with the buffer solution. Transfer to a dark bottle, store in a refrigerator and protect from light. The reagent should be colourless when used; discard after 1 week.

Procedure
(a) Place 5 mL of buffer-substrate solution into each of two test tubes for each sample to be tested (test and blank).
(b) Stopper the tubes and warm to 37°C in a covered water bath.
(c) Add 1 mL of the milk sample to one tube of buffer-substrate (test).
(d) Add 1 mL of boiled milk to the second tube of buffer-substrate (blank).
(e) Mix the contents of the tubes and incubate at 37°C for exactly 2 h.
(f) Mix again and examine both tubes in a Lovibond colour comparator using disc APTW or APTW 7 in daylight or daylight-type illumination. Revolve the disc until the test sample is matched. Record readings falling between two standards by affixing a plus or minus sign in front of the figure of the nearest standard. The reading is in µg of *p*-nitrophenol/mL of milk.

continued

Interpretation

The standard specified in the Milk (Special Designations) Regulations 1989 [6] was 10 µg p-nitrophenol/mL. Levels below this were considered satisfactory. However this level was probably assigned because it was the lowest level that could be detected with confidence. The presence of any yellow coloration indicates underpasteurization and if any phosphatase activity is detected sufficient raw milk is present to cause illness if pathogens are also present. Further investigations at the dairy should be undertaken to establish the source of the raw milk.

Method 4 Peroxidase test (Storch test)

The peroxidase enzyme present in raw milk is inactivated at 75–80°C. If the milk has been overheated (>75°C) during pasteurization, inactivation of the enzyme will occur and give a negative peroxidase test. The test has no public health or hygiene significance; its only value is as a quality test. The method is described in Commission Decision 91/180/EEC [5].

Principle

The peroxidase enzyme decomposes hydrogen peroxide. The atomic oxygen liberated oxidizes the colourless 1,4-phenylenediamine into the purple indophenol. The colour intensity is proportional to the concentration of the enzyme.

Equipment

Test tubes

Graduated pipettes or pipettor and tips, to deliver 10 mL and 0.1 mL.

Reagents

1,4-phenylenediamine solution 2%: dissolve in warm water and make up to 100 mL. Keep tightly closed and store in a cool, dark place. Discard if a sediment forms.

Hydrogen peroxide solution: dilute 9 mL of hydrogen peroxide 30% in water and make up to 100 mL. To stabilize, add 0.1 mL of concentrated sulphuric acid. Keep tightly closed. If kept in a cool, dark place without contact with organic compounds the solution is stable for 1 month.

Procedure

(a) Transfer 5 mL of milk sample into a clean test tube with a suitable closure.
(b) Add 5 mL of 1,4-phenylenediamine solution.
(c) Add two drops of hydrogen peroxide solution.
(d) Mix well, then examine for production of a blue colour within 30 s. If this occurs, report the result as positive. If no blue colour is produced, report the result as negative. If the colour production occurs later than 30 s after the addition of the reagents the reaction is unspecific.

Interpretation

Properly pasteurized milk that has not been overheated should give a positive peroxidase test.

7.2 Untreated milk

Untreated milk for drinking that is sold directly to the ultimate consumer by a producer of raw milk must satisfy a 30°C colony count test and a coliform test. This applies to milk from cows, goats and sheep. If cows' milk is to be exported to other European Union (EU) countries, it must also satisfy a *Staphylococcus aureus* test and *Salmonella* must be absent in 25 mL. Untreated milk to be used for making dairy products must satisfy a 30°C colony count test and a test for *S. aureus*. The methods for *S. aureus* and *Salmonella* are the same as those described in Section 6.14, method 1 and Section 6.12, method 1, respectively.

Sampling

Samples of untreated milk should be transported at a temperature between 0°C and 4°C; however, if the examination will take place within 24 h a storage temperature of between 0°C and 6°C is acceptable. The time between sampling and analysis should not exceed 36 h.

Method 1 Colony count

The reference procedure described in Commission Decision 91/180/EEC [5] for the colony count test on liquid milk is a pour plate method.

> **Special note**
> For routine purposes, other methods of colony counting such as spiral plating (Section 5.4) are acceptable. If results are required for referee purposes the pour plate method should be used.

Equipment
Water bath at 44–47°C
Incubator at 30±1°C
Pipettes or pipettors and tips, to deliver 1 mL.

Reagents
Peptone saline solution (maximum recovery diluent)
Milk plate count agar.

Procedure
Mix the contents of the sample container thoroughly by inverting the container 25 times before removing a sample portion.

(a) Prepare serial 10-fold dilutions of the milk to 10^{-3} in peptone saline solution.
(b) Proceed as for the method described for the pre-incubated plate count for pasteurized milk, steps (c)–(g) of Section 7.1, method 1.
(c) Incubate the plates at 30±1°C for 72±3 h.

continued

Calculation

(d) Calculate the colony count as described in Section 7.1, method 1 steps (i)–(k).

Interpretation

The standard specified for drinking milk in the Dairy Products (Hygiene) Regulations [2] is 2.0×10^4 cfu/mL. Counts below this are satisfactory. Other standards apply if the milk is to be pasteurized or used for production of dairy products [2].

Method 2 Coliform test

Procedure

Proceed as for pasteurized milk using violet red bile agar, steps (a)–(i) of Section 7.1, method 2.

Calculation

Calculate the coliform count per mL by totalling the coliform colonies in the three plates and dividing by three.

Interpretation

Coliform counts below 100 cfu/mL are satisfactory [2].

Method 3 *Cryptosporidium* detection

If it is necessary to examine untreated milk for the presence of *Cryptosporidium* the sample should be sent to the appropriate reference facility (see Appendix C).

7.3 Ultra heat treated and sterilized milk

The Dairy Products (Hygiene) Regulations 1995 [2] require a colony count test to be performed after pre-incubation of samples at 30°C. If heat-resistant spores are likely to cause a problem this pre-incubation may be performed at 55°C. The Regulations only apply to samples taken at the heat-treatment plant after ultra heat treatment (UHT) or sterilization. Since the products are effectively 'sterile' the test is aimed at detecting the presence of any viable organisms. There should be no detectable organisms when sampled or during the shelf-life of the product.

Method 1 Colony count (ultra heat treated and sterilized milk)

Equipment
Incubator at $30\pm1°C$
Incubator at $55\pm1°C$ (optional)
Water bath at $44–47°C$
Pipettes or pipettor and tips, to deliver 1 mL.

Media
Milk plate count agar.

Procedure
(a) Incubate the intact container at $30\pm1°C$ for 15 days (or $55°\pm1°C$ for 7 days).
(b) Mix the contents thoroughly by inverting the container 25 times. Open the container and aseptically transfer two 1 mL aliquots to separate sterile Petri dishes.
(c) Add 15–18 mL of molten milk plate count agar tempered to $44–47°C$ to each plate. Mix the contents of the Petri dishes and allow to set.
(d) Add 15–18 mL of agar to an empty Petri dish as a sterility control.
(e) Invert the set plates and incubate at $30\pm1°C$ for 72 ± 3 h.
(f) Count any visible colonies.
(g) Calculate the count per mL by totalling the colonies in the two plates and dividing by two.

Up to 100 cfu/mL of sample are allowed in order to avoid test failures due to contamination introduced in the laboratory during testing. The product should not contain any viable organisms.

Interpretation
Counts of less than or equal to 100 cfu/mL are considered satisfactory [2].

7.4 Dairy products

For most dairy products, current legislation requires tests for *Escherichia coli* and examination for the presence of *Listeria monocytogenes* and *Salmonella*. Tests for *Staphylococcus aureus* are also included for cheese products. Associated guidelines also require coliform and aerobic colony counts. Three methods are specified for the enumeration of *E. coli* but no method is specified for coliforms in dairy products because the levels are guideline criteria and are not standards. A summary of appropriate diluents for use in the preparation of the sample homogenates is shown in Table 7.1.

Table 7.1 Diluents for use in sample preparation of milk and dairy products.

Product	Diluent
Milk	0.1% peptone/0.85% saline solution
Liquid milk products	0.1% peptone/0.85% saline solution
Cheese and processed cheese	2% sodium citrate solution pH 7.5 *or* dipotassium hydrogen phosphate solution pH 7.5
Frozen milk products including edible ices	0.1% peptone/0.85% saline solution
Butter	0.1% peptone/0.85% saline solution
Custards, desserts, fresh cream	0.1% peptone/0.85% saline solution
Fermented milks and soured cream	Dipotassium hydrogen phosphate solution pH 7.5
Dried milk powder	Dipotassium hydrogen phosphate solution pH 7.5
Dried sweet whey, dried buttermilk, lactose	0.1% peptone/0.85% saline solution
Acid casein, lactic casein, acid whey powder	Dipotassium hydrogen phosphate solution pH 8.4
Caseinate	Dipotassium hydrogen phosphate solution pH 7.5

Method 1 Coliforms and presumptive *Escherichia coli*—most probable number using 4-methylumbelliferyl-β-D-glucuronide (MUG)

The method described below corresponds to the method in BS ISO 11866-2:1997 [10] but has been modified by the inclusion of Durham tubes for the detection of gas in tubes of the medium to allow detection of coliforms. The method has the sensitivity necessary to satisfy both the standard and guideline values specified for each type of product.

Equipment
Incubator at $30 \pm 1°C$
Ultraviolet lamp 360–366 nm
Test tubes or bottles; check for autofluorescence before use
Durham tubes.

Media and reagents
Lauryl tryptose broth (lauryl sulphate broth) containing 0.01% 4-methylumbelliferyl-β-D-glucuronide (MUG) and 0.01% tryptophan: dispensed in 10 mL volumes in test tubes or bottles containing an inverted Durham tube (LTMUG).

Double strength lauryl tryptose broth containing 0.02% MUG and 0.02% tryptophan: dispensed in 10 mL amounts in tubes or bottles containing an inverted Durham tube.

continued

Brilliant green bile broth (BGBB): dispensed in test tubes or bottles containing an inverted Durham tube.

Kovac's indole reagent.

0.5 M sodium hydroxide solution.

Procedure

> Note: it is essential to perform the various stages of this method in the exact sequence described.

(a) Prepare a 10^{-1} homogenate in a suitable diluent (Table 7.1) and further decimal dilutions in peptone saline diluent.

(b) If a low level of detection is required (<10 cfu/g or mL) add 10 mL of the test sample if liquid, or 10 mL of the 10^{-1} suspension, to each of three tubes containing double strength LTMUG.

(c) Add 1 mL of the test sample if liquid, or 1 mL of the 10^{-1} suspension, to each of three tubes containing single strength LTMUG.

(d) Add 1 mL of each further dilution, as required, to each of three tubes containing single strength LTMUG.

(e) Carefully mix the inoculum and the medium, taking care not to introduce air into the Durham tubes.

(f) Incubate all inoculated tubes at 30°C for 48±2 h.

(g) Examine at 24±2 h and 48±2 h for the presence of gas. Tubes showing gas production contain presumptive coliforms.

(h) At the time of gas detection, subculture each tube showing the presence of gas to BGBB. Also subculture tubes of double strength medium which do not show gas after 48 h. If gas detection occurs at 24 h, reincubate the LTMUG tubes.

(i) Incubate the BGBB tubes at 30°C for 24±2 h, then examine for the presence of gas. If gas is detected, the presence of coliforms is considered confirmed.

> Experience has shown that organisms other than coliforms, notably *Bacillus* spp., may produce gas in BGBB. It is not a requirement of the regulations, but the subculture of tubes showing gas production is recommended to confirm the presence of coliforms.

(j) Count the number of positive tubes at each dilution and use tables to obtain the most probable number (MPN)/g or mL for coliforms (see Section 5, Table 5.7, pp. 121–2).

(k) At 48 h, after appropriate subculture to BGBB has been performed, add 1 mL of 0.5 M sodium hydroxide solution.

(l) Examine the tubes under ultraviolet light for the presence of blue-white fluorescence and record results.

(m) When the tubes have been examined for fluorescence, add 0.5 mL of Kovac's indole reagent, mix well and examine after 1 min. A red colour in the alcoholic phase indicates the presence of indole. Tubes showing fluorescence and formation of indole are positive for the presence of presumptive *E. coli*.

(n) Count the number of positive tubes at each dilution and use tables (Section 5, Table 5.7, pp. 121–2) to obtain the MPN/g or mL for presumptive *E. coli*.

Method 2 Presumptive *Escherichia coli* — most probable number

This method is described in BS ISO 11866-1 : 1997 [11]. It is not suitable for coliform detection in dairy products because incubation of the primary medium takes place at 37°C, not 30°C. The method is a nine-tube (3,3,3) test as described in Section 6.6, method 3 (pp. 152–3) using lauryl tryptose medium containing Durham tubes for gas detection.

Method 3 Presumptive *Escherichia coli* — direct enumeration using membranes

This method is identical to the method described in Section 6.6, method 5 (pp. 153–4). It is fully described in BS ISO 11866-3 : 1997 [12].

Method 4 *Staphylococcus aureus*

The procedure described in Section 6.14, method 1 (p. 174) is suitable.

Method 5 *Salmonella*

The procedure described in Section 6.12, method 1 or method 2, (pp. 169–70) is most appropriate. The pH of the pre-enrichment broth may need adjustment to neutrality before incubation (see Table 6.10, p. 170).

Method 6 *Listeria monocytogenes*

The Dairy Products (Hygiene) Regulations [2] require the absence of *L. monocytogenes* in either 1 g or 25 g of product, depending on the type of product. An enrichment procedure is therefore necessary and enumeration is not required. The procedures described in Section 6.10, methods 1 and 2 are appropriate (pp. 163–5).

Liquid milk-based products

This group of products includes pasteurized cream, yoghurt and milk-based drinks. Current legislation [2] specifies the absence of *Listeria monocytogenes* in 1 g and *Salmonella* in 25 g. The Guidance Notes [4] also give guideline levels for coliforms. Five samples taken at the same time from the producer's or heat treatment premises should be examined for statutory purposes. Use Section 7.4, method 1 steps (a)–(j). As the guideline value for m (the threshold value for the number of bacteria, see Section 3.10) is 0, three tubes of 10 mL of the 10^{-1}

homogenate in double strength LTMUG are required in addition to three tubes of 1 mL of the 10^{-1} homogenate and three tubes of 1 mL of the 10^{-2} dilution.

Results are satisfactory if coliforms are not detected and unsatisfactory if more than five coliforms/mL or g are obtained.

Pasteurized cream

Pasteurized cream sampled at the heat treatment premises must satisfy the phosphatase test and give a negative reaction in the peroxidase test in addition to the requirements above.

The peroxidase test is identical to the method described in Section 7.1, method 4.

Method 7 Phosphatase test for cream

In order to aid pipetting, a small amount of cream may be taken off after mixing and warmed in a 37°C water bath for 1–2 min.

If testing for microbial phosphatase is required, the sample should be heated at 66 ± 1°C for 30 min instead of 63°C before re-testing for phosphatase due to the higher cream content. If testing for reactivation is required, follow the appropriate method described below.

Method 7a Spectrophotometric method

Reagents
Zinc sulphate solution: dissolve 4.5 g zinc sulphate ($ZnSO_4.7H_2O$) in 25 mL of deionized water, warming if necessary. Cool, then make up to 100 mL with water.

Treat fresh cream in the same way as fresh milk and examine using Section 7.1, method 3a.

For old or slightly sour cream use 8 mL of the barium borate-hydroxide buffer plus 2 mL of water in place of 10 mL of buffer and substitute 1 mL of zinc sulphate solution for the zinc-copper precipitant.

If phosphatase activity is detected examine for reactivation by pre-treating the sample as described in Section 7.1, method 3b and then re-test for phosphatase activity by Section 7.1, method 3a [13,14].

Method 7b Fluorimetric method

Examine according to Section 7.1, method 3b. Use a separate dedicated channel of the fluorimeter for each cream type (single, whipping, double, etc.).

Method 7c Colourimetric test

This method was described in full in Statutory Instrument No. 1509 [15], which has now been revoked. However it may be useful for screening purposes. Samples showing evidence of tainting or souring should not be tested.

Reagents
As for Section 7.1, method 3c, and in addition:
30% (w/v) zinc sulphate solution
15% (w/v) potassium ferrocyanide solution
40% (w/v) magnesium chloride ($MgCl_2.6H_2O$) solution.

Procedure
(a) Pipette 15 mL of the buffer-substrate solution into each of two test tubes, stopper them and pre-warm the contents by placing in a water bath at $37\pm0.5°C$.
(b) Add 2 mL of cream to one tube, replace stopper and mix thoroughly.
(c) Add 2 mL of previously boiled cream (of the same type as the sample) to the second tube to act as a blank; mix thoroughly.
(d) Incubate the tubes for 120 min in the water bath at $37\pm0.5°C$.
(e) Remove the tubes from the water bath and mix the contents thoroughly.
(f) Add 0.5 mL of zinc sulphate solution to each tube.
(g) Replace stoppers, mix thoroughly and leave to stand for 3 min.
(h) Add 0.5 mL of potassium ferrocyanide solution to each tube and mix thoroughly.
(i) Filter the contents of each tube through separate filter papers (e.g. Whatman No. 4 0) and collect the clear filtrates into clean tubes.
(j) Place the blank and test filtrates in the comparator and examine using disc APTW or APTW 7 in daylight or daylight-type illumination. Revolve the disc until the test sample is matched. Record readings falling between two standards by affixing a plus or minus sign in front of the figure of the nearest standard. The reading is in µg of p-nitrophenol/mL of cream.

Interpretation
As for milk, the test is considered satisfactory if the cream gives a reading of 10 µg or less of p-nitrophenol/mL. If phosphatase is detected, further testing for reactivation is necessary.

Reactivation
If the cream does not satisfy the test, examine as follows:

(k) Transfer 10 mL of cream into each of two clean test tubes.
(l) Add nothing to one tube (the control) and to the other add a volume of magnesium chloride solution according to the butterfat content of the cream:

continued

	Fat content (%)	Magnesium chloride solution (mL)
Clotted cream	55	0.20
Double cream	48	0.25
Whipping cream	35	0.35
Single cream	18	0.50
Half cream	12	0.56

Other percentages by extrapolation.

(m) Stopper the tubes, mix by inversion and incubate for 60 min at $37\pm0.5°C$ in a water bath.
(n) Invert occasionally during incubation.
(o) Remove test tubes and transfer 2 mL from each to two clean test tubes.
(p) Repeat the test as described in steps (a)–(j) of this method.
(q) If the intensity of the colour of the filtrate from the tube containing magnesium is higher than the control then proceed as follows.
(r) Dilute the filtrate one in four with the buffer-substrate solution and again compare with the filtrate of the control.
(s) If the colour is equal to or more intense than that of the undiluted control, the original positive phosphatase result is void and reactivation has taken place. If the colour is less intense than that of the undiluted control then the original result stands since reactivation of enzyme has not been demonstrated.

Ultra heat treated and sterilized cream

These products are required to satisfy a colony count test after pre-incubation of an unopened sample container. The test is the same as that described in Section 7.3, method 1.

Untreated (raw) cream

Testing of untreated cream is not covered in the regulations or guidance notes. Similar tests to those for untreated milk should be performed. The coliform test should be performed as described in Section 7.4, method 1 steps (a)–(j) using 10^{-1}, 10^{-2} and 10^{-3} dilutions. Coliform counts below 100 cfu/mL are satisfactory.

Pasteurized milk-based drinks

In addition to the tests already described, a phosphatase test is appropriate (but not specified in current legislation). The fluorimetric method described in Section 7.1, method 3b can be used for all drinks including deeply coloured ones.

In order to achieve the required sensitivity when performing the coliform test, use 10 mL volumes as well as 1 mL volumes of the 10^{-1} dilution.

Yoghurt and other fermented products

Tests applicable to these products are described under the 'Liquid milk-based products' heading above. Use dipotassium hydrogen phosphate solution pH 7.5 as the diluent for preparation of the sample homogenate.

Ultra heat treated and sterilized milk-based drinks

See 'ultra heat treated and sterilized cream' above.

Frozen milk-based products including ice-cream

Current legislation requires the absence of *Salmonella* in 25 g and *Listeria monocytogenes* in 1 g. The guidance notes specify colony count and coliform tests. Examination for *Escherichia coli* is not required. The sample may be thawed immediately before testing by placing in a water bath at $37 \pm 1°C$ until just molten.

Method 8 Colony count

As this is a guideline parameter and not a standard, any of the methods described in Section 5.3–5.6 are suitable. Milk plate count agar should be used with incubation at $30 \pm 1°C$ for 72 ± 3 h.

Interpretation
Refer to Section 3 for criteria. Colony counts below 10^5 cfu/g are satisfactory; counts exceeding 5×10^5 cfu/g are unsatisfactory.

Method 9 Coliform test

Procedure
(a) Prepare 10^{-1}, 10^{-2} and 10^{-3} dilutions of sample in peptone saline diluent.
(b) Proceed through steps (c)–(i) of Section 7.4, method 7.
(c) Compute the MPN from Section 5, Table 5.7 (pp. 121–2).

Interpretation
Refer to Section 3.10 for criteria. If fewer than 10 coliforms/g are detected the results are satisfactory. If more than 100 coliforms/g are present the results are unsatisfactory.

Powdered milk-based products

For statutory purposes, 10 samples of milk powder or five samples of other powdered milk-based products should be examined for *Salmonella*. Coliform guideline levels are also specified [4]. Section 7.4, method 7, above, is suitable. There is no requirement to examine for *Escherichia coli*. The appropriate diluents for use in preparation of the sample are shown in Table 7.1.

Cheese

The microbiological criteria for cheese depend upon the type of cheese (hard, soft or fresh) and the type of milk used (raw, thermised or pasteurized). These criteria can be found in Section 3 (p. 38). All specifications require the absence of *Salmonella* in 25 g and the absence of *Listeria monocytogenes* in 1 g for hard cheese or 25 g for other cheese types. Levels for *Staphylococcus aureus* are specified for all cheese types except hard cheese made from pasteurized milk. Levels for *Escherichia coli* are specified for all soft cheese regardless of milk type and also guideline levels for coliforms in soft cheese made from heat treated milk. Section 7.4, method 1 is appropriate.

Fresh cheese is regarded as soft cheese that is not subjected to a maturation period. As permitted levels for coliforms and *E. coli* are high it is necessary to test sample dilutions from 10^{-1} to 10^{-5}.

Levels for *E. coli* below 100 cfu/g are satisfactory for soft cheese made with heat treated milk. If the milk used was raw or thermised levels below 10000 cfu/g are considered satisfactory, but in practice much lower levels are frequently achieved.

The sample homogenate should be prepared in either 2% sodium citrate solution pH 7.5 or dipotassium hydrogen phosphate pH 7.5 (see Table 7.1). Buffered peptone water used for pre-enrichment of the sample for *Salmonella* testing should be pre-warmed to 45°C to help disperse the fat. If the cheese contains a high fat content the use of a surfactant can aid isolation (see Section 6, Table 6.10, p. 170).

7.5   References

1   Council of the European Communities. Directive No. 92/46/EEC. Laying down the health rules for the production and placing on the market of raw milk, heat treated milk and milk based products. *Official J Eur Communities* 1992; **L268**: 1–32.

2   England & Wales. *The Dairy Products (Hygiene) Regulations 1995. Statutory Instrument No. 1086*. London: HMSO, 1995.

3   Food Safety Act 1990 Code of Practice No. 18. *Enforcement of the Dairy Products (Hygiene) Regulations 1995 and the Dairy Products (Hygiene) (Scotland) Regulations ('The Regulations')*. London: HMSO, 1995.

4   Ministry of Agriculture, Fisheries and Food, Department of Health, Scottish Office, Welsh Office. *Dairy Products (Hygiene) Regulations 1995 — Guidance Notes*. 1995.

5   European Commission. 91/180/EEC. Commission decision laying down certain methods of analysis and testing of raw milk and heat treated milk. *Official J Eur Communities* 1991; **L93**: 1–48.

6   Great Britain. *The Milk (Special Designations) Regulations 1989. Statutory Instrument No. 2383*. London: HMSO, 1989.

7   British Standards Institution (BSI). BS 4285. *Microbiological Examination for Dairy Purposes. Section 3.7 Enumeration of Coliform Bacteria*. London: BSI, 1987.

8   British Standards Institution (BSI). BS EN ISO 11816-1. *Milk and Milk Products. Determination of Alkaline Phosphatase Activity using a Fluorimetric Method. Part 1: Milk and Milk-based Drinks*. London: BSI, 2000.

9   Association of Official Analytical Chemists (AOAC). Official Method No. 961.08. Phosphatase (reactivated and residual) in milk. In: *AOAC Official Methods of Analysis*, 16th edn. Dairy Products, Arlington VA: AOAC, 1995, p. 36.

10 British Standards Institution (BSI). BS ISO 11866-2. *Milk and Milk products. Enumeration of Presumptive Escherichia coli. Part 2. Most Probable Number Technique Using 4-methylumbelliferyl-β-D-glucuronide (MUG)*. London: BSI, 1997.

11 British Standards Institution (BSI). BS ISO 11866-1. *Milk and Milk Products. Enumeration of Presumptive Escherichia coli. Part 1. Most Probable Number Technique*. London: BSI, 1997.

12 British Standards Institution (BSI). BS ISO 11866-3. *Milk and Milk Products. Enumeration of Presumptive Escherichia coli. Part 3. Colony-count Technique at 44°C Using Membranes*. London: BSI, 1997.

13 Association of Official Analytical Chemists (AOAC). Official Method No. 950.41. Phosphatase (residual) in cream. In: *AOAC Official Methods of Analysis*, 16th edn. Dairy Products, Arlington VA: AOAC, 1995, p. 47.

14 Association of Official Analytical Chemists (AOAC). Official Method No. 965.27. Phosphatase (reactivated and residual) in cream. In: *AOAC Official Methods of Analysis*, 16th edn. Dairy Products, Arlington VA: AOAC, 1995, p. 47.

15 Great Britain. *The Milk and Dairies (Heat Treatment of Cream) Regulations 1983. Statutory Instrument No. 1509*. London: HMSO, 1983.

8 Eggs and egg products

8.1 Shell eggs
8.2 Bulk liquid egg

8.1 Shell eggs

The following methods are recommended for the examination of shell eggs for salmonellae on the basis of their successful use. Whenever possible an attempt should be made to quantify the numbers of organisms present.

> Disposable gloves should be worn during the examination of shell eggs.

Documentation

Record the following:
- The source of the eggs (i.e. shop, supermarket, farm gate, etc.).
- The type and size of the eggs (i.e. battery or free-range, small, medium, large, etc.).
- The name of the packer or producer.
- The packing and sell-by dates.
- The presence of visible cracks and/or faecal material adhering to the shell.

Equipment
Incubator set at $37 \pm 1°C$
Incubator set at $41.5 \pm 1°C$.

Media
Buffered peptone water (BPW)
Rappaport Vassiliadis soya peptone broth (RVS)
Selective agars: xylose lysine desoxycholate agar (XLD) and a second medium of choice, e.g. modified brilliant green agar (BGA), manitol lysine crystal violet bile agar (MLCB), a chromogenic agar, etc.

Method 1 Individual eggs: examination without shell disinfection (Fig. 8.1)

Procedure

(a) Crack the egg against the top of a sterile screw-capped jar or disposable plastic 250 mL container holding 180 mL BPW and drop the contents into it.

(b) Homogenize the mixture by shaking the container.

> The use of BPW is optional as homogenized egg is a good culture medium. BPW prevents coagulation of the egg during incubation.

(c) Drop the shell into a further 180 mL BPW contained in a separate screw-capped jar.

(d) Incubate the BPW cultures at 37°C for 18±2 h.

(e) Subculture the BPW containing egg contents to XLD and a second medium of choice and proceed with isolation of salmonellae as described in steps (c)–(f) of Section 6.12, method 1.

(f) Subculture 0.1 mL of BPW containing the shells to 10 mL of RVS broth. Incubate at 41.5°C for 20–24 h and proceed with the isolation of salmonellae as described in steps (c)–(f) of Section 6.12, method 1.

A modified procedure to separate yolk and albumen is as follows:

1 Proceed as described in step (a) but with an empty jar or container.

2 Aspirate the albumen with a sterile 10 mL pipette and transfer to a tared sterile container. Weigh the transferred albumen and add nine times the weight of BPW, then mix. This forms a 1/10 homogenate. Continue as described above. Report the final result in relation to the weight examined.

3 Repeat step 2 above with the yolk using a fresh sterile pipette.

4 Proceed with the isolation of salmonellae as described in steps (d) and (e).

Method 2 Individual eggs: examination with shell disinfection (Fig. 8.2)

Procedure

(a) Wipe the shell with a large sterile cotton wool swab moistened with BPW and then drop the swab into 180 mL of BPW in a sterile screw-capped jar or disposable 250 mL container.

(b) Wipe the shell with a large isopropyl alcohol impregnated wipe or cotton wool ball soaked in 70% industrial methylated spirit (IMS), or immerse the egg in IMS. Remove and allow to dry completely.

(c) Crack the egg against the top of a sterile jar or disposable plastic 250 mL container holding 180 mL of BPW and drop the contents of the egg into it. Discard the shell.

(d) Incubate the BPW cultures at 37°C for 18±2 h.

continued

(e) Subculture the BPW containing egg contents to XLD and a second medium of choice and follow the procedure for isolation of salmonellae described in steps (c)–(f) of Section 6.12, method 1.

(f) Subculture 0.1 mL BPW containing the swab from the shell to 10 mL RVS broth. Incubate at 41.5°C for 20–24 h and proceed with the isolation of salmonellae described in steps (c)–(f) of Section 6.12, method 1.

A modified procedure to separate yolk and albumen is as follows:

1 Proceed as described in steps (a)–(c) but drop the yolk and albumen into separate sterile 60 mL or 250 mL containers.

2 Aspirate the albumen with a sterile 10 mL pipette and transfer to a tared sterile container. Weigh the quantity and add nine times the weight of BPW, then mix. Proceed as described in steps (d) and (e) of method 1. Report the final result in relation to the weight examined.

3 Repeat step 2 above with the yolk using a fresh sterile pipette.

4 Proceed with the isolation of salmonellae as described in steps (d) and (e) of method 1.

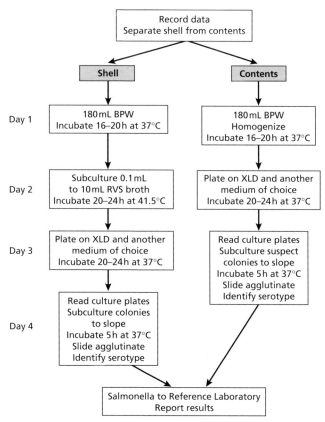

Fig. 8.1 Examination of individual shell eggs without shell disinfection.

Method 3 Batched eggs: examination without shell disinfection (Fig. 8.3)

> Disposable gloves should be changed after each batch of six eggs.

Procedure

(a) Break the contents of six eggs into a tared stomacher bag. Weigh the contents and then homogenize. Add an equal weight of BPW. Alternatively mix the egg contents vigorously with an equal weight of BPW in a sterile wide-necked container.

(b) Decant, if necessary, into a sterile flask of 1 L capacity or a large wide-necked screw-capped container and incubate at 37°C for 18±2 h.

(c) Put the shells into a sterile screw-capped jar containing 180 mL BPW and incubate at 37°C for 18±2 h.

(d) Subculture 0.1 mL of BPW shell culture to 10 mL RVS broth and incubate at 41.5°C for 20–24 h.

(e) Proceed from steps (b) and (d) above with the isolation of salmonellae as described in steps (c)–(f) of Section 6.12, method 1.

Method 4 Batched eggs: examination with shell disinfection (Fig. 8.4)

Procedure

(a) Wipe the shells of six eggs with a large sterile cotton wool swab moistened with BPW and then drop the swab into 180 mL BPW contained in a sterile screw-capped jar or disposable container of 250 mL capacity. Incubate at 37°C for 18±2 h.

(b) Wipe the shells with a large wipe impregnated with isopropyl alcohol or a cotton wool ball soaked in 70% IMS, or immerse the eggs in IMS. Allow to dry completely.

> Disposable gloves should be changed before proceeding further.

(c) Break the six eggs into a tared stomacher bag and weigh. Homogenize the contents then add an equal weight of BPW. Alternatively mix the egg contents vigorously with an equal weight of BPW in a sterile wide-necked container. Discard the shells.

(d) Decant the egg mixture, if necessary, into a sterile flask of 1 L capacity or a large wide-necked screw-capped container and incubate at 37°C for 18±2 h.

(e) Subculture 0.1 mL of the shell swab culture to 10 mL of RVS broth and incubate at 41.5°C for 20–24 h.

(f) Proceed from steps (a) and (d) above with the isolation of salmonellae as described in steps (c)–(f) of Section 6.12, method 1.

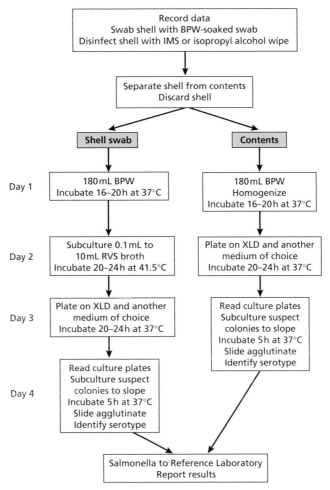

```
                    ┌─────────────────────────────────────────────┐
                    │              Record data                    │
                    │    Swab shell with BPW-soaked swab          │
                    │ Disinfect shell with IMS or isopropyl alcohol wipe │
                    └─────────────────────────────────────────────┘
                                      │
                    ┌─────────────────────────────┐
                    │  Separate shell from contents │
                    │         Discard shell         │
                    └─────────────────────────────┘
```

	Shell swab	Contents
Day 1	180 mL BPW Incubate 16–20 h at 37°C	180 mL BPW Homogenize Incubate 16–20 h at 37°C
Day 2	Subculture 0.1 mL to 10 mL RVS broth Incubate 20–24 h at 41.5°C	Plate on XLD and another medium of choice Incubate 20–24 h at 37°C
Day 3	Plate on XLD and another medium of choice Incubate 20–24 h at 37°C	Read culture plates Subculture suspect colonies to slope Incubate 5 h at 37°C Slide agglutinate Identify serotype
Day 4	Read culture plates Subculture suspect colonies to slope Incubate 5 h at 37°C Slide agglutinate Identify serotype	

```
                    ┌─────────────────────────────────────────────┐
                    │  Salmonella to Reference Laboratory         │
                    │            Report results                   │
                    └─────────────────────────────────────────────┘
```

Fig. 8.2 Examination of individual shell eggs with shell disinfection.

8.2 Bulk liquid egg

Raw (unpasteurized) and pasteurized liquid egg should be transported to the laboratory and examined separately to ensure no cross-contamination occurs.

Raw bulk liquid egg

Sampling

Take samples from the raw egg balance tank immediately before pasteurization. This will enable the most representative results on levels of contamination to be obtained. If the balance tank has a sample tap, allow some of the egg to run to waste to minimize contamination from the tap before taking the sample into a sterile disposable container. Use sterile disposable dippers to take samples from

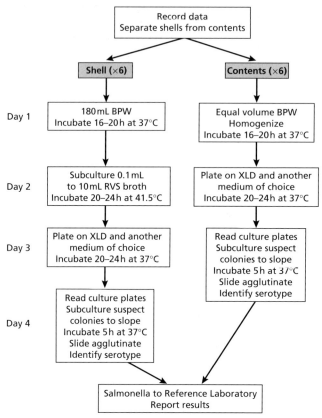

Fig. 8.3 Examination of batched shell eggs without shell disinfection.

balance tanks without sample taps. Most processing plants will not allow glass jars to be brought into the plant.

On arrival at the laboratory, defrost samples of frozen egg in a refrigerator at 0–4°C or at room temperature for 2–3 h. Examine raw egg in 25 mL samples.

Many samples of raw egg are likely to contain at least one *Salmonella* spp. Where a sample is positive for salmonellae, a most probable number (MPN) estimation may be performed as described in Section 6.12, method 6.

Method 1 Enrichment culture for *Salmonella* spp.

Procedure

(a) Add 25 mL of the raw liquid egg to a jar containing 225 mL of BPW plus 5 mg of novobiocin/L and 10 mg of cefsulodin/L.

(b) Incubate at 37°C for 18±2 h, then subculture 0.1 mL to 10 mL of RVS broth.

(c) Incubate RVS broth for 20–24 h at 41.5°C and subculture on XLD and a second medium of choice. Proceed with isolation of salmonellae as described in steps (c)–(f) of Section 6.12, method 1.

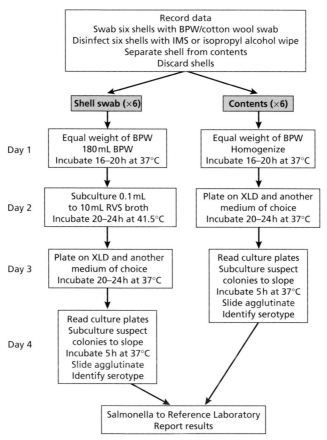

Fig. 8.4 Examination of batched shell eggs with shell disinfection.

Pasteurized bulk liquid egg

Council Directive 89/437/EEC [1], on hygiene and health problems affecting the production and the placing on the market of egg products, specifies the tests to be performed on heat treated liquid egg and egg products when sampled at the production premises. The microbiological tests are a mesophilic aerobic colony count (30°C), Enterobacteriaceae count and absence of *Staphylococcus aureus* in 1 g and *Salmonella* in 25 g or mL. For statutory purposes internationally recognized methods of examination should be used. The provisions of this directive have been implemented in the UK in the Egg Products Regulations 1993 [2]. In addition to the microbiological criteria, these regulations specify an alpha-amylase test to ensure that the product is adequately pasteurized (see Method 7).

Sampling

Take the sample from the pasteurized egg holding tank as close to the pasteurizer as possible by the procedure agreed on site. Samples of frozen egg should be defrosted in a refrigerator at 0–4°C or room temperature for 2–3 h on arrival at the laboratory.

Method 2 Examination for *Salmonella* spp.

Examine a 25 g or 25 mL portion of sample by Section 6.12, methods 1, 2 or 3.

Method 3 Enumeration of *Salmonella* spp.

Procedure

(a) Take a sufficient quantity of sample to test 6×18 mL by the multiple tube method (Section 5.7, method 1).

(b) Add 18 mL to each of six jars containing 180 mL of BPW.

(c) Incubate for 18 ± 2 h at 37°C.

(d) Subculture 0.1 mL from each jar to separate 10 mL volumes of RVS broth.

(e) Incubate for 20–24 h at 41.5°C and subculture on XLD and a second medium of choice. Proceed with the isolation of salmonellae as described in steps (c)–(f) of Section 6.12, method 1.

(f) From the number of jars shown to contain salmonellae, calculate the MPN of the organisms/g of sample from Table 5.5 (p. 119). The MPN of organisms present may be estimated in the range from one to >10 per 100 mL.

Method 4 Aerobic colony count

UK legislation allows the use of either a pour plate technique or a surface spread technique. Methods 5.3, 5.4 and 5.6 are suitable. Incubate the plates at 30°C for 72 ± 3 h.

Method 5 Enterobacteriaceae

Examine the sample by the method described in Section 6.7, method 1.

Method 6 *Staphylococcus aureus*

The legislation requires absence of *Staphylococcus aureus* in 1 g; therefore an enrichment method is required (although the UK legislation specifies a colony count technique). Section 6.14, method 4 is suitable for detection by enrichment.

Method 7 Alpha-amylase test

This is a test for the efficiency of the pasteurization process. The time/temperature combination used for the process should inactivate the enzyme alpha-amylase present in the egg so the starch added during the test will not be broken down and will give a blue coloration with iodine. The presence of large numbers of *Bacillus* spp. may cause a false 'fail' result due to the presence of bacterial amylases. The test is only applicable to whole liquid egg.

> Glassware (flasks, tubes, pipettes) for use in this test should not be used for any other purpose and should be kept separate from other glassware. It should be carefully and thoroughly cleaned to remove substances that may interfere with the test.

Reagents
Fresh starch solution: weigh out analytical quality soluble starch to the equivalent of 0.7 g dry starch. Mix with a small quantity of cold water to produce a thin cream. Transfer this to about 50 mL of boiling water and boil for 1 min. Cool rapidly. Add three drops of toluene and make the volume up to 100 mL with water. Store at 4°C. Discard the solution 14 days after preparation.

0.001 M iodine solution: prepare a stock 0.1 M solution by dissolving 3.6 g of potassium iodide in 20 mL of water. Add 1.27 g of iodine and make up to 100 mL with water. This solution is stable for a period of 6 months. Just before use, prepare a working solution by diluting 1 mL of stock solution to 100 mL with water.

15% (w/v) trichloracetic acid solution.

Procedure
(a) Weigh 15 g of liquid egg into a flask and add 2 mL of fresh starch solution.
(b) Mix well and incubate in a water bath at 44±0.5°C for 30 min
(c) Allow mixture to cool, then transfer 5 mL to a test tube containing 5 mL of 15% trichloracetic acid solution. Mix well.
(d) Add 15 mL distilled water. Mix well.
(e) Either filter the mixture through Whatman® no. 12 fluted filter paper, discarding the first few drops of filtrate, or centrifuge the mixture. Transfer 10 mL of clear filtrate or supernatant to a test tube containing 2 mL of 0.001 M iodine solution.
(f) Examine the colour of the solution. A blue-violet colour indicates the presence of starch and thus the absence of alpha-amylase. To quantify the colour use (i) a spectrophotometric standard with an optical density of 0.15 when compared against water in 1 cm cells at a wavelength of 585 μm, or (ii) a disc 4/26 in a Lovibond® colour comparator. If the test solution colour is greater than three on the disc it indicates the presence of starch and thus the destruction of the alpha-amylase by the heat treatment applied to the egg.

Controls
Include control samples with every batch of tests. Raw liquid egg serves as a positive control and boiled liquid egg as a negative control.

8.3 References

1 Commission of the European Communities. Directive 89/437/EEC. Hygiene and health problems affecting the production and the placing on the market of egg products. *Off J Eur Communities* 1989; L212, 22.7.89, 87–100.

2 Great Britain. *Statutory Instrument 1993 No. 1520. The Egg Products Regulations.* London: HMSO, 1993.

9 Live bivalve molluscs and other shellfish

Council Directive 91/492/EEC [1] sets out the designation of production areas of bivalve molluscs based on levels of *Escherichia coli* or faecal coliforms/100 g of flesh and intravalvular liquid. A three-dilution, five-tube most probable number (MPN) method is specified for testing without precise details, but other bacteriological methods of equivalent accuracy are permitted. In the UK testing for *E. coli* is performed because it is considered to be a more specific indicator of faecal pollution than faecal coliforms. The microbiological criteria for the classification of shellfish harvesting areas are shown in Table 9.1.

In addition to the classification criteria, diarrhoetic shellfish poison (DSP) must be absent from the shellfish flesh and levels of paralytic shellfish poison (PSP) must be below 80 μg/100 g of flesh. If these levels are exceeded fishing is prohibited in that harvesting area until compliance is achieved. Since the publication of the Directive another shellfish poison known as amnesic shellfish poison (ASP) has been identified; levels of ASP should be below 20 μg/g of flesh [2].

Testing for DSP, PSP and ASP is normally performed by reference laboratories. Routine monitoring of shellfish harvesting areas in the UK for marine biotoxins is a statutory responsibility of the Food Standards Agency who can advise on the specialist laboratories currently contracted to undertake this task. In England the reference facility for outbreak related samples is the Food Safety Microbiology Laboratory, Central Public Health Laboratory. Tel: 020 8200 4400, ext. 3521/4113. The UK National Reference Laboratory for biotoxins is the Fisheries Research Services (FRS) Marine Laboratory, Aberdeen AB11 9DB. Tel: 01224 876544.

An end-product standard is defined for shellfish intended for immediate human consumption. For faecal coliforms and *E. coli* this is given as category A in Table 9.1. In addition, the shellfish should meet the standards defined above for biotoxins and *Salmonella* should be absent in 25 g of shellfish flesh. The Directive recognized the absence of routine virus testing procedures and this is still true today. However consumption of molluscs containing viruses, in particular Norwalk-like virus (NLV; also known as small round structured virus or SRSV) is the most common cause of illness from this type of food. At present, methods for the direct detection of viral pathogens (NLV and hepatitis A virus or HAV) in shellfish are all based on the polymerase chain reaction (PCR). However,

Table 9.1 Classification of harvesting areas.

Category	Escherichia coli/100 g	Faecal coliforms/100 g	Interpretation
A	<230	<300	May go for direct consumption
B	90% of samples not to exceed 4600	90% of samples not to exceed 6000	Must be depurated or relayed to meet Category A (may also be heat treated by approved method)
C	Must not exceed 46 000*	Must not exceed 60 000	Must be relayed for long period (>2 months) to meet Category A or B (may also be heat treated by approved method)
D	>46 000*	>60 000	Prohibited (may also be prohibited on health grounds rather than monitoring results)

*Figures not included in EEC regulations.

processing of shellfish extracts to recover low levels of contaminating virus and to remove PCR inhibitors is difficult. Currently these methods are complex, poorly standardized and restricted to specialist facilities [3]. The relationship between the levels of E. coli and the presence of virus particles in depurated shellfish is poor, but studies have shown a much better relationship between the levels of certain types of phage, in particular F-specific RNA bacteriophage [4], and the risk of viral contamination. Phage detection methods are much simpler to perform than virus detection methods and might be incorporated more easily into routine examination of live bivalve molluscs.

Testing for viral contamination (NLV and HAV) is also currently performed by reference facilities. The Enteric Virus Unit at the Central Public Health Laboratory, Tel. 0208 200 4400, and other peripheral Public Health Laboratory Service (PHLS) laboratories can advise on analysis of clinical samples associated with shellfish outbreaks. The UK National Reference Laboratory for bacteriological and viral contamination of shellfish is the Centre for Environment, Fisheries and Aquaculture Science (CEFAS), Weymouth DT4 8UB. Tel: 01305 206600.

Method 1 Multiple tube method for *Escherichia coli*

This method is the standard procedure used in the UK [5]. Minerals modified glutamate broth is used for the first stage of the test based on the detection of acid production followed by detection of β-glucuronidase activity at 44°C using a chromogenic agar for confirmation of the presence of *Escherichia coli*.

continued

A pooled sample of at least six shellfish are required for testing to overcome the variability associated with individual shellfish. Additional shellfish should be submitted by the sampling authority to allow for rejections. All samples should be stored dry at 4°C and examined preferably within 6 h of collection but no later than 24 h after collection. Samples should not be frozen.

Sample size
Oysters/clams 10–15
Mussels 15–30
Cockles 30–50.

Equipment
Stomacher (optional)
Rotary blender (optional)
Shucking knives
Balance with resolution 0.1 g or greater
Incubators at 37 ± 1°C and 44 ± 1°C.

Reagents
0.1% peptone solution (in water), pH 7.2 ± 0.2
0.1% peptone/0.85% sodium chloride solution
Minerals modified glutamate medium, double and single strength
5-bromo-4-chloro-3-indolyl β-D-glucuronide (BCIG) agar. Tryptone bile agar containing 144 μmol/L 5-bromo-4-chloro-3-indolyl-β-D glucuronic acid (e.g. 0.075 g/L of cyclohexylammonium salt).

Control cultures
NCTC 9001	*Escherichia coli*	Positive
NCTC 13216	*Escherichia coli*	β-glucuronidase weak positive
NCTC 9528	*Klebsiella aerogenes*	β-glucuronidase negative

Sample preparation
(a) Select at least 10 oysters and clams, 15 mussels or 30 cockles. Discard any gaping shellfish and those with obvious signs of damage.
(b) Clean the molluscs by scraping, scrubbing and washing under cold running water of potable quality and allow to drain on clean paper towels.
(c) Open the molluscs with a flamed and cooled shucking knife, as follows:

Oysters/clams
Insert the knife between the two shells towards the hinge end of the shellfish, push further into the shellfish and prise open the upper shell. Allow any liquor to drain into a sterile weighed bag or beaker. Push the blade through the shellfish and sever the muscle attachments by slicing across. Remove the upper shell and scrape the contents of the lower shell into the sterile bag or beaker. Repeat for at least 10 oysters/clams to obtain the required weight and add to the same bag or beaker.

continued

Mussels/cockles

Insert the knife between the shells through the byssal opening of the shellfish and separate the shells by twisting the knife. Collect any liquor in a weighed sterile bag or beaker. Cut the muscle between the two shells and scrape the contents into the sterile bag or beaker. Repeat for a minimum of 15 mussels or 30 cockles to obtain the required weight, adding the contents to the same bag or beaker.

Preparation of homogenate

Using stomacher

(d) Place the bag containing the shellfish meat and liquor inside two more bags to prevent puncture from shell.

(e) Place the bag in the stomacher and operate the machine for 2–3 min.

(f) Transfer 50 g of the homogenate to another stomacher bag and add approximately 100 mL from a measured 450 mL volume of 0.1% peptone solution.

(g) Place the bag in the stomacher and operate the machine for 2–3 min. Add the remainder of the 0.1% peptone solution and mix well. This gives the 10^{-1} dilution.

or:

Using blender

(d) Weigh the shellfish flesh and liquor and add two parts by mass of 0.1% peptone solution.

(e) Homogenize mixture in a rotary blender for sufficient time to achieve 15 000–20 000 revolutions. The duration should not exceed 2.5 min.

(f) Stand for 30 s.

(g) Swirl briefly, then transfer 30 mL of the homogenate to a measured 70 mL of 0.1% peptone solution and mix well. This gives the 10^{-1} dilution.

Preparation of dilutions

(h) Prepare a 10^{-2} dilution by transferring 1 mL of 10^{-1} dilution to 9 mL of 0.1% peptone/0.85% sodium chloride solution. Further dilutions may also be required when raw molluscs are being examined for classification of shellfish harvesting areas, i.e. 10^{-3} and 10^{-4}.

Procedure

(i) Prepare 15 tubes of minerals modified glutamate medium, five containing 10 mL of double strength medium and 10 containing 10 mL of single strength medium.

(j) Add 10 mL of 10^{-1} dilution to each of the five tubes containing double strength medium.

(k) Add 1 mL of 10^{-1} dilution to each of five tubes of single strength medium.

(l) Add 1 mL of 10^{-2} dilution to each of five tubes of single strength medium.

(m) Repeat step (l) with further dilutions if necessary.

(n) Incubate all tubes at 37°C for 24±2 h.

(o) Examine all tubes for acid production, signified by a colour change to yellow. The presence of any acid, regardless of quantity, is regarded as a positive result. Absence of acid production after 24±2 h constitutes a negative result for *E. coli*.

continued p. 237

Table 9.2 Most probable number (MPN) of organisms [5]. Tables for multiple tube method using 5×1 g, 5×0.1 g, 5×0.01 g.

1 g	0.1 g	0.01 g	MPN/100 g
Category A (<230 Escherichia coli)			
0	0	0	<20
0	0	1	20
0	1	0	20
1	0	0	20
1	0	1	40
1	1	0	40
1	2	0	50
2	0	0	40
2	0	1	50
2	1	0	50
2	1	1	70
2	2	0	70
2	3	0	110
3	0	0	70
3	0	1	90
3	1	0	90
3	1	1	130
3	2	0	130
3	2	1	160
3	3	0	160
4	0	0	110
4	0	1	140
4	1	0	160
4	1	1	200
4	2	0	200
5	0	0	220
Category B (>230 E. coli, <4600 E. coli)			
4	2	1	250
4	3	0	250
4	3	1	310
4	4	0	320
4	4	1	380
5	0	1	290
5	0	2	410
5	1	0	310
5	1	1	430
5	1	2	600
5	1	3	850
5	2	0	500
5	2	1	700
5	2	2	950
5	2	3	1200
5	3	0	750

Table 9.2 *continued.*

1 g	0.1 g	0.01 g	MPN/100 g
5	3	1	1100
5	3	2	1400
5	3	3	1750
5	3	4	2100
5	4	0	1300
5	4	1	1700
5	4	2	2200
5	4	3	2800
5	4	4	3450
5	5	0	2400
5	5	1	3500
Category C (>4600 E. coli, <46 000 E. coli)			
5	5	2	5400
5	5	3	9100
5	5	4	16 000
5	5	5	>18 000*

*Needs further dilutions to clarify classification.

Table 9.3 Most probable number (MPN) of organisms [5]. Tables for multiple tube method using 5×0.1 g, 5×0.01 g, 5×0.001 g.

0.1 g	0.01 g	0.001 g	MPN/100 g
Category A (<230 Escherichia coli)			
0	0	1	200
0	1	0	200
1	0	0	200
Category B (>230 E. coli, <4600 E. coli)			
1	0	1	400
1	1	0	400
1	2	0	500
2	0	0	400
2	0	1	500
2	1	0	500
2	1	1	700
2	2	0	700
2	3	0	1100
3	0	0	700
3	0	1	900
3	1	0	900
3	1	1	1300
3	2	0	1300

Table 9.3 *continued.*

0.1 g	0.01 g	0.001 g	MPN/100 g
3	2	1	1600
3	3	0	1600
4	0	0	1100
4	0	1	1400
4	1	0	1600
4	1	1	2000
4	2	0	2000
4	2	1	2500
4	3	0	2500
4	3	1	3100
4	4	0	3200
4	4	1	3800
5	0	0	2200
5	0	1	2900
5	0	2	4100
5	1	0	3100
5	1	1	4300
Category C (>4600 E. coli, <46 000 E. coli)			
5	1	2	6000
5	1	3	8500
5	2	0	5000
5	2	1	7000
5	2	2	9500
5	2	3	12 000
5	3	0	7500
5	3	1	11 000
5	3	2	14 000
5	2	3	17 500
5	3	4	21 000
5	4	0	13 000
5	4	1	17 000
5	4	2	22 000
5	4	3	28 000
5	4	4	34 500
5	5	0	24 000
5	5	1	35 000
Prohibited (>46 000 E. coli)			
5	5	2	54 000
5	5	3	91 000
5	5	4	160 000
5	5	5	>180 000

Table 9.4 Most probably number (MPN) of organisms [5]. Tables for multiple tube method using 5×0.01 g, 5×0.001 g, 5×0.0001 g.

0.01 g	0.001 g	0.0001 g	MPN/100 g
Category B (>230 Escherichia coli, <4600 E. coli)			
0	0	1	2000
0	1	0	2000
1	0	0	2000
1	0	1	4000
1	1	0	4000
2	0	0	4000
Category C (>4600 E. coli, <46 000 E. coli)			
1	2	0	5000
2	0	1	5000
2	1	0	5000
2	1	1	7000
2	2	0	7000
2	3	0	11 000
3	0	0	7000
3	0	1	9000
3	1	0	9000
3	1	1	13 000
3	2	0	13 000
3	2	1	16 000
3	3	0	16 000
4	0	0	11 000
4	0	1	14 000
4	1	0	16 000
4	1	1	20 000
4	2	0	20 000
4	2	1	25 000
4	3	0	25 000
4	3	1	31 000
4	4	0	32 000
4	4	1	38 000
5	0	0	22 000
5	0	1	29 000
5	0	2	41 000
5	1	0	31 000
5	1	1	43 000
Prohibited (>46 000 E. coli)			
5	1	2	60 000
5	1	3	85 000
5	2	0	50 000
5	2	1	70 000
5	2	2	95 000
5	2	3	120 000

Table 9.4 *continued.*

0.01 g	0.001 g	0.0001 g	MPN/100 g
5	3	0	75 000
5	3	1	110 000
5	3	2	140 000
5	3	3	175 000
5	3	4	210 000
5	4	0	130 000
5	4	1	170 000
5	4	2	220 000
5	4	3	280 000
5	4	4	345 000
5	5	0	240 000
5	5	1	350 000
5	5	2	540 000
5	5	3	910 000
5	5	4	1 600 000

(p) Subculture each tube showing acid production to a section of BCIG agar, and streak to obtain isolated colonies.

(q) Incubate the BCIG agar plates at 44°C for 20–24 h.

(r) Examine the plates for the presence of blue colonies, typical of β-glucuronidase positive *E. coli*.

(s) Consider tubes that yield growth of blue colonies on BCIG agar as positive for the presence of *E. coli*.

Calculation

(t) For each dilution, count the number of positive tubes.

(u) If dilutions of 10^{-3} or higher were used, select the highest dilution having five positive tubes and the next two higher dilutions. If no dilution contains five positive tubes, select the three highest dilutions amongst which at least one positive result was obtained.

(v) Use the number of positive tubes at each dilution selected to determine the MPN by reference to the MPN table for the appropriate dilution range (Tables 9.2–9.4). 10 mL of the 10^{-1} dilution is equivalent to 1 g of flesh, 1 mL of the 10^{-1} dilution is equivalent to 0.1 g of flesh, etc.

Method 2 *Salmonella* spp.

The sample should be prepared for examination as described in steps (a)–(c) in method 1. Homogenize the sample as described in steps (d)–(g) using either a stomacher or a blender, but use buffered peptone water instead of 0.1% peptone solution. Then proceed as described in Section 6.12, method 2.

Method 3 Phage detection

F-specific RNA bacteriophages are bacterial viruses that have analogous morphology and genetic structure to human pathogenic viruses (NLV, enteroviruses and HAV) found in sewage. This, allied to their abundance in sewage and ease of enumeration, make them a good indicator of viral contamination in the marine environment. Their presence in shellfish is indicative of sewage pollution and potential contamination by human pathogenic viruses. They are particularly useful indicators of potential viral contamination in shellfish after treatment where traditional bacterial indicators are removed more readily than human viruses. F-specific RNA bacteriophages are capable of infecting a specified F-pili producing bacterial host strain. Infection produces visible plaques on a confluent lawn grown under appropriate culture conditions with the infectious process being inhibited in the presence of ribonuclease (RNase) in the plating media

Principle of method

A culture of host strain is mixed with a small volume of molten nutrient medium. Shellfish homogenate is added and the mixture flooded on a solid nutrient agar base and allowed to set. This is then incubated at 37°C during which time the host multiplies to produce a confluent lawn. Visible plaques form where bacteriophage is present. It is assumed that each plaque is derived from one bacteriophage. Where necessary, simultaneous examination of parallel plates with added RNase for confirmation by differential counts is carried out. The results are expressed as the number of plaque forming units (pfu)/100 g of shellfish [6].

Sample size

As for method 1.

Equipment

As for method 1, and in addition:
Centrifuge
Water bath at $45 \pm 2°C$
Spectrophotometer
Colony counter
Sterile glassware.

Reagents

1.0% calcium-glucose solution
12.5% w/v nalidixic acid solution
Tryptone yeast extract glucose broth (TYGB)
Tryptone yeast extract glucose 2% agar (TYGA2) as plates
Tryptone yeast extract glucose 1% agar (TYGA1) in 100 mL volumes
100% w/v RNase (store at –20°C)
0.1% peptone solution (negative control)
MacConkey agar
Glycerol
Chloroform.

continued

Microbiological reference materials

Salmonella typhimurium strain WG49, phage type 3 Nal^r (F′ 42 lac:Tn5), NCTC 12484.

> To prepare a working culture of *S. typhimurium* WG49, inoculate TYGB and incubate for 18±2 h at 37°C. Subculture to MacConkey agar and incubate at 37°C for 18±2 h; then select five to seven lactose positive colonies and inoculate into 100 mL of pre-warmed TYGB. Incubate for 5±1 h at 37°C, then add 20 mL glycerol. After mixing thoroughly aliquot into plastic vials and freeze at −70°C.

Bacteriophage MS2 NCO12487 (for positive control; obtainable from NCTC) (see Appendix C).

> Positive MS2 controls are produced by inoculating an exponentially growing culture of *S. typhimurium* WG49 with MS2 NCO12487. Incubate at 37°C. After 4–5 h add 5±1 mL of chloroform to lyse bacterial cells, then incubate at 5±3°C for 18±2 h. Centrifuge the mixture to remove cell debris. The MS2 culture is then titrated with *S. typhimurium* WG49. The dilution required to give 30–500 plaques is calculated and aliquots stored at −70°C.

Sample preparation

(a) Prepare the sample as described in method 1. Prepare the homogenate using a blender, as described in steps (d) and (e) of method 1, to produce a 1/3 homogenate.

(b) Centrifuge 30–50 mL of homogenate, prepared as above, at 2000±200 g for 5 min at room temperature.

(c) Make any decimal dilutions, if required, by adding 1±0.1 mL of supernatant to 9±0.2 mL of 0.1% peptone solution.

Agar overlay preparation

(d) Melt TYGA1 then cool to 45°C in the water bath.

(e) Add 1±0.1 mL of 1.0% calcium-glucose solution per 100±2 mL of TYGA1. If high levels of background bacteria are expected add 400±2 μL of 12.5% w/v nalidixic acid solution.

(f) Aliquot 2.5±0.1 mL of TYGA1 for each replicate sample into bijoux held at 45°C in the water bath. (If DNA plaques are expected, for example in samples from faecally polluted areas, perform confirmatory tests in the presence of 100±1 μL 100% w/v RNase).

Preparation of host

(g) Add 1±0.1 mL of calcium-glucose solution to 100±1 mL of TYGB at 37°C.

(h) Inoculate this medium with 1±0.1 mL of *S. typhimurium* WG49 working culture.

(i) Incubate at 37°C for 4±2 h to achieve a cell density of 7–40×10^7 cfu/mL at 600 nm, using sterile TYGB as the blank.

Assay

(j) Immediately after incubation add 1±0.1 mL of WG49 host culture to all test bijoux followed by 1±0.1 mL of the sample under test. Mix contents by inverting the bijoux.

continued

(k) Pour the prepared contents of each bijou over the surface of individual TYGA2 plates and distribute evenly by circular movement of the Petri dish. Repeat with appropriate positive and negative controls.

(l) Incubate TYGA2 plates at 37°C for 18 ± 4 h. Count pfu within 4 h or store at 5 ± 3°C for up to 48 h.

(m) Count all plaques on each plate except those exhibiting typical DNA phage morphology, i.e. plaques of approximately 6 mm diameter with a clear lysis zone in the centre. Where dilutions have been made select plates with about 30–300 pfu.

Expression of results

Calculate the number of pfu/100 g as follows:

$$C_{pfu} = \frac{N - N_{RNase} \times F}{n}$$

Where:

C_{pfu} is the confirmed number of F-specific RNA bacteriophages, expressed as pfu in 1 mL of undiluted sample

N is the total number of plaques

N_{RNase} is the total number of plaques counted with RNase

n is the number of replicates

F is the dilution factor.

As shellfish flesh samples are diluted 1/3 during the homogenization step, the above result represents the number of bacteriophages in 0.3 g of shellfish. To express results per 100 g multiply the value obtained by 300. If further dilutions were made (step (c)) also multiply by the appropriate dilution factor.

If no plaques are present express the result as <30 pfu/100 g shellfish flesh.

Interpretation

Shellfish containing levels of F-specific RNA bacteriophage of <100 pfu/100 g shellfish flesh and intravalvular fluid are unlikely to be contaminated with viruses causing gastroenteritis.

9.1 References

1 Council of the European Communities. Directive No. 91/492/EEC on shellfish hygiene. Classification and monitoring of shellfish harvesting water. *Off J Eur Communities* 1991; **L268**: 1–14.

2 Council of the European Communities. Directive 97/61/EC of 20 October 1997 amending the annex to Directive 91/492/EEC laying down the health conditions for the production and placing on the market of live bivalve molluscs. *Off J Eur Communities* 1997; **L295**: 35–6.

3 Lees D. Viruses and bivalve shellfish (review). *Int J Food Microbiol* 2000; **59**: 81–116.

4 Dore WJ, Henshilwood K, Lees DN. Evaluation of F-specific RNA bacteriophage as a candidate human enteric virus indicator for bivalve molluscan shellfish. *Appl Environ Microbiol* 2000; **66**: 1280–5.

5   Donovan TJ, Gallacher S, Andrews NJ, *et al.* Modification of the standard method used in the United Kingdom for counting *Escherichia coli* in live bivalve molluscs. *Comm Dis Public Health* 1998; **1**: 188–96.

6   ISO 10705-1 (BS 6068-4 Part 11 1996). *Water Quality. Microbiological Methods. Detection and Enumeration of Bacteriophages. Part 1: Enumeration of F-specific RNA Bacteriophages.* Geneva: International Organization for Standardization (ISO), 1995.

10 Confirmatory biochemical tests

The identity of an organism may be confirmed by demonstrating its ability to perform a number of biochemical reactions, each species conforming to a recognizable result pattern.

Most of the media used in the tests detailed in this section can be obtained from commercial sources, usually in powder form, and require reconstituting and sterilizing before use. Some of the reagents prescribed in the tests may not be available commercially, and so methods for the preparation of these have been included in this section.

This section does not cover the entire range of biochemical and other identification tests encountered in food microbiology, but it brings together a number of those most commonly used and a few which are specific to a particular group of organisms. Rapid multi-test micro-methods, as discussed briefly at the start of Section 6, are not included. A fuller range of identification tests can be found in *Cowan and Steel's Manual for the Identification of Medical Bacteria* [1].

Positive and negative controls should be included in each batch of tests. The reference strains of control organisms are listed in the test methods where appropriate.

10.1 Acid production from sugars [1]

Examples of sugars include glucose, salicin, mannose, xylose and rhamnose.

Control organisms

Control organisms for sugar reactions may vary according to individual laboratory preference. Stock cultures should be kept of organisms that have known positive and negative reactions in each sugar.

Reagents

Peptone water (1% peptone, 0.5% NaCl)

10% sugar solutions

Andrade's indicator solution (or equivalent).

Procedure

(a) Prepare a 10% solution of the required sugar and sterilize at 115°C for 10 min. Use a small autoclave to avoid prolonged heating which would denature the carbohydrate. If this is not available, sterilize by filtration.

(b) To 90 mL sterile peptone water add 10 mL of the required sterile 10% sugar solution and 1–2 mL of Andrade's indicator solution. Alternatively a peptone water Andrade base may be used.

(c) Transfer 4–5 mL volumes aseptically to sterile bijoux bottles or test tubes. An inverted Durham tube may be incorporated to check for gas production. Incubate overnight at 37°C to check for sterility.

(d) Inoculate a pure culture of the test organism into the bottle or tube of peptone water sugar and incubate at 37°C (30°C for some organisms, e.g. *Yersinia* spp.) for up to 7 days.

(e) Observe the development of a pink coloration which indicates the production of acid and, if a Durham tube is included, the presence/absence of gas in the tube.

10.2 CAMP test (for *Listeria*)

The CAMP (Christie, Atkins, Munch–Petersen) test demonstrates the enhancement of haemolysis of some strains of *Listeria* spp. by *Staphylococcus aureus* and *Rhodococcus equi* [1–3].

Control organisms

NCTC 11994	*Listeria monocytogenes*	CAMP test (*S. aureus*) positive
NCTC 11846	*Listeria ivanovii*	CAMP test (*S. aureus*) negative
NCTC 11846	*Listeria ivanovii*	CAMP test (*R. equi*) positive
NCTC 11994	*Listeria monocytogenes*	CAMP test (*R. equi*) negative

Procedure

(a) Prepare two plates by overlaying about 10 mL of nutrient agar with a thin layer (3–4 mL) of 5% sheep blood agar.

continued

(b) Across the centre of one plate streak the recommended standard strain of *S. aureus* (NCTC 1803) and across the centre of the other the recommended standard strain of *R. equi* (NCTC 1621).

(c) Inoculate the test organism on each plate by streaking at right angles to within 1–2 mm of the standard organisms.

(d) Incubate the plates at 37°C for 18 h.

(e) Examine for enhancement of haemolysis of the test organism by either, both or neither of the standard strains where the two cultures are closest together. This appears as a completely clear area shaped like an arrow head. Plate XIV (facing p. 150) shows both standard strains on a single plate. The slight enhancement of haemolysis of *L. monocytogenes* with *R. equi* is not uncommon but should not be interpreted as a positive result. Enhancement should be as a clear arrow as shown for *L. ivanovii*.

> The zones of haemolysis produced vary with different strains of *Listeria* spp. and interpretation of positive reactions requires practice. Freshly poured plates give the best results and it is essential to have a control organism on each plate.

10.3 Catalase production

This test detects the production of the enzyme catalase [1], which will split hydrogen peroxide with the production of gas bubbles. The test can be difficult to interpret as some species are only weakly reactive. However, as with *Listeria*, if adequate controls are included the test is straightforward and an essential part of the identification procedure.

Control organisms

NCTC 11047	*Staphylococcus epidermidis*	Positive
NCTC 775	*Enterococcus faecalis*	Negative

> To avoid false positive results in this test the following precautions should be taken.
> - Glassware has to be clean.
> - Blood agar media should not be used.
> - Pseudo-catalase reactions may occur in the presence of low concentrations of glucose (e.g. as in plate count agar). These reactions can be avoided by using media containing 1% glucose.

Procedure

(a) Inoculate the test organisms on a slope of nutrient agar and incubate at 37°C for 24 h.

continued

Either

(b) Using a pasteur pipette, gently run 2–3 drops of 3% hydrogen peroxide down the slope of the medium so that it covers the test growth.

(c) Examine immediately and observe the production of gas bubbles which indicate a positive reaction. Examine again after 5 min.

Or:

(b) Place a drop of hydrogen peroxide on a glass microscope slide.

(c) With a bacteriological loop, gently rub a colony of the test organism into the hydrogen peroxide.

(d) Observe for the production of gas bubbles (use a safety cabinet to safeguard against aerosols).

Alternative method

1 Inoculate a tube of nutrient broth with the test organism and incubate at 37°C overnight.

2 Add 1 mL of 3% hydrogen peroxide to the culture and examine immediately and after 5 min for the presence of gas bubbles.

10.4 Coagulase test

Coagulase tests demonstrate the ability of strains of *Staphylococcus aureus* to produce substances which will coagulate plasma. With a few exceptions, coagulases are not produced by other members of the genus *Staphylococcus*.

Plasma

Allow the plasma to reach room temperature before use.

Types of plasma suitable for method 1 and method 2 include human, rabbit, horse and pig. Avoid the use of human plasma if possible, but if other types are not available obtain the human plasma direct from the blood transfusion service and ensure that it has been tested to screen out human immunodeficiency virus (HIV) and is not hepatitis positive.

Plasma which contains citrate as the sole anticoagulant should not be used as organisms that can utilize citrate may give a false positive reaction if the test organism is not a pure culture.

Before routine use check new batches of plasma for their ability to give a strong reaction.

Method 1 Tube test

The tube coagulase test [1,3] detects 'free' coagulase, and is stipulated in standard methods for detection of *S. aureus* [4].

continued

Control organisms

NCTC 6571   *Staphylococcus aureus* (Oxford strain)   Weak positive

NCTC 8532   *Staphylococcus aureus*   Positive

NCTC 11047   *Staphylococcus epidermidis*   Negative

Procedure

(a) Place 0.5 mL of plasma (diluted 1 : 10 in saline) in a 75 mm × 12 mm test tube.

(b) Add 0.1 mL of an 18–24 h nutrient broth culture of the test organism and incubate at 37°C, preferably in a water bath.

(c) Examine after 1 h, 3 h and 6 h incubation for the formation of a clot (see Plate XV, facing p. 150).

(d) Leave overnight at room temperature and examine again for clot formation.

(e) Record formation of a clot as a positive reaction.

Method 2 Slide test

The slide coagulase test [1] is a rapid test that detects clumping factor (or 'bound' coagulase). If negative results are obtained, they should be confirmed by the tube test (method 1) or desoxyribonuclease (DNase) testing (Section 10.5).

Control organisms

NCTC 6571   *Staphylococcus aureus* (Oxford strain)   Positive

NCTC 11047   *Staphylococcus epidermidis*   Negative

Procedure

(a) Emulsify a colony from a non-selective plate culture of the test organism in two separate drops of saline on a microscope slide to produce a creamy suspension.

(b) Mix a loopful of undiluted plasma into one of the suspensions and examine for microscopic clumping occurring within 5–10 s. This indicates the presence of bound coagulase; delayed clumping does not constitute a positive result.

(c) Examine the second suspension to ensure absence of autoagglutination.

Commercial latex test kits are available that are used in a manner similar to method 2.

10.5   Desoxyribonuclease production

Strains of *Staphylococcus aureus* produce a heat-stable desoxyribonuclease (DNase), or thermonuclease. While other *Staphylococcus* spp. occasionally produce DNase, they are not heat stable. The DNA molecule is hydrolysed to a mixture of mono- and polynucleotides by the action of enzymes (DNases) produced by microorganisms. Agar containing DNA can be used to demonstrate the production of microbial DNase [1,5]. Colonies producing DNase are surrounded by a clear zone when plates are flooded with hydrochloric acid, or a pink zone against a blue background when flooded with toluidine blue solution [6].

This test may be used in addition to the coagulase test (Section 10.4) for the confirmation of *S. aureus*. Alternatively, the method described below is useful as a screening test but will also detect strains of *Staphylococcus* that produce heat labile DNase. Confirmation of DNase positive colonies by coagulase testing is therefore necessary.

Control organisms

Gram positive organisms:

NCTC 6571	*Staphylococcus aureus* (Oxford strain)	Positive
NCTC 11047	*Staphylococcus epidermidis*	Negative

Gram negative organisms:

NCTC 11935	*Serratia marcescens*	Positive
NCTC 11934	*Edwardsiella tarda*	Negative

Procedure

(a) Prepare an initial solution of DNA of known concentration in distilled water.

(b) Add sufficient of this solution to nutrient agar immediately before autoclaving to give a final concentration of 2 mg/mL (DNase agar). Sterilize the medium at 121°C for 15 min and pour plates as soon as the medium cools to 50°C. Alternatively use a commercially available complete medium.

(c) Prepare plates containing 15–20 mL of agar.

(d) Place a small spot or a streak of each test colony on the surface of the DNase agar plate and incubate for 18–24 h at 37°C.

(e) Add 2–3 mL of 1 M (10%) hydrochloric acid or 0.1% toluidine blue solution to the plate and rock until the surface is completely covered.

(f) Remove the excess liquid after approximately 30 s.

(g) The medium will become opaque with clear zones around the growth of any organisms that produce DNase if hydrochloric acid is used. If toluidine blue solution is used the medium turns blue with the formation of pink zones around positive strains (see Plate XVI, facing p. 150).

It is advantageous to incorporate dyes into the medium which can distinguish DNA hydrolysis and thus avoid the use of acid in step (e). Toluidine blue and methyl green form coloured complexes with polymerized DNA, the colour changes as the DNA is hydrolysed.

10.6 Gram reaction

The Gram reaction is a primary identification procedure used to determine the ability of a microorganism to retain the first stain used in the procedure when a decolorizing agent such as ethanol or acetone is added [1,7]. Gram positive organisms retain the stain but Gram negative organisms are decolorized. The Gram reaction is a stable characteristic but Gram positivity may be lost as cells age. A Gram negative reaction may be false either due to the age of the culture or to excessive decolorization with powerful solvents. Thus a positive result has more significance than a negative result. When possible the procedure should be performed on a young culture (18–24 h old).

Control organisms

| NCTC 10447 | *Staphylococcus epidermidis* | Positive |
| NCTC 9001 | *Escherichia coli* | Negative |

Reagents

Crystal violet (1% aqueous solution)
Lugols iodine (1% iodine, 2% potassium iodide)
Acetone/alcohol mixture: 20% acetone/80% methylated spirit
Safranin solution (0.5% aqueous solution).

Procedure

(a) Using a sterile loop prepare a light suspension of organisms in sterile distilled water on a clean microscope slide.
(b) Air dry the film and then heat fix by passing the slide twice through a gas flame. DO NOT OVERHEAT.
(c) Allow to cool.
(d) Place the slide on a staining rack and flood with crystal violet solution.
(e) Leave for 30 s before washing off with running tap water.
(f) Flood the slide with Lugols iodine solution.
(g) Leave for 30 s before washing off with running tap water.
(h) To decolorize, run the acetone/alcohol over the film and wash off immediately with running tap water.
(i) Flood the slide with safranin solution.
(j) Leave for 1 min before washing off with running tap water.
(k) Gently blot the film dry or allow to air dry.
(l) Place a drop of immersion oil on the film and examine under the microscope using the ×100 oil immersion lens.
(m) Microorganisms that appear dark purple are Gram positive; those that are pink are Gram negative.
(n) Record the reaction to the Gram procedure and the appearance of the organisms (shape and any other particular features).

10.7 Haemolysis (e.g. for *Listeria*)

When growing on blood agar media some organisms can produce haemolysins which diffuse into the medium and affect the red blood cells. This effect may appear as β-haemolysis, a green zone with the blood cells still intact, or as beta-haemolysis, a clear colourless zone where the cells are completely lysed [1].

Horse blood cells are most commonly used to demonstrate this effect but more reliable results may be obtained with sheep blood cells. When recording results of haemolysis tests the report should state the type (animal species) of blood cells used.

Control organisms

NCTC 11994   *Listeria monocytogenes*   Positive
NCTC 11288   *Listeria innocua*   Negative

Procedure

(a) Inoculate a blood agar plate with the test organism using a loop in the normal manner ensuring that the organism is spread sufficiently to produce single colonies. Incubate overnight (18–24 h) at 37°C.

(b) Examine the plate for visible zones of haemolysis around the colonies. Transmitted light improves contrast.

10.8   Hippurate hydrolysis (for campylobacters)

Campylobacter jejuni can hydrolyse hippurate to form glycine and benzoic acid [1,8,9]. The production of glycine can be detected by the addition of a ninhydrin solution to the test medium.

Control organisms

NCTC 11322   *Campylobacter jejeuni*   Positive
NCTC 11366   *Campylobacter coli*   Negative

Reagents

Ninhydrin: 3.5% solution in equal parts acetone and butanol. Store in the dark at room temperature.

Sodium hippurate: 5% aqueous solution. Distribute in 0.5 mL volumes and store at −20°C.

Procedure

(a) Grow the test organism on blood agar for 18–24 h at 37°C in a microaerobic atmosphere.

(b) Transfer a 2 mm loopful of the colonial growth from this plate to 2 mL of distilled water. Mix the organisms to suspend and add 0.5 mL of sodium hippurate solution.

(c) Incubate in a water bath at 37°C for 2 h.

(d) Add 1 mL of ninhydrin solution and leave for 2 h at room temperature (or 10 min at 37°C).

(e) A positive reaction is shown by the development of a purple colour which indicates the formation of glycine (see Plate XVII, facing p. 150).

10.9 Hydrogen sulphide test (for salmonellae, campylobacters and yersiniae)

The production of hydrogen sulphide is a feature of the normal metabolic action of many microorganisms. Triple sugar iron (TSI) agar slopes are used in the identification of enteric pathogens. This medium turns black if the test organism produces hydrogen sulphide [1].

In general, many *Salmonella* spp. are hydrogen sulphide positive, while *Yersinia* spp. are negative. In *Campylobacter* spp. hydrogen sulphide production is variable between and within species.

Control organisms

NCTC 11934	*Edwardsiella tarda*	Positive
NCTC 12145	*Campylobacter jejuni*	Positive
NCTC 7475	*Proteus rettgeri*	Negative
NCTC 11168	*Campylobacer jejuni*	Negative

Procedure
(a) Prepare tubes of TSI agar as slopes with a generous butt.
(b) Using a straight wire inoculate the test organism deep into the butt of the medium and streak up the slope.
(c) Incubate for 18–24 h at 37°C for salmonellae and 30°C for yersiniae. For campylobacters, incubate in a reduced oxygen, increased carbon dioxide atmosphere for up to 3 days.
(d) Examine for blackening of the medium (see Plate XVIII, facing p. 150).

Rapid test for *Campylobacter*
(a) Suspend a large loopful (5 mm) of growth from an 18–24 h blood agar culture, incubated at 37°C in not more than 7% oxygen, in the upper third of 3–4 mL of ferric bisulphite pyruvate (FBP) medium in a small screw-capped tube.
(b) Incubate closed at 37°C for 2 h.
(c) Examine for blackening of the medium.

10.10 Indole test

The ability of certain microorganisms to break down the amino-acid tryptophan, with the production of indole, is an important characteristic used in the classification and identification of bacteria. The presence of indole in the growth medium can be detected by the addition of an indole reagent (e.g. Kovac's); a pink coloration is produced in the reagent [1].

Control organisms

NCTC 9001   *Escherichia coli*   Positive
NCTC 11935   *Serratia marcescens*   Negative

Reagent

Kovac's reagent: dissolve 5 g of *p*-dimethyl aminobenzaldehyde in 75 mL of analytical grade amyl alcohol. The reagent will dissolve more rapidly if warmed gently in a water bath at 55°C. Cool and add 25 mL of concentrated hydrochloric acid. Mix gently and store at 4°C.

Procedure

(a) Inoculate a tube of peptone water, tryptone water or broth containing 0.03% tryptophan with a pure culture of the test organism and incubate at 37°C for up to 48 h. Some tests may require incubation at 30°C or 44°C.

(b) Add 5–10 drops (0.2 mL) of Kovac's reagent, shake and allow to stand for up to 10 min. A pink coloration at the surface indicates the presence of indole.

10.11 Motility test (for listerias and other organisms) [1]

Control organisms

NCTC 11994   *Listeria monocytogenes*   Positive at 21°C
NCTC 11934   *Edwardsiella tarda*   Positive at 37°C
NCTC 8574   *Shigella sonnei*   Negative
or:
NCTC 9528   *Klebsiella aerogenes*   Negative

Procedure

(a) Prepare small tubes of nutrient broth.

(b) Inoculate with the test organism and incubate at the appropriate temperature. For *Listeria* spp. this should be 21°C for 4–6 h.

(c) Place a drop of the broth on the surface of a glass microscope slide and cover with a glass cover slip.

(d) Examine by optical microscopy for motility of the test organism. *Listeria* spp. exhibit a typical 'tumbling' motility at 21°C but not at 37°C.

> A 'hanging drop' preparation may help microscopic examination. Place a drop of the test culture on a glass cover slip and invert over a thin ring of Vaseline® or Plasticine® on a glass microscope slide

10.12 Nitrate reduction

Nitrate reduction may be shown by detection of one of the breakdown products or by demonstration of the disappearance of nitrate from the medium. The products of reduction range from nitrite to gaseous nitrogen. The objective of the first test is to show the presence of nitrite; if this is not detected the medium is then tested for the presence of residual nitrate. If no residual nitrate can be detected it indicates that the nitrite has been further broken down. For organisms that do not appear to reduce nitrate, a reducing agent (zinc dust) is then added. If a red colour develops this signifies that the nitrate has not been reduced. If no red colour is produced then there is no nitrate present and the nitrite has been further reduced [1].

Control organisms

| NCTC 7464 | *Bacillus cereus* | Positive |
| NCTC 9001 | *Escherichia coli* | Negative |

Reagents

Nitrate broth or *nitrate motility medium.*

Nitrite reagents: A. 5-amino-2-naphthalene-sulphonic acid (0.1% solution in 15% by volume acetic acid). B. Sulfanilic acid (0.4% solution in 15% by volume acetic acid).

Zinc dust.

Procedure

(a) Inoculate tubes of nitrate broth or nitrate motility medium (stab inoculation) with the test strain and incubate for up to 5 days at 30°C.
(b) Mix equal volumes of nitrite reagents A and B just before use.
(c) To each tube of nitrate broth or nitrate motility medium showing growth add 0.2–0.5 mL of the reagent mixture.
(d) Formation of a red colour confirms the reduction of nitrate to nitrite.
(e) If there is no red colour after 15 min add a small amount of zinc dust and allow to stand for 15 min.
(f) If a red colour develops after the addition of zinc dust then no reduction of nitrate has taken place.
(g) If there is no red colour there is no nitrate present, the nitrite has been further reduced.

10.13 O129 sensitivity

The pteridine derivative O129 (2,4-diamino-6,7-di-isopropyl pteridine phosphate) specifically inhibits the growth of *Vibrio* spp., although the number of strains showing resistance seems to be increasing. Resistance can be demonstrated by placing discs of the reagent on plates previously seeded with the organisms and incubating. A zone of inhibition indicates sensitivity to the reagents [1,10].

Control organisms

| NCTC 10885 | *Vibrio parahaemolyticus* | Positive (sensitive) |
| NCTC 10662 | *Pseudomonas aeruginosa* | Negative (resistant) |

Reagents
O129 discs: 10 µg and 150 µg
Blood agar plates
Sterile saline (0.85% sodium chloride).

Procedure
(a) Prepare a light suspension of the test organism in saline.
(b) Inoculate the surface of a blood agar plate with this suspension.
(c) Using sterile forceps place discs containing 10 µg and 150 µg of O129 reagent on the plate.
(d) Incubate the plates at 37°C for 18–24 h.
(e) Examine for inhibition of growth of the test organism around the discs.
(f) Record as sensitive (S) or resistant (R).
(g) Include control strains with each set of tests. The following results should be obtained:

V. parahaemolyticus:	10 µg R	150 µg S
Ps. aeruginosa:	10 µg R	150 µg R

10.14 Oxidase test

The test to detect the production of cytochrome c oxidase by microorganisms is used to categorize them into groups at an early stage of their identification [1].

Control organisms

| NCTC 10662 | *Pseudomonas aeruginosa* | Positive |
| NCTC 9001 | *Escherichia coli* | Negative |

Reagent
Oxidase reagent [1]:
Either:
(a) Freshly prepared each day: dissolve 0.1 g of tetramethyl *p*-phenylene diamine dihydrochloride in 10 mL of distilled water. Addition of 1% ascorbic acid and storage in the dark extends the life of the reagent to 4 to 5 days. Discard if a purple coloration develops.
Or:

continued

(b) Prepared from stable basal solution [11]:
   Ethylene diamine tetraacetic acid (EDTA) disodium salt 1 g
   Sodium thiosulphate pentahydrate 0.5 g
   Distilled water 100 mL
   Dilute 10 mL of basal solution to 100 mL with distilled water. Add 0.2 g of tetra-methyl p-phenylene diamine dihydrochloride.

> Prepared in this way, the basal solution is stable for 6 months and the reagent for 2–4 weeks at 4°C. Discard if a purple coloration develops.

Procedure
(a) Moisten a piece of filter paper in a Petri dish with two or three drops of oxidase reagent.
(b) Using a wooden stick, glass rod or platinum loop (do not use a nichrome bacteriological loop), transfer a colony of the test organism to the filter paper and rub it on the area moistened with oxidase reagent.
(c) Observe for the development of a dark purple coloration indicating the production of oxidase.

10.15 Spore stain

The ability to form spores is a characteristic used to confirm the identity of some species of bacteria. The combination of spore morphology and biochemical tests has long been used for the identification of *Bacillus* spp. These organisms can be divided into groups on the basis of the shape, size and location of the spores within the vegetative cells. These can be determined either by the use of phase contrast microscopy or with a spore stain. A simple procedure that does not involve heating is described [12].

Control organisms

| NCTC 7464 | *Bacillus cereus* | Positive |
| NCTC 9001 | *Escherichia coli* | Negative |

Reagents
10% aqueous malachite green solution
0.5% aqueous safranin solution.

Procedure
(a) Prepare a film of the test organism on a clean microscope slide.

continued

(b) Flood the slide with aqueous malachite green solution and leave to stand for 40–45 min.
(c) Wash under running tap water.
(d) Flood the slide with 0.5% aqueous safranin solution.
(e) Leave for 15 s and rinse under running tap water.
(f) Gently blot the film dry or allow to air dry.
(g) Bacterial bodies stain red, spores green.
(h) Record the position and shape of the spores and whether they distend the bacterial cell.

10.16 Urease test

Urease activity is shown by the production of ammonia from a solution of urea. The change in pH can be demonstrated by the addition of an indicator to the medium [1].

Control organisms

NCTC 7475	*Proteus rettgeri*	Positive
NCTC 11935	*Serratia marcescens*	Negative

Procedure
(a) Prepare tubes of Christensen's urea medium. These may be as agar slopes or broths.
(b) Inoculate a slope or broth with the test organism and incubate at 30°C or 37°C. The test can often be read after 5–6 h incubation in a water bath.
(c) Observe for a pink coloration of the medium which denotes the production of urease.

10.17 Voges Proskaüer test (for listeriae and other organisms) [1]

Control organisms

NCTC 11994	*Listeria monocytogenes*	Positive
or:		
NCTC 11935	*Serratia marcescens*	Positive
NCTC 9001	*Escherichia coli*	Negative
or:		
NCTC 7475	*Proteus rettgeri*	Negative

Reagents

5% α-naphthol solution in ethanol (the colour of the reagent should not be darker than straw colour)

40% potassium hydroxide solution.

Procedure

(a) Prepare tubes containing 5 mL of glucose phosphate broth.

(b) Inoculate with a pure culture of the test organism and incubate at 37°C for 48 h.

(c) Add 0.6 mL of α-naphthol solution and 0.2 mL of potassium hydroxide solution.

(d) Shake vigorously and observe for the development of a pink/red coloration.

(e) Slope the tubes and leave at room temperature for 1 h. Examine again for pink/red coloration before declaring the test negative.

10.18 References

1 Barrow GI, Feltham RKA, eds. *Cowan and Steel's Manual for the Identification of Medical Bacteria*, 3rd edn. Cambridge: Cambridge University Press, 1993.

2 BS EN ISO 11290-1 (BS 5763 Part 18). *Microbiology of Food and Animal Feeding Stuffs — Horizontal Method for the Detection and Enumeration of Listeria monocytogenes. Part 1. Detection Method*. Geneva: International Organization for Standardization (ISO), 1997.

3 McLauchlin J. The identification of *Listeria* species. *DMRQC Newsletter* 1988; **3**: 1–3. (Internal publication of the Public Health Laboratory Service (PHLS).)

4 BS EN ISO 6888-1. *Microbiology of Food and Animal Feeding Stuffs — Horizontal Method for the Enumeration of Coagulase-positive Staphylococci. Technique Using Baird–Parker Agar Medium*. Geneva: International Organization for Standardization (ISO), 1999.

5 Jeffries CD, Holtman DF, Guse DG. Rapid method for determining the activity of microorganisms on nucleic acids. *J Bacteriol* 1957; **73**: 590–1.

6 Streitfeld MM, Hoffmann EM, Janklow HM. Evaluation of extracellular deoxyribonuclease activity in *Pseudomonas*. *J Bacteriol* 1962; **84**: 77–80.

7 ISO 7218 (BS 5763 Part 0). *Microbiology of Food and Animal Feeding Stuffs — General Rules for Microbiological Examinations*. Geneva: International Organization for Standardization (ISO), 1996.

8 Hwang MN, Ederer GM. Rapid hippurate hydrolysis method for presumptive identification of group B streptococci. *J Clin Microbiol* 1975; **1**: 114–15.

9 Skirrow MB, Benjamin J. Differentation of enteropathogenic campylobacter. *J Clin Path* 1980; **33**: 1122.

10 Furniss AL, Lee JV, Donovan TJ. *The Vibrios. Public Health Laboratory Service Monograph Series No. 11*. London: HMSO, 1997.

11 Daubner I, Mayer J. Die anwendung des oxydase-testes bie der hygienisch-bakteriologischen wasseranalyse. *Arch Hyg Bakt* 1968; **152**: 302–5.

12 Holbrook R, Anderson JM. An improved selective and diagnostic medium for the enumeration of *Bacillus cereus* in foods. *Can J Microbiol* 1980; **26**: 753–9.

Appendix A: Quick reference guide to the microbiological tests

Appendix A

Quick reference guide to the microbiological tests

Key

◆ The tests marked with this symbol are, in the terminology defined in Section 3 of this manual, 'statutory' tests

◀ The tests marked with this symbol are 'recommended' tests

■ The tests marked with this symbol are 'supplementary' tests

	1 Colony count (aerobic)	2 Other specified count (e.g. pre-incubated)	3 Aeromonas spp.	4 B. cereus and Bacillus spp.	5 Brucella spp.	6 Campylobacter spp.	7 Clostridia	8 Coliforms (30°C)	9 Coliforms	10 Enterobacteriaceae	11 Enterococci	12 Escherichia coli	13 Lactobacilli and other lactic acid bacteria	14 Listeria monocytogenes	15 Pseudomonas spp.	16 Salmonella spp.	17 Shigella spp.	18 Staphylococcus aureus	19 Vibrio spp.	20 Yeasts and moulds	21 Yersinia spp.	22 Peroxidase	23 Phosphatase	24 Alpha-amylase	25 Aw	26 pH	27 Can examination	28 Cryptosporidium	29 Direct microscopic smear	30 Shelf-life
Animal feeds	◀			◀			◆			◆						◆		◀												
Baby foods	■			◀			◀		◀			◀				◀		◀												
Bakery products, confectionary	◀								◀			◀				■				◀									■	
Brine—bacon curing	◀	◀	◀	◀			◀		◀	◀		◀	◀			◀		◀	◀						◀	◀	◀		◀	
Canned food	■			◀				◆				◆		◆		◆		◀												
Cereals and rice	◀	◆		■				◀				◀		◀		■		■												
Coconut																◀														
Dairy products – cheese	◆	◆						◆				◆		◆		◀		◆				◆	◆			◀				
– cream (untreated)		◆												◀		◆		◀			■									
– cream (pasteurized)		◆				◀		◆						◆		◆		■			■	◆	◆						■	
– cream (UHT)		◆																												
– ice-cream	◆	◆		◀	■	◀	◆	◆				◀		■		◆		■												
– ice-cream (UHT mix)		◆		■	■	■						■		■		◆					■		◆				■			
– milk (liquid) – untreated	◆						◀	◀				◀		◆		◆		◆			■	◆	◆		◀	◀			■ ◀	
– pasteurized																		■												
– sterilized																														
– UHT		◆																												
– milk-based drinks – pasteurized		◆						◆				◀		◆		◆		◆			■		◆							
– sterilized or UHT																														
– milk (dried)	◀			◀								◀		◆		◆		◆		◀										■
– yoghurt	■							◆				◀		◆		◆		■		◀										
Dried foods	◀			◀				◆	◀	◀		◀		◆		◀	◀	◆		◀					◀					

Eggs	– shell
	– raw bulk liquid
	– pasteurized bulk liquid
	– albumen, liquid
	– albumen, crystalline
	– powdered
	– preserved by other methods
Fish and other seafood	– raw fish
	– cooked fish
	– crustaceans (raw)
	– crustaceans (cooked)
	– molluscs (raw)
	– molluscs (cooked)
	– preserved
Frozen lollies	
Fruit juice, beverages and slush drinks	– fruit juice
	– carbonated soft drinks
	– slush drinks
Gelatin	
Mayonnaise and sauces	
Meat	– red, sausage, poultry (raw)
	– cooked
	– cooked meat pies
	– cured meats
	– processed non-cured meats
Pre-cooked foods	– ready-to-eat foods
	– cook–chill, cook–freeze
Surfaces and containers	– hands
	– food surfaces and equipment
	– cloths
	– containers
Vegetables and fruit	– fresh
	– blanched and frozen
Water	– potable, including that used in food production
	– natural mineral water
	– bottled spring/drinking water

Column reference numbers: 1–30

* For pH > 4.5.   † For products containing ice-cream or milk.

Appendix B: Investigation and microbiological examination of samples from suspected food poisoning incidents

Introduction

Whenever a food poisoning incident is suspected every effort should be made to obtain accurate histories of food consumption from the individuals who have developed symptoms. Remnants of uneaten food associated with the incident should be taken from both the place of preparation and that of consumption. At the earliest opportunity as much detail as possible should be collected concerning the method of preparation, the cooking and the storage of all implicated food items, as memories are short. Even small delays in obtaining this information can hamper an epidemiological investigation.

Food-borne infections vary in their mode of action on the gastrointestinal tract. Those in which the infecting organism has multiplied to a large extent in the foodstuff before ingestion will have a shorter incubation period than those in which growth within the intestine has to occur before symptoms are experienced. Pre-formed toxin, in food, is likely to act on the stomach and cause rapid onset vomiting. The toxins of *Clostridium botulinum* are absorbed and produce more serious sequelae by affecting the central nervous system. The longest incubation times are associated with those organisms that subsequently invade the blood stream after entering the lower intestine. Intermediate delay periods of onset occur where the mode of action is by way of enterotoxins liberated only when the organisms begin to either lyse or sporulate.

Knowledge of the clinical details of the illness and the presentation of symptoms provide vital clues as to the likely food poisoning organism (Tables B.1 (infections) and B.2 (intoxications)).

It is rarely practicable or necessary to culture for all pathogens in all samples. Relevant tests will be selected in the light of available clinical and epidemiological information. For example a pathogen may already have been isolated from human specimens examined in parallel with the food. The residue of samples should be stored under refrigeration for possible further examination.

Figure B.1 illustrates a scheme to be considered when a suspect food arrives in the laboratory. Much of the work may be omitted or postponed if the clinical information gives a clear lead or if the pathogen has already been isolated from the patient. Detailed methods for the isolation and identification of the various

Table B.1 Microbiological food-borne infections: usual incubation periods and symptoms. Reproduced with permission, from [1].

Causative organism	Incubation period	Symptoms
Salmonella spp.	12–48 h	Diarrhoea, vomiting, fever, abdominal pain lasting for several days
Salmonella typhi	12–20 days	Fever, septicaemia and other systemic symptoms
Campylobacter jejuni/coli	2–5 days	Fever and malaise often precede abdominal pain and profuse diarrhoea (often bloody)
Escherichia coli		
EPEC, EIEC, ETEC, EaggEC	10–72 h (depending on group)	Diarrhoea, vomiting, fever, malaise
VTEC serotype O157	12–60 h	Haemorrhagic colitis, haemolytic uraemic syndrome
Shigella spp.	1–4 days	Abdominal cramps, diarrhoea and fever, dysentery
Yersinia enterocolitica	1–7 days (can be shorter)	Abdominal pain, fever, headache, diarrhoea, malaise and vomiting
Vibrio parahaemolyticus	12–24 h	Profuse diarrhoea, leading to dehydration, vomiting and fever
Vibrio cholerae-O1 and non-O1	48–72 h	Profuse watery diarrhoea
Aeromonas spp.	8–36 h	Diarrhoea, malaise
Clostridium perfringens	8–18 h	Abdominal pain, diarrhoea, nausea, rarely vomiting or fever
*Bacillus licheniformis**	2–14 h	Predominantly diarrhoea, vomiting occasionally, abdominal pain
*Bacillus cereus**	8–16 h	Predominantly diarrhoea with occasional vomiting
Listeria monocytogenes	1–7 days 1–10 weeks	Diarrhoeal symptoms (rare) Meningitis, fever, septicaemia, abortion
NLV	12–48 h (may be as long as 72 h)	Nausea, projectile vomiting, diarrhoea lasting 1–2 days
Cryptosporidium parvum	1–2 weeks	Diarrhoea, bloating
Cyclospora cayetanensis	1–2 weeks	Watery diarrhoea lasting 1–8 weeks, abdominal pain, bloating

*Members of the *Bacillus* group produce illness with a range of symptoms and incubation periods. The full mechanism of action has not been fully elucidated and so the *Bacillus* spp. included in this table have been allocated on the basis of their main symptom.

EaggEC, enteroaggregative *Escherichia coli*; EIEC, enteroinvasive *E. coli*; EPEC, enteropathogenic *E. coli*; ETEC, enterotoxigenic *E. coli*; NLV, Norwalk-like viruses (also known as small round structured viruses, SSRV); VTEC, verocytotoxin producing *E. coli*.

Table B.2 Microbiological food-borne intoxications: usual incubation periods and symptoms. Reproduced with permission, from [1].

Causative organism	Incubation period	Symptoms
Staphylococcus aureus	2–6 h	Severe vomiting, abdominal pain, diarrhoea, occasionally severe dehydration leading to collapse
*Bacillus cereus**	1–5 h	Acute vomiting; diarrhoea also common
*Bacillus subtilis**	1–14 h (can be as short as 10 min)	Vomiting and diarrhoea
Clostridium botulinum	12–36 h	Fatigue, lassitude, dizziness, involvement of central nervous system causing blurred vision, difficulty with speech and breathing

*Members of the *Bacillus* group produce illness with a range of symptoms and incubation periods. The full mechanism of action has not been fully elucidated and so the *Bacillus* spp. included in this table have been allocated on the basis of their main symptom.

food poisoning organisms from food are to be found elsewhere in this manual.

Aerobic colony counts (total viable counts) and enumeration of indicator organisms (Enterobacteriaceae and *Escherichia coli*), expressed as colony forming units (cfu)/g, are complementary to the examination for specific food poisoning organisms. They may give an indication of whether effective hygiene and temperature control procedures have been applied during preparation, transportation and storage. Even microscopic examination of simple stained smears from homogenized food suspensions can reveal relative numbers of morphological types of organisms. It can also be useful as a rapid screening test when staphylococcal food poisoning is suspected.

The following notes on individual microorganisms are provided as an aid to laboratory workers in selecting relevant procedures and follow-up tests.

Organisms causing food-borne infections

Salmonella

With a few important exceptions, e.g. *S. enterica subsp.* Typhi, *S.* Dublin and *S.* Choleraesuis, salmonellae show little host specificity and most can cause gastroenteritis when ingested by humans. In the investigation of outbreaks efforts should be directed towards demonstrating a common Salmonella type in patients and food and in establishing the reason for the presence of salmonellae in food. Incubation time is usually 12–48 h or longer since multiplication has to occur in the intestine.

Isolation of salmonellae from stool specimens in acute cases is usually possible by direct plating on suitable selective agars, although enrichment may

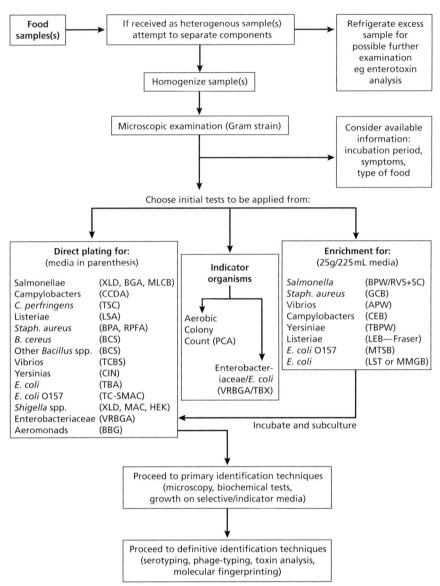

Fig. B.1 Suggested scheme for the examination of food specimens from food poisoning outbreaks [1].

Culture media:

APW, alkaline peptone water; BCS, bacillus cereus selective agar (e.g. PEMBA or MYP); BGA, brilliant green agar; BPA, Baird Parker agar; BPW, buffered peptone water; CEB, campylobacter enrichment broth; CCDA, cefoperazone charcoal desoxycholate agar; CIN, cefsulodin-irgasan novobiocin agar; HEK, Hektoen agar; GCB, Giolitti Cantoni broth; DCA, desoxycholate citrate agar; LEB, listeria enrichment broth (e.g. Fraser broth); LSA, listeria selective agar (e.g. Oxford); LST, lauryl sulphate tryptose broth; MAC, MacConkey agar; MLCB, mannitol lysine crystal violet bile agar; MMGB, minerals modified glutamate broth; MTSB, modified trypticase soya broth; PA, Preston agar; PCA, plate count agar; RPFA, rabbit plasma fibrinogen agar; RVS, Rappaport Vassiliadis soya peptone broth; SC, selenite-cystine broth; SEB, shigella enrichment broth; TC–SMAC, tellurite-cefixime sorbitol MacConkey agar; TBA, tryptone bile agar; TBPW, tris buffered peptone water; TBX, tryptone bile agar supplemented with BCIG; TCBS, thiosulphate citrate bile-salt sucrose agar; TSC, tryptose sulphite cycloserine agar; VRBGA, violet red bile glucose agar; XLD, xylose lysine desoxycholate agar.

be necessary for diagnosis of carriers and asymptomatic cases. Opinions differ on the number of *Salmonella* organisms that need to be ingested to form an infecting dose. In some outbreaks large numbers have been found in the implicated food while in others there is every indication that infection has resulted from ingestion of fewer than 100 salmonellae. In many food and milk-borne outbreaks the organisms cannot be recovered from the implicated source by direct plating techniques. For this reason many enrichment protocols have been described for the isolation of salmonellae from food, and many comparisons of these methods have been made. No single procedure has been found to be suitable for the recovery of all salmonellae from all types of food. Most of the methods described involve primary enrichment in non-selective broth, to allow recovery of sublethally injured organisms, followed by secondary enrichment in elective or selective broths. Secondary enrichment broths are subcultured after incubation on to selective agars. Suspect Salmonella colonies are checked for purity and their identity confirmed by biochemical and serological tests.

Salmonella Typhi and the *S.* Paratyphi A, B and C are worthy of special mention. These serotypes are host adapted to humans, but can be transmitted in food. The usual source of these organisms in food is by contamination from an infected food worker or by direct contamination from human sewage. The traditional techniques used for isolation of *Salmonella* from food may not be suitable for the detection of these host-adapted serotypes. Use of media containing brilliant green or malachite green dyes and methods using elevated temperatures (41.5°C) are particularly unsuitable. Procedures using other enrichment media (e.g. tetrathionate broth [formulations without brilliant green] or selenite) incubated at 37°C for 24–48 h and subcultured to xylose lysine desoxycholate agar (XLD) and bismuth sulphite agars are more likely to be successful. These organisms are categorized as Hazard Group 3 pathogens and therefore all work undertaken with high-risk samples and known positive cultures should be carried out in a Containment Level 3 laboratory.

Salmonellae are identified initially according to the serological reactions of their somatic O and flagellar H antigens. Strain diversity can also be demonstrated within each serotype. To assist in epidemiological investigations special methods of strain identification have been developed for some of the commoner Salmonella serotypes. For example, phage typing is available for *S.* Typhimurium, *S.* Enteritidis, *S.* Hadar and *S.* Virchow. Antimicrobial resistance patterns are also valuable, especially for characterization of strains of *S.* Typhimurium that have acquired multiple resistance. Application of molecular fingerprinting techniques has become commonplace. The gold standard is pulsed field gel electrophoresis (PFGE) [2] and single enzyme amplified fragment length polymorphism (SAFLP) is also proving to be a valuable technique [3].

Campylobacter jejuni (C. coli)

Campylobacter jejuni is now well recognized as the major cause of bacterial gastroenteritis in humans, but the epidemiology and mode of transmission of the organism has still not been fully determined. The route of infection is by ingestion and the incubation period is usually 2–5 days. Bloody diarrhoea with fever and abdominal pain are commonly the predominant features of the illness.

In several large outbreaks milk (either untreated or inadequately pasteurized) and water (from drinking water supplies or from recreational exposure) have been shown conclusively to be the vehicles of transmission. In the majority of sporadic cases the vehicle is not identified even when a particular food item is suspected. There are, however, strong associations between cases and either the handling of raw poultry or consumption of undercooked poultry.

It has been demonstrated that as few as 500 *Campylobacter* organisms can be an infective dose. Isolation of the organism from food and environmental sources is, therefore, attempted by enrichment culture. Enrichment broths are incubated at either 37°C or 41.5°C, or a combination of the two temperatures to allow recovery of sublethally damaged organisms, for 48–72 h and then subcultured on to selective agar media. These are further incubated under microaerobic conditions at 37°C or 41.5°C for 48–72 h. Suspect *Campylobacter* colonies on these media may be confirmed by giving a positive oxidase test and showing typical cell morphology by modified Gram stain and motility by either phase contrast or dark-field microscopy. Cultures may be identified and subdivided more fully into biotypes using several methods [4].

To aid epidemiological investigations and surveillance further characterization is necessary. In the UK this is currently achieved by a combination of serotyping and phage typing supplemented by molecular fingerprinting techniques [5–7]. PFGE and restriction fragment length polymorphism (RFLP) methods are most frequently used although gene sequence typing is now being introduced.

Escherichia coli

The historical association of acute gastroenteritis in infants below the age of 3 years with a number of serotypes of *Escherichia coli* is well founded. These serotypes, which are not specifically related to the production of verocytotoxin or identifiable enterotoxins, are usually designated enteropathogenic *E. coli* (EPEC). Outbreaks that were quite common in hospitals and nurseries a few decades ago are now very infrequent and this may be due to improvements in standards of hygiene.

A different group of *E. coli* serotypes produce an invasive type of diarrhoea similar to that caused by *Shigella dysenteriae* in which actual invasion of the colonic mucosa with ulceration occurs. Food-related outbreaks are infrequent, but when they do occur there appears to be no predilection for any particular age group. These are known as enteroinvasive *E. coli* (EIEC).

People who travel from countries with a high standard of hygiene to areas of the world with poor hygiene, particularly those with a tropical climate, frequently fall victim to travellers' diarrhoea in which the most common cause is enterotoxigenic *E. coli* (ETEC). The source of the organism is contaminated food or water but the indigenous population are largely unaffected owing to immunity acquired by previous exposure. ETEC also invade and colonize the surface of the intestinal mucosa and then produce enterotoxins (similar to cholera toxins) that may be heat labile and/or heat stable.

Enteroaggregative *E. coli* (EaggEC) are so called because of their ability to adhere to HEp-2 cells in tissue culture in a characteristic manner. EaggEC have been associated with sporadic cases of diarrhoea and food-borne outbreaks in the UK. Another group of *E. coli* are the diffusely adherent *E. coli* (DEAC) but the pathogenicity of these organisms is poorly understood.

Direct plating on selective media such as MacConkey agar can be used for the isolation of these organisms from clinical cases but it is usually necessary to send faecal specimens to a reference laboratory for diagnosis and confirmation.

Isolation of these groups of *E. coli* from food can be done successfully by a combination of direct plating on selective media, such as MacConkey agar or violet red bile-salt lactose agar, and enrichment in minerals modified glutamate or lauryl sulphate tryptose broths. Isolates are confirmed by growth and indole production at 44°C. Demonstration of β-glucuronidase activity is frequently used for confirmation of *E. coli* isolated from food but this characteristic is not exhibited by all *E. coli* strains that cause gastrointestinal disease.

Many serogroups of *E. coli* produce toxins specific for vero cells in tissue culture. There are two main toxins VT1 and VT2 and, because they are closely related to shiga toxins found in *Shigella dysenteriae*, they are also known as ST1 and ST2. These verocytotoxins are associated with human cases presenting with diarrhoeal symptoms, haemorrhagic colitis and haemolytic uraemic syndrome. Hence, strains that produce these toxins are designated verocytotoxin producing *E. coli* (VTEC) or shiga toxin producing *E. coli* (STEC). Not all serogroups that produce verocytotoxins cause disease in humans although they are widely distributed in food-chain animals.

The major human pathogen in this group of verocytotoxin producing *E. coli* is serotype O157:H7. Isolation from clinical specimens is done by direct plating on cefixime-tellurite sorbitol MacConkey (TC-SMAC) agar incubated at 37°C for 24 h. Strains of this serotype are more readily detected by their lack of ability to ferment sorbitol in sorbitol MacConkey agar. Colonies are usually confirmed by latex agglutination with anti-O157 reagent and sent for confirmation of toxin production to a reference laboratory.

Gastrointestinal disease has been linked with many different foods but mainly with red meat and dairy products. Isolation of the VTEC O157 from foods is achieved by a combination of enrichment in modified trypticase soya broth (MTSB) incubated at 41.5°C for 24 h, immunomagnetic separation and plating onto CT-SMAC. Suspect colonies are confirmed as presumptive positive VTEC O157 by biochemical and latex agglutination tests. (Note: VTEC O157 isolates are usually β-glucuronidase negative.) Tests for toxin production and toxin typing usually require the facilities of a reference laboratory. For the epidemiological investigation of outbreaks and sporadic cases additional characterization of isolates is needed. These tests, undertaken by the reference laboratory, include phage typing, toxin gene typing and PFGE.

VTEC are now categorized as Hazard Group 3 pathogens and therefore all work undertaken with high-risk samples and known positive cultures should be performed in a Containment Level 3 laboratory.

Shigella **spp.**

This genus includes *Shigella dysenteriae*, *S. boydii*, *S. flexneri* and *S. sonnei*. These are host-adapted organisms and only infect humans and other primates. Infection with these organisms may produce a range of symptoms; the most severe cases develop dysentery, but milder forms may result in a self-limiting diarrhoeal disease. The infective dose is known to be low and the organisms can be spread via contaminated food and water, contact with contaminated environmental surfaces and by flies. Person-to-person spread is also important in institutional outbreaks. Food-borne transmission is usually the result of contamination of ready-to-eat foods by human sewage. Outbreaks of infection with *S. sonnei* and *S. flexneri* have been associated with contaminated salad vegetable crops and fruit.

Isolation from suspect food products is achieved by a combination of direct plating onto a suitable selective medium and by enrichment culture. The enrichment broths currently available are not specific for isolation of *Shigella* spp. but also grow other Gram negative enteric organisms.

Isolates should be referred to a reference laboratory for confirmation, specialist serotyping, phage typing (*S. sonnei*) and molecular typing.

Yersinia enterocolitica

Yersinia enterocolitica has been associated with a variety of human clinical disorders including diarrhoea, abscesses, septicaemia, arthritis, skin rash and symptoms similar to those of appendicitis. The organism has also been implicated in food poisoning where symptoms of abdominal pain, fever, vomiting and diarrhoea have been reported. The incubation period in food poisoning incidents is usually 24–36h but can be longer. The organism can multiply in foods stored for prolonged periods at refrigeration temperatures (4°C) and also in acidic foods (pH 4.8). In such foods it may be found at high and therefore presumably hazardous levels.

The successful isolation of *Y. enterocolitica* from food and environmental samples is achieved by the use of enrichment techniques followed by plating onto selective media. A number of different enrichment procedures have been described and there is still debate on which enrichment and isolation procedure should be used to achieve the best recovery. One of the most productive has been enrichment in simple buffer solutions incubated at low temperatures, 4–9°C, for periods of up to 14 days with periodic subculture of the enrichment broth onto cefsulodin-irgasan-novobiocin (CIN) agar for incubation at 30°C overnight. However, this prolonged incubation period is impractical and successful recovery using incubation at 21°C and 25°C has been described.

For epidemiological purposes a biotyping scheme that subdivides *Y. enterocolitica* into five biochemical groups has been described. Further subdivision of the species is possible using a serotyping scheme based on the somatic antigens and by phage typing. There are at least 58 serotypes of which serotypes O3, O8, O9 and O5,27 have been most commonly associated with human illness.

Vibrio parahaemolyticus

Vibrio parahaemolyticus, a halophilic Gram negative organism, was first recognized as a food poisoning organism in Japan. It has assumed prominence there as the commonest cause of food poisoning associated with the consumption of raw or processed seafoods in summer. In the United Kingdom the organisms should be considered and sought in all cases or outbreaks of gastroenteritis where seafoods are implicated and also in persons who have recently travelled abroad.

Enumeration of *V. parahaemolyticus* in foods should be attempted by inoculating and spreading dilutions of food suspensions on to the surface of plates of selective media followed by incubation overnight at 37°C. In addition a portion (25 g) of the food should be added to a suitable alkaline enrichment broth then incubated at 37°C followed by 41.5°C and subcultured after 6 h and 18–24 h on to selective agar plates. Following incubation suspect colonies are picked from the plates; those which produce oxidase and catalase and are sensitive to vibriostatic agent O129 (2,4-diamino-6,7-di-iso-propylpteridine) are classed as vibrios. Further identification of *V. parahaemolyticus* and its differentiation from other organisms is dependent on biochemical tests.

Serological typing of *V. parahaemolyticus* is important in epidemiological investigations: all strains have identical H antigens, but so far 11 'O' and 53 'K' antigens have been recognized, allowing identification of 54 different types.

Vibrio cholerae O1 and non-O1 cholera vibrios

Traditionally, cholera and other choleraic infections caused by these organisms have not been considered in relation to food microbiology because the mode of transmission is primarily by water either directly or indirectly. The global movement of food products has created the potential for transmission of cholera to non-endemic areas. The Food Safety Act now embraces water used in the food industry so it is appropriate that mention is made of these organisms with regard to foods that come from an aqueous environment, or are washed in or irrigated with water that may be contaminated. Wet fish and non-acid fruits and vegetables should be examined when cholera infection is present in the place of origin of such foods. The same media and techniques are used as for the detection of *V. parahaemolyticus*, but each organism has different cultural, biochemical and serological characteristics.

Aeromonas

The majority of clinicians and food microbiologists have yet to be fully convinced that this group of Gram negative bacilli are an established cause of food poisoning in humans. These organisms are present in all natural waters and moist environments and, not unexpectedly, in food submitted for laboratory examination, especially that stored at low ambient temperatures where *Aeromonas* spp. are still able to multiply rapidly.

Normal healthy humans rarely carry *Aeromonas* spp. in their faeces and when they do the strains appear to be similar to those in the environment. There is, however, growing evidence that individuals who have experienced incapacitating gastrointestinal symptoms, predominantly of diarrhoea, following the consumption of foods which can be heavily contaminated with *Aeromonas* spp. and in whom no other bacterial cause has been found, often yield heavy growths of these organisms if faeces are cultured on appropriate laboratory media. Enrichment in liquid media containing antibiotics is often employed since *Aeromonas* spp. tend to be inherently resistant to many antibiotics. They are also resistant to the chemical compounds used as disinfectants, including chlorine. It may well be that, rather than being the primary pathogens, *Aeromonas* spp. grow selectively and opportunistically in the gut of individuals in whom the balance of the natural flora is disturbed for some reason.

From knowledge of the pathogenicity of *Aeromonas* spp. it is not possible to give a precise incubation time for symptoms to develop although some guidance is given with the 8–36 h in Table B.1. It is important, however, to try to ascertain from the history of the food the likely source and to determine the particular item in which the number of *Aeromonas* organisms ingested would have been greatest. Outbreaks of enteritis due to aeromonads are unknown in the UK and the investigation of a sporadic case is often unrewarding.

Aeromonas hydrophila and *A. sobria* are the species most commonly isolated from meat products while *A. caviae* is more often associated with fish and fish products. Serotyping at a reference laboratory (available for strains from humans with or foods associated with gastroenteric infection) may lead to the elucidation of more of the epidemiology of infections due to these organisms.

Clostridium perfringens

Clostridium perfringens food poisoning outbreaks usually occur following the ingestion of large numbers (10^6 or more/g) of the organism in the suspected food. Investigation of the food preparation techniques will almost invariably reveal that the food has been held in conditions that allow spore germination and subsequent proliferation, i.e. in the temperature range 20–55°C for at least several hours. Onset of symptoms is usually 8–18 h depending on the quantity of food ingested.

Clostridium perfringens is readily isolated from stool specimens by direct plating onto neomycin blood agar incubated anaerobically at 37°C overnight. When examining specimens from outbreaks it is useful to determine the spore count following alcohol shock treatment of a faecal suspension. Investigation of faecal specimens for *C. perfringens* enterotoxin can be done by tissue culture and immunoassay methods, but this is best done at a reference laboratory.

Isolation and enumeration of *C. perfringens* in suspected foods is important in the microbial assessment of the food. The current preferred method is a pour plate technique using tryptose sulphite cycloserine (TSC) agar incubated anaerobically at 37°C overnight. Black colonies, indicative of sulphite reducing clostridia, should be confirmed by inoculation into motility-nitrate and lactose-gelatine media. The numbers of vegetative *C. perfringens* decline rapidly in refrigerated foods; enrichment using cooked meat broth or reinforced clostridial medium may therefore be indicated if there has been a significant delay before examination in a food poisoning investigation.

To confirm the link between implicated food and cases it is important to characterize the isolates. It is useful to send multiple colony picks to a reference laboratory for serotyping and molecular fingerprinting using SAFLP.

Listeria monocytogenes

Listeria monocytogenes is widely distributed in nature and is the causative organism of several forms of human disease. While it is undoubtedly food-borne, *L. monocytogenes* is rarely associated with outbreaks of gastrointestinal disease. Infection with *L. monocytogenes* is manifested in many ways, from symptomless carriage to fatal septicaemia or meningitis. The initial isolate of *L. monocytogenes* is therefore usually made in pure culture from blood or cerebrospinal fluid and culture of intestinal content may be unproductive. Listeriosis in pregnancy is of importance because of the ability of the organism to cross the placenta to infect the foetus, resulting in neonatal infection or abortion. The predisposing factors which enable the organism to gain entry to the blood stream are not clearly understood, but immunosuppression associated with malignancies and reduced immunocompetence at the extremes of life are important, as is the number of *L. monocytogenes* bacteria ingested with food.

Although the infective dose of *L. monocytogenes* is unknown it is likely to vary greatly between individuals possibly owing to other predisposing factors such as immune status. However, on the basis of the frequency with which foods harbour low numbers of the organism and of the small numbers of reported cases of food-borne listeriosis it would be reasonable to suggest that the infective dose is high. In the rare instances where incriminated foods have been available from cases of listeriosis, the levels of *L. monocytogenes* recorded have been greater than 10^3/g. Foods containing greater than 100 cfu/g should be considered to be potentially hazardous to health.

As a result of epidemiological studies of outbreaks of listeriosis in the 1980s, dairy products have been established as one of the commonest sources of infection. Laboratory studies have failed to show that *L. monocytogenes* survives normal pasteurization processes. The consumption of dairy products containing unpasteurized or under-pasteurized milk such as soft cheeses, fresh cream and ice-cream before development of symptoms in infected individuals has been documented. Other implicated foods include meat pâtés, coleslaw, chicken, turkey, fin fish and shellfish. With knowledge of the history of the food it may be possible to target those items eaten from the categories listed above. Although the optimal temperature for growth is 34–35°C, *L. monocytogenes* continue to multiply at low temperatures when other flora are inhibited. Long shelf-life food products that have been held at refrigeration temperature for prolonged periods may therefore be more suspect than fresh foods.

Enumeration of *L. monocytogenes* in food suspensions is important and is achieved by plating directly onto plates of a suitable listeria selective agar (LSA) medium. Enrichment protocols to detect low numbers of *Listeria* include primary and secondary enrichment steps with subsequent subculture to LSA. For the isolation of *L. monocytogenes* culture media are incubated at 35–37°C; this temperature may inhibit the growth of other species of *Listeria* that have not been implicated in illness. Identification of *L. monocytogenes* and other species is by biochemical tests.

For the confirmation of outbreaks it is essential to send isolates to a reference laboratory for identification and subtyping using serotyping, phage typing and PFGE. Epidemiological studies suggest that certain recognizable serotypes, notably 1/2a, 1/2b and 1/4b, which occur more frequently in human disease, may be more pathogenic.

Organisms causing food-borne intoxications

Staphylococcus aureus

Staphylococcal food poisoning is a food-borne intoxication, and results from the ingestion of food in which *Staphylococcus aureus* has already grown to high numbers and produced exotoxin(s). There are currently 12 different staphylococcal enterotoxins (SEs) that can be detected either by immunoassay or by the polymerase chain reaction (PCR). The short incubation period and symptoms experienced closely resemble those seen with many chemical intoxicants. Bacteriological evidence is, therefore, essential for the confirmation of staphylococcal food poisoning outbreaks.

Diagnosis of human cases of staphylococcal food poisoning is straightforward and *S. aureus* can be isolated directly from stool samples by direct plating onto a selective agar. In outbreaks large numbers of *S. aureus* can be isolated from suspected foods and it is important to enumerate the organisms using selective agar media incubated at 37°C for 24–48 h. If the food is known or suspected to have been handled or stored in a manner which may have affected the viability of the organisms, then enrichment broth culture followed by plating onto selective agar should be used for isolation. Traditionally, media containing high salt concentrations such as salt meat broth have been used, but these can be very inhibitory to stressed cells. Presumptive colonies from the selective agar cultures should be confirmed as *S. aureus* by a coagulase test or commercial equivalent and by desoxyribonuclease (DNase) production.

Isolates from food samples, clinical specimens and from food handlers should be further characterized by special tests carried out at the reference laboratory. These include phage typing, toxin typing and PFGE. Conclusive proof of a staphylococcal outbreak is provided by detection of indistinguishable strains from food and cases, by confirming the production of enterotoxin and, when possible, by detecting enterotoxin in the implicated food.

Bacillus cereus and other *Bacillus* spp.

Bacillus cereus food poisoning usually results from the ingestion of food containing large numbers (10^6–10^8/g) of the organism and pre-formed toxin (emetic type) and is therefore an intoxication. A less common diarrhoeal type of food poisoning is associated with infection followed by toxin production predominantly in the intestine. Vomit and faeces should both be examined if possible. Isolation from these samples is achieved by direct plating onto *B. cereus* selective agar (BCS), e.g. polymyxin pyruvate egg yolk mannitol bromothymol blue agar (PEMBA) or phenol red egg yolk polymyxin agar (PREP or MYP) agar incubated at 30–37°C overnight. Both of these BCS agars contain mannitol and egg yolk emulsion. *Bacillus cereus* is distinguished from other *Bacillus* species by: (i) production of blue or turquoise to peacock blue colonies on PEMBA or pink colonies on MYP (PREP) due to the inability of *B. cereus* to ferment mannitol; and (ii) production of a zone of opacity around the bacterial growth due to lecithinase activity.

As large numbers of *B. cereus* are required to cause illness, isolation and enumeration in the examination of food samples associated with outbreaks can usually be achieved by direct plating onto the surface of BCS agar incubated aerobically at 30–37°C for 24 h. Selective enrichment is rarely necessary and the significance of *B. cereus* recovered by enrichment techniques is dubious.

Further confirmation of isolates requires biochemical tests. A serotyping scheme is available for *B. cereus* that is based on agglutination with sera raised against the H (flagellar) antigens. Serotyping, tests for toxin production and molecular finger printing methods are valuable in confirming outbreaks and are available from the reference laboratory.

Other members of the genus *Bacillus*, notably those of the *B. subtilis*–*licheniformis* group, have also been implicated in outbreaks of food poisoning.

Initial isolation and enumeration procedures are similar to those for *B. cereus*. Biochemical tests are necessary for confirmation; unlike *B. cereus* these organisms do ferment mannitol and do not produce lecithinase.

Clostridium botulinum

The name *Clostridium botulinum* is used to describe several phenotypically different clostridia that produce extremely potent exotoxins. These toxins are classified as A, B, C, D, E, F and G. The toxins cause a neuroparalytic illness, commonly referred to as botulism. *Clostridium botulinum* producing toxin types A, B, E and F are associated with botulism in humans.

The classical food-borne illness results from the ingestion of food in which *Clostridium botulinum* has multiplied and produced one of the neurotoxins. In view of the severity of the illness, rapid identification of the food source is essential in order to prevent further cases. Suspected foods, together with any containers, should be examined without delay. If a commercially manufactured product is suspected, as much information as possible about the product, such as brand name, batch code and package size, should be obtained. A health hazard warning may need to be issued pending the results of the laboratory examinations.

Serum and faecal specimens should be collected from suspect cases and sent immediately for toxin testing. Suspected foods together with rinses from containers should be examined for the presence of toxin and cultured by direct and enrichment methods using specialist media. Enumeration of organism is not usually considered necessary. In view of the potency of the neurotoxins, isolates of *C. botulinum* or suspected foods should be referred to a reference laboratory for these specialist tests.

Confirmation of a case of botulism is dependent on detecting neurotoxin in the clinical specimens. Food poisoning is confirmed by demonstration of toxin production by the isolates from the food together with the presence of toxin in the suspected food. Currently the only reliable method for the detection of biologically active toxin is the mouse bioassay. Although immunodiffusion tests and immunoassay techniques have been developed they lack sensitivity; they do not confirm the presence of functionally active toxin and hence cannot be used diagnostically.

Protozoa and viruses

It should be remembered that not all food-borne gastrointestinal disease is caused by bacterial pathogens. Both protozoa and viruses must be considered if the symptoms suggest the possibility and there is absence of one of the usual suspects.

Cryptosporidium parvum and *Cyclospora* spp. have been associated with food-borne transmission and outbreaks of disease. The foods implicated are usually salad vegetables or soft fruits that have been contaminated by sewage polluted water. However, meat and milk have also been implicated in outbreaks of cryptosporidiosis [8].

Norwalk-like viruses (NLVs), previously known as small round structured viruses (SRSV), have been transmitted via food but this is usually due to contamination from a food handler excreting the virus. Shellfish are also recognized as a source of these viruses and become contaminated during filtration of sewage-infected water. Other viruses such as hepatitis A and rotavirus may also be associated with food-borne transmission [9]. Examination of clinical specimens and suspect foods require specialized techniques for detection which are outside the scope of this manual.

References

1 Department of Health. *Management of Outbreaks of Food-borne Illness. Guidance Prepared by a Department of Health Working Group*. London: Department of Health, 1994.
2 Threlfall EJ, Powell NG, Rowe B. Differentiation of salmonellae by molecular methods for epidemiological investigations. *PHLS Microbiol Digest* 1994; **11**: 199–202.
3 Peters TM, Threlfall EJ. Single-enzyme amplified fragment length polymorphism and its applicability for *Salmonella* epidemiology. *System Appl Microbiol* 2002; **24**: 400–4.
4 Bolton FJ, Wareing DRA, Skirrow MB, Hutchinson DN. Identification and biotyping of campylobacters. In: Board RG, Jones D, Skinner FA, eds. *Identification Methods in Applied and Environmental Microbiology. Society for Applied Bacteriology Technical Series No. 29*. 1992: 151–61. Oxford: Blackwell Scientific Publications.
5 Frost JA, Oza AN, Thwaites RT, Rowe B. Serotyping scheme for *Campylobacter jejuni* and *Campylobacter coli* based on direct agglutination of heat stable antigens. *J Clin Microbiol* 1998; **36**: 335–9.
6 Thwaites RT, Frost JA. Drug resistance in *Campylobacter jejuni*, *C.coli* and *C.lari* isolated from humans in England and Wales. *J Clin Pathol* 1999; **52**: 812–14.
7 Frost JA, Kramer JM, Gillanders SA. Phage typing of *Campylobacter jejuni* and *C.coli*. *Epidemiol Infect* 1999; **123**: 47–55.
8 Nichols GL. Food-borne protozoa. *Br Med Bull* 1999; **55**: 209–35.
9 Appleton H. Control of food-bone viruses. *Br Med Bull* 2000; **56**: 172–83.

Appendix C: UK reference facilities, Public Health Laboratory Service external quality assurance schemes and culture collection

The following list of reference facilities was correct at the time of publication of this manual but will inevitably require revision periodically.

Aeromonas hydrophila (offered as special, i.e. non-routine diagnosis, for isolates from blood only)
Laboratory of Enteric Pathogens
Public Health Laboratory Service (PHLS) Central Public Health Laboratory
61 Colindale Avenue
London NW9 5HT
Tel: 020 82004400, ext. 3173

***Bacillus* spp.** (identification)
Food Safety Microbiology Laboratory
PHLS Central Public Health Laboratory
61 Colindale Avenue
London NW9 5HT
Tel: 020 82004400, ext. 3505/3521

Bacillus cereus (serotyping and enterotoxins)
Food Safety Microbiology Laboratory
PHLS Central Public Health Laboratory
61 Colindale Avenue
London NW9 5HT
Tel: 020 82004400, ext. 3505/3521

***Brucella* spp.** (identification and serology)
Brucella spp. Special Diagnostic Services
Liverpool Public Health Laboratory
University Hospital Aintree
Lower Lane
Liverpool L9 7AL
Tel: 0151 5294900

***Campylobacter* spp.** (identification and typing)
Laboratory of Enteric Pathogens
PHLS Central Public Health Laboratory
61 Colindale Avenue
London NW9 5HT
Tel: 020 82004400, ext. 3772

Can analysis
Campden and Chorleywood Food Research Association
Chipping Campden
Gloucestershire GL55 6LD
Tel: 01386 832000
Leatherhead Food Research Association
Randalls Road
Leatherhead
Surrey KT22 7RY
Tel: 01372 376761

Chemical analysis
Laboratory of the Government Chemist
Queens Road
Teddington
Middlesex TW11 0LY
Tel: 020 89437000
or:
Local Public Analyst
(refer to local telephone directory)

***Clostridium* spp.** (identification)
Anaerobe Reference Unit
University Hospital of Wales
Heath Park
Cardiff CF14 4XW
Tel: 029 20742171

Clostridium botulinum (isolation, identification and toxin detection)
Food Safety Microbiology Laboratory
PHLS Central Public Health Laboratory
61 Colindale Avenue
London NW9 5HT
Tel: 020 82004400, ext. 4933/4116

Clostridium perfringens (serotyping and enterotoxins)
Food Safety Microbiology Laboratory
PHLS Central Public Health Laboratory
61 Colindale Avenue
London NW9 5HT
Tel: 020 82004400, ext. 3521/4116

Cryptosporidium spp. (identification and typing)
Cryptosporidium Reference Unit
Swansea Public Health Laboratory
Singleton Hospital
Sketty
Swansea SA2 8QA
Tel: 01792 285055, ext. 5051

Escherichia coli (identification and serotyping, enterotoxin and verocytotoxin)
Laboratory of Enteric Pathogens
PHLS Central Public Health Laboratory
61 Colindale Avenue
London NW9 5HT
Tel: 020 82004400, ext. 3173

Fish and shellfish toxins (ciguatera, diarrhoetic shellfish poisoning (DSP), paralytic shellfish poisoning (PSP), scombrotoxin)
Food Safety Microbiology Laboratory
PHLS Central Public Health Laboratory
61 Colindale Avenue
London NW9 5HT
Tel: 020 82004400, ext. 4933/4116

Listeria spp. (identification)
Food Safety Microbiology Laboratory
PHLS Central Public Health Laboratory
61 Colindale Avenue
London NW9 5HT
Tel: 020 82004400, ext. 3505/3521

Listeria monocytogenes (typing)
Food Safety Microbiology Laboratory
PHLS Central Public Health Laboratory
61 Colindale Avenue
London NW9 5HT
Tel: 020 82004400, ext. 3505/3521

Mycotoxins
Section Head, Mycotoxins
Central Science Laboratory
Sand Hutton
York YO41 1LZ
Tel: 01904 462000

Red kidney bean (haemagglutinins)
Food Safety Microbiology Laboratory
PHLS Central Public Health Laboratory
61 Colindale Avenue
London NW9 5HT
Tel: 020 82004400, ext. 4933/4116

Salmonella spp. (serotyping and phage typing)
Laboratory of Enteric Pathogens
PHLS Central Public Health Laboratory
61 Colindale Avenue
London NW9 5HT
Tel: 020 82004400, ext. 3132

Shigella spp. (serotyping)
Laboratory of Enteric Pathogens
PHLS Central Public Health Laboratory
61 Colindale Avenue
London NW9 5HT
Tel: 020 82004400, ext. 3173

Staphylococcus aureus (enterotoxin)
Food Safety Microbiology Laboratory
PHLS Central Public Health Laboratory
61 Colindale Avenue
London NW9 5HT
Tel: 020 82004400, ext. 3521/3505

Staphylococcus aureus (typing and extended toxin testing)
Laboratory of Hospital Infection
PHLS Central Public Health Laboratory
61 Colindale Avenue
London NW9 5HT
Tel: 020 82004400, ext. 4224/4227

Streptococcus spp. (identification and typing)
Respiratory and Systemic Infection Laboratory
PHLS Central Public Health Laboratory
61 Colindale Avenue
London NW9 5HT
Tel: 020 82004400, ext. 4288/4289

Vibrio spp. (identification and typing)
Laboratory of Enteric Pathogens
PHLS Central Public Health Laboratory
61 Colindale Avenue
London NW9 5HT
Tel: 020 82004400, ext. 3173

Virological

Enteric, Respiratory and Neurological Virus
    Laboratory
PHLS Central Public Health Laboratory
61 Colindale Avenue
London NW9 5HT
Tel: 020 82004400, ext. 3018

Yersinia **spp.** (serology and serotyping)
Laboratory of Enteric Pathogens
PHLS Central Public Health Laboratory
61 Colindale Avenue
London NW9 5HT
Tel: 020 82004400, ext. 3173

Shellfish associated (testing and virological
problems)
Centre for Environment, Fisheries and
    Aquaculture Science (CEFAS)
Weymouth Laboratory
Barrack Road
The Nothe
Weymouth
Dorset DT4 8UB
Tel: 01305 206600

PHLS external quality assessment schemes

Food microbiology
PHLS food and *Legionella* external quality
    assessment (EQA) schemes

Food Safety Microbiology Laboratory
PHLS Central Public Health Laboratory
61 Colindale Avenue
London NW9 5HT
Tel: 020 82004400, ext. 4117/4119

National Collection of Type Cultures (NCTC)
Central Public Health Laboratory
61 Colindale Avenue
London NW9 5HT
Tel: 020 82004400, ext. 3774

Virus isolation scheme
Reading Public Health Laboratory
South Block
Royal Berkshire Hospital
London Road
Reading RG1 5AN
Tel: 0118 9877730

Water microbiology (indicator organisms)
PHLS water EQA scheme
Public Health Laboratory
Institute of Pathology
Newcastle General Hospital
Westgate Road
Newcastle-upon-Tyne NE4 6BE
Tel: 0191 2724585

Appendix D: Bibliography

Australian Institute of Food Science and Technology (AIFST) (NSW Branch) Food Microbiology Group. *Food-borne Microorganisms of Public Health Significance*, 5th edn. North Ryde, NSW, Australia: CSIRO, 1997.

Banwart GI. *Basic Food Microbiology*, 2nd edn. New York: Van Norstrand Reinhold, 1989.

Corry JEL, Curtis GDW, Baird RM. *Culture Media for Food Microbiology*. London: Elsevier Science, 1995.

Davies A, Board R. *The Microbiology of Meat and Poultry*. London: Blackie Academic and Professional, 1998.

Doyle MP, ed. *Food-borne Bacterial Pathogens*. New York: Marcel Dekker, 1989.

Doyle MP, Beuchat LR, Montville TJ, eds. *Food Microbiology. Fundamentals and Frontiers*. Washington, D.C.: American Society of Microbiology (ASM) Press, 1997.

Hayes PR, Forsythe SJ. *Food Hygiene, Microbiology and HACCP*, 3rd edn. London: Elsevier Science, 1999.

Heijden K van der, Younes M, Fishbein L, Miller S, eds. *International Food Safety Handbook. Science, International Regulation and Control*. New York: Marcel Dekker, 1999.

Hersom AC, Hulland ED. *Canned Foods. Thermal Processing and Microbiology*, 7th edn. Edinburgh: Churchill Livingstone, 1980.

Hui YH, *et al.* eds. *Food-borne Disease Handbook*, 2nd edn. *Vol. 1 Bacterial Pathogens. Vol. 2 Viruses, Parasites, Pathogens and HACCP. Vol. 3 Plant Toxicants. Vol. 4. Seafood and Environmental Toxins*. New York: Marcel Dekker, 2001.

International Commission on Microbiological Specifications for Foods. *Microorganisms in Foods. 1. Their Significance and Methods of Enumeration*, 2nd edn. Toronto: University of Toronto Press, 1978.

International Commission on Microbiological Specifications for Foods. *Microbial Ecology of Foods. Vol. 1 Factors Affecting Life and Death of Microorganisms*. London: Academic Press, 1980.

International Commission on Microbiological Specifications for Foods. *Microorganisms in Food. 2. Sampling for Microbiological Analysis and Specific Applications*, 2nd edn. Oxford: Blackwell Scientific, 1986.

International Commission on Microbiological Specifications for Foods. *HACCP in Microbiological Safety and Quality*. Oxford: Blackwell Scientific, 1988.

International Commission on Microbiological Specifications for Foods. *Microorganisms in Foods. 5. Microbiological Specifications of Food Pathogens*. London: Blackie Academic and Professional, 1996.

International Commission on Microbiological Specifications for Foods. *Microorganisms in Foods. 6. Microbial Ecology of Food Commodities*. London: Blackie Academic and Professional, 1998.

Jay JH. *Modern Food Microbiology*, 6th edn. New York: Chapman and Hall, 2000.

Lancet. *A Lancet Review. Food-borne Illness*. London: Edward Arnold, 1991.

Lightfoot NF, Maier EA, eds. *Microbiological Analysis of Food and Water. Guidelines for Quality Assurance*. Amsterdam: Elsevier, 1998.

Lund B, Baird-Parker A, Gould GW. *Microbiological Safety and Quality of Food* (2 vols). Kluwer Academic/Plenum Publishing, 1999.

Mitchell RT. *Practical Microbiological Risk Assessment*. Oxford: Chandos Publishing Ltd, 2000.

Mossel DAA, Corry JEL, Struijk CB, Baird RM. *Essentials of the Microbiology of Foods. A Textbook for Advanced Studies*. Chichester: John Wiley and Sons, 1995.

National Research Council (US) Food Protection Committee. *Subcommittee on Microbiological Criteria. An Evaluation of the Role of Microbiological Criteria for Foods and Food Ingredients*. Washington, D.C.: National Academy Press, 1985.

Ryser ET, Marth EH. *Listeria, Listeriosis and Food Safety*, 2nd edn. New York: Marcel Dekker, 1999.

Samson RA, Hocking AD, Pitt JI, King AP. *Modern Methods in Food Mycology*. Amsterdam: Elsevier, 1992.

Sutherland JP, Varnum AH, Evans MG. *A Colour Atlas of Food Quality Control*. London: Wolfe Publishing, 1986.

Tui AT, ed. *Handbook of Natural Toxins. Vol. 7. Food Poisoning*. New York: Marcel Dekker, 1992.

US Food and Drug Administration. *Bacteriological Analytical Manual*, 8th edn, Revision A. Gaithersburg, MD: Association of Official Analytical Chemists (AOAC), 1998.

Vanderzant C, Splitsoesser DF, eds. *Compendium of Methods for the Microbiological Examination of Foods*, 3rd edn. Washington, D.C.: American Public Health Association, 1992.

Varnum AH, Evans MC. *Food-borne Pathogens. An Illustrated Text*. London: Wolfe Publishing, 1991.

Useful websites

Association of Public Analysts: www.the-apa.org.uk
Campden and Chorleywood Food Research Association: www.campden.co.uk
Centre for the Environment, Fisheries and Aquaculture Science: www.cefas.co.uk
Chartered Institute of Environmental Health: www.cieh.org.uk
Department of the Environment, Food and Rural Affairs: www.defra.gov.uk
Department of Health: www.doh.gov.uk
Drinking Water Inspectorate: www.dwi.gov.uk
Environment Agency: www.environment-agency.gov.uk
European Commission: www.europa.eu.int
Food Standards Agency: www.food.gov.uk
Health and Safety Executive: www.hse.gov.uk
Her Majesty's Stationery Office: www.hmso.gov.uk
Institute of Food Science and Technology: www.ifst.org.uk
Local Authorities Coordinating Body of Food and Trading Standards: www.lacots.com
Public Health Laboratory Service: www.phls.co.uk
Scottish Centre for Infection and Environmental Health: www.show.scot.nhs.uk/scieh
Veterinary Laboratories Agency: www.defra.gov.uk/corporate/vla/default/htm
World Health Organization: www.who.int/home-page/

Index